Proceedings of the
XXIV International Congress on Electrocardiology

ELECTROCARDIOLOGY '97

Bratislava, Slovak Republic 24–28 June 1997

Proceedings of the
XXIV International Congress on Electrocardiology

ELECTROCARDIOLOGY '97

Bratislava, Slovak Republic 24–28 June 1997

Editors

Ljuba Bacharova

Institute for Heart Research, Slovak Academy of Sciences

Peter W Macfarlane

University of Glasgow

World Scientific

Singapore • New Jersey • London • Hong Kong

Published by

World Scientific Publishing Co. Pte. Ltd.

P O Box 128, Farrer Road, Singapore 912805

USA office: Suite 1B, 1060 Main Street, River Edge, NJ 07661

UK office: 57 Shelton Street, Covent Garden, London WC2H 9HE

British Library Cataloguing-in-Publication Data
A catalogue record for this book is available from the British Library.

ELECTROCARDIOLOGY '97

ISBN 981-02-3380-9

This book is printed on acid-free paper.

Printed in Singapore by Uto-Print

PREFACE

ELECTROCARDIOLOGY 1997 contains the Proceedings of the 24th International Congress on Electrocardiology (the 38th International Symposium on Vectorcardiography) which was held in Bratislava, Slovak Republic, 24th-28th June, 1997. The main aims of the Annual Congress have been to gather together scientists, from all Continents, working in the interdisciplinary field of electrocardiology and to encourage meaningful and fruitful discussions in order to stimulate the exchange of current knowledge.

We believe that this book will contribute to consolidation of knowledge in the highly complex field of electrocardiology and will facilitate a multidisciplinary approach to further studies. It should serve as a valuable reference for basic scientists, practising, clinical and investigative cardiologists as well as postgraduate students. We trust it will stimulate the curiosity of readers to gain further insight into this exciting area of medical research.

This book continues the series Electrocardiology 1991, 1992, 19.., with a similar format being adopted as previously. The Editors would like to thank World Scientific Publishing in Singapore for their assistance during its preparation.

We would also like to take this opportunity to thank the local organising committee for the work undertaken in connection with organising the International Congress.

Ljuba Bachárová
Peter W. Macfarlane
Editors

The XXIVth International Congress on Electrocardiology was organized under the auspices of the International Society of Electrocardiology

CONTENTS

II. Computer Modeling

III. Heart Rate Regulation and Rhythm Disturbances

IV. Body Surface Potential Mapping

V. Computer Assisted Electrocardiography

I. Basic Electrophysiology and Electropharmacology

HETEROGENEITY IN SENSITIVITY OF CARDIAC MYOCYTES TO ISCHEMIA AS A SUBSTRATE FOR ARRHYTHMOGENESIS IN ISCHEMIA AND REPERFUSION

J. SLEZAK, N. TRIBULOVA, T. RAVINGEROVA, J. STYK, A. ZIEGELHOEFFER, L. OKRUHLICOVA
Inst. Heart Research SAS, Dubravská cesta 9, Bratislava, Slovak Republic

O. SLEZAKOVA
Faculty of Medicine UK, Sasinkova 2, Bratislava, Slovak Republic

Differences in sensitivity of specific parts of the heart and regional variations in response to ischemic injury can present an important culprit of cardiac arrhythmias. Histochemical localization and activities of glycolytic, oxidative and hydrolytic enzymes were studied together with ultrastructure of myocardial cells in right and left ventricles, atria, nodal tissue and Purkynje system in isolated perfused rat hearts under control as well as different experimental conditions including calcium paradox, ischemia, reperfusion and oxygen-free radicals. Histochemical reaction for glycogen phosphorylase as well as acetylcholine esterase was more intense in the nodal tissue and Purkynje fibers, whereas oxidative enzymes showed intense reaction in contractile cells of the ventricles. Calcium paradox caused more histochemical enzyme changes in the subepicardial layer. Ischemia-reperfusion had more damaging effect in the subendocardial layer. Oxygen-free radicals caused transmurally focal injuries. This pattern of histochemical changes also correlated with ultrastructural injury in these regions. Ventricular muscle suffered marked decrease, whereas atrial muscle showed a relatively less decrease in different histochemical enzyme activities. Purkynje fibers were the least affected tissue in this respect. The differential changes were most sensitively reflected by glycogen phosphorylase followed by lactate dehydrogenase, alkaline phosphatase, isocitrate dehydrogenase and β-hydroxybutyrate dehydrogenase. Transmural heterogeneity in ventricular histochemical response to injuries may be multifactorial originating from the functional, metabolic, and flow differences in subepicardial and subendocardial regions of the ventricle. Differences in sensitivity to ischemia produce foci of myocytes with different stages of injury which can be identified as a major factor in genesis of arrhythmia and ventricular fibrillation.

1 Introduction

It has been shown that different parts of the heart under physiological conditions reveal superspecialization of different areas (compartments) reflected by biochemical, functional, structural, and histochemical differences. These are even more pronounced under pathological conditions[1-23].

In the present study, we report regional variations in the histochemical localization of certain glycolytic, oxidative, and hydrolytic enzymes in isolated perfused rat hearts.

2 Material and Methods

Isolated perfused rat hearts were subjected to calcium paradox (CaP), postischemic reperfusion (REP) or oxygen free radicals (OFR).

CaP - was introduced by 3 min. calcium depletion followed by calcium repletion.

REP - ischemia lasting 30 min was followed by 15 min reperfusion.

OFR - bolus application of the OFR generating system followed by perfusion for 15 min.

After the respective protocols, samples were taken from different regions of the control as well as experimental hearts and processed for histochemical as well as ultrastructural studies.

The time-course of changes in coronary flow (CF), contractile activity of the heart (max dP/dt) and heart rate (HR) during CaP, REP, and OFR perfusion were compared with their respective controls.

Differences in the sensitivity of various regions of the heart to conditions of calcium paradox (CaP), ischemia reperfusion (REP), and injury caused by reactive oxygen free radical species (OFR) with respect to physiologic, histochemical, and ultrastructural changes were examined.

3 Results

- The most severe enzyme histochemical changes were found in Ca paradox injury
- Decrease in enzymatic activities was more pronounced in the right ventricle in comparison to the left ventricle.
- The decrease in enzyme activities was smaller in atrial muscle comparing with ventricles.
- The smallest decrease of enzyme activities was observed in the conduction system.
- Ultrastructural analysis showed good correlation with histochemical findings.
- The differences in enzyme activities in the ventricle, atria and conduction system relate to functional, structural and metabolic heterogeneity of different parts of the heart.

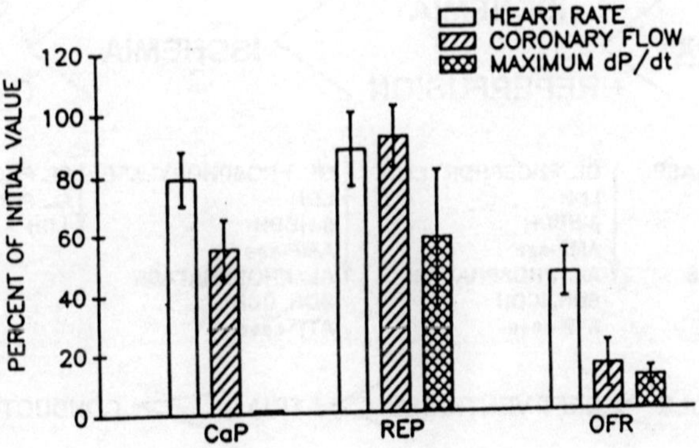

Figure 1: Changes in HR, CF, and maximum dP/dt in isolated hearts subjected to calcium paradox (CaP), ischemia-reperfusion (REP) and oxygen-free radicals (OFR).

Table1: Histochemical changes in glycogen phosphorylase under different experimental conditions.

Experimental condition	Ventricles			Atria	Conducting System
	Muscle Region	Left	Right		
CONTROL	Epi	+++	+++	++++	++++
	Endo	+++	+++		
CaP	Epi	-	-	++	+++
	Endo	+++	-		
REP	Epi	+++	+++	+++	++++
	Endo	-	-		
OFR	Epi	++	++	++++	++++
	Endo	++	++		

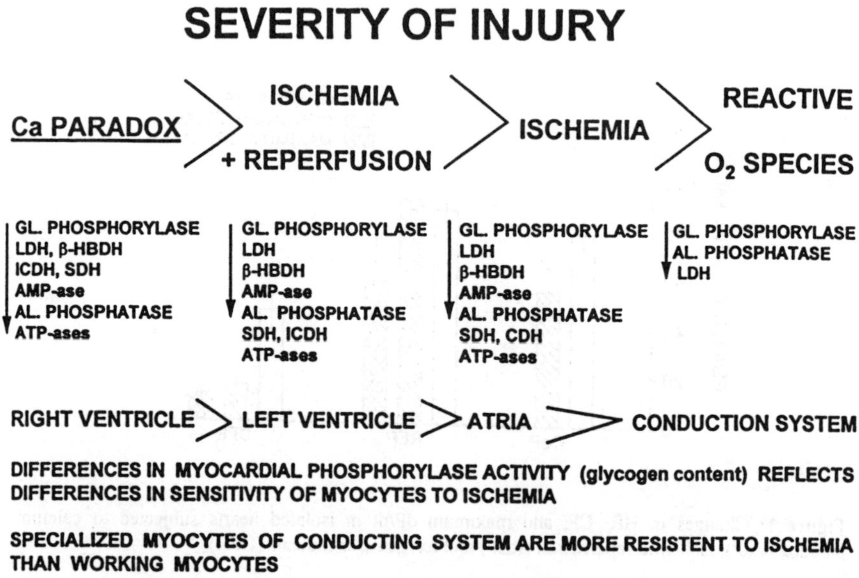

4 Conclusion

It can be concluded that differences in enzyme activities in different parts of the heart reflect functional, structural and metabolic heterogeneity of the different functional parts of the heart muscle. This should be considered, in particular under stress of pathological conditions, where differences in sensitivity to ischemia may produce foci of myocytes with different stages of injury. These can be identified as a major factor in genesis of arrhythmia and ventricular fibrillation.

Acknowledgment

This work was supported by VEGA SAV grant and Canadian and Manitoba Heart and Stroke Foundations.

References

1. Fawcett and N.S. McNutt, *J. Cell. Biol.* **42,** 1 (1969).
2. B.Korecky, L.H.Michael, in ed. N.S.Dhalla, G.Rona *Recent advances in studies on cardiac structure and metabolism. myocardial biology.* (University Park Press, Baltimore, 4, 77-87, 1974).
3. McNutt and D.W.Fawcet, *J.Cell.Biol.*, **42**, 46 (1969).
4. K.Schror *et al., J.Mol.Cell.Cardiol.* **11**, 45-55 (1979).
5. N.S.Dhalla et al., *Proceedings of the Society for Experimental Biology and Medicine,* **119**, 1147-50 (1965).
6. N.S.Dhalla et al., *Can.J.Physiol.Pharmacol*, **5,** 360-7 (1980).
7. A.G.Mulder et al., *Am.J.Physiol.***186**, 309-12 (1956).
8. P .Braveny and J.Sumbera, *Scripta Medica* **41**, 241-8 (1968).
9. T.F.McDonald and D.P.Macleod, *J.Mol.Cell.Cardiol.* **5,** 149-59 (1973).
10. K.H.Teoh et al., *Thorac.Cardiovasc.Surg*. **96**, 725-9 (1988).
11. D.Franzen et al., *Am.J.Physiol.* **254**, H-344-H53 (1988).
12. H.Fujiwara et al., *Circ.Res.* **51**, 6, 683-93 (1982).
13. J.I.E.Hoffman, *Progr.Cardiovasc.Dis.* **29**, 429-64 (1987).
14. E.S.Kirk and C.R.Honig, *Am.J.Physiol.* **207**, 661-8 (1964).
15. J.A.Leipala et al., *J.Mol.Cell.Cardiol.* **21**, 841-8 (1989).
16. B.I.Levy et al., *Pflugers Arch.* **407**, 388-95 (1986).
17. H.N.Sabbah et al., *Am.J.Physiol.* **240**, H-920-H6 (1981).
18. A.F.M.Schaapherder et al., *Basic Res.Cardiol.* **85**, 33-44 (1990).
19. P.D.Stein et al., *Am.J.Physiol.* **238**, H-625-H30 (1980).
20. J.Slezak et al., *Gen.Physiol.Biphys.* **6,** 491-512, (1987).
21. J.Slezak and M.Klobusicka, *Folia Morphologica* **17**, 2, 165-170 (1969).
22. J.Slezak et al., *Laboratory Investigation* **67**, 3, 322 (1992).
23. N.Tribulova et al., *Bratislavske lekarske Listy* **92**, 934-44 (1991).

THE ANTIARRHYTHMIC-DEFIBRILLATORY EFFECT OF d-SOTALOL IN MONOLAYER OF RAT CARDIO MYOCYTES

M. MANOACH, D. VARON, A. SHAINBERG[1], T. ZINMAN[1], A.ISAAC, N. TRIBULOVA[2]

Department of Physiology, Tel Aviv Medical School, Tel Aviv, Israel, [1]Department of Life Sciences, Bar Ilan University, Israel, [2]Institute for Heart Research, Slovak Academy of Sciences Bratislava, Slovak Republic

Calcium ions have been implicated in the mechanisms of ventricular arrhythmias. Impairment of intercellular coupling by calcium overload is considered to facilitate ventricular fibrillation (VF) and to suppress its self termination. According to our hypothesis, any compound that decreases intracellular calcium concentration $[Ca^{2+}]i$ during VF can serve as defibrillating drug. In this study, we examined the effect of d-sotalol on calcium overload in cultured, spontaneously beating rat cardiomyocytes. The changes of $[Ca^{2+}]i$ were measured by indo-1 method and the intercellular synchronization by image analysis. The results showed that increase in $[Ca^{2+}]o$ from 1.9 mM to 3.9 mM increased $[Ca^{2+}]i$ from 100 nM to 320 nM and transformed the synchronized cell movement to an asynchronous one. Administration of $5x\ 10^{-6}$ M d-sotalol decreased the $[Ca^{2+}]i$ to its basic level and restored the synchronized activity. In summary: Our results showed that increase in $[Ca^{2+}]i$ known to caused inhibition of intercellular coupling, that could lead to arrhythmia and fibrillation while d-sotalol prevented this effect. These results support our hypothesis, that class III antiarrhythmic compounds with positive inotropic effect, increase intercellular synchronization, by decreasing $[Ca^{2+}]i$, most probably by increasing the cAMP dependent Ca^{2+} uptake in the sarcoplasmic reticulum and therefore can act as a defibrillating compound.

Introduction

Calcium homeostasis in cardiac myocytes results from integrated function of transsarcolemal Ca^{2+} influx and efflux pathway. It is modulated by membrane potential, and intracellular Ca^{2+} uptake and release, caused predominantly by the sarcoplasmic reticulum (SR) function[1]. Intracellular Ca^{2+} homeostasis in cardiac myocytes is of great functional importance for diastolic resting state of the contractile elements, for excitation-contraction-coupling and for the force of contraction modulated by variations in the magnitude of the calcium transient[1]. It is widely accepted that impaired intracellular Ca^{2+} homeostasis might be a crucial factor for the initiation of ventricular arrhythmias and fibrillation (VF)[2]. It has been shown that in isolated spontaneous beating myocytes, elevation of free intracellular Ca^{2+} ($[Ca^{2+}]i$) induced premature beats, rapid asynchronized beating rate, tachyarrhythmia as well as chaotic or fibrillating beating activity in small roups of myocytes[3,4]. Fast pacing,tachycardia and VF themselves increase $[Ca^{2+}]i$ [5]. Moreover, in the presence of elevated $[Ca^{2+}]i$ appearance of spontaneous arrhythmias could severely enhance $[Ca^{2+}]i$ overload[3]. Extremely rapid Ca^{2+} transients were observed during ventricular fast pacing, tachycardia and VF[5]. It is possible that these rapid Ca^{2+} transient functions cause $[Ca^{2+}]i$ overload through insufficient Ca^{2+} removal by the SR[5]. Disturbances in Ca homeostasis may enable the persistence of this type of arrhythmia[2] while the absence of Ca overload or reduction of $[Ca^{2+}]i$ reversed the arrhythmias and lead to a spontaneous defibrillation[2,3].

On the basis of our previous studies on the mechanisms involved in spontaneous defibrillation[6,7], we have hypothesized[8] that self defibrillation requires high degree of intercellular synchronization. Therefore, any compound that exhibits positive inotropy effect, increases cAMP level, decreases or prevents $[Ca^{2+}]i$ overload, during VF, and thereby increases intercellular coupling can serve as a defibrillating compound. Recently, it has been found that pretreatment with d-sotalol and tedisamil (class III antiarhythmic compounds) prevents sustained VF in human and experimental animals and helps the heart to defibrillate by itself[9,10]. The defibrillating ability and positive inotropic effect have been related to the prolongation of action potential duration and refractory period due to the inhibition of K^+ ionic currents[11,12]. However, the effect of d-sotalol and tedisamil on calcium homeostasis have not been evaluated. Following our above mentioned hypothesis[8], we suggested that this defibrillating effect should be connected with changes in intercellular coupling and synchronization through effect on $[Ca^{2+}]i$. The aim of the present studies was, therefore, to examine the effect of d-sotalol on free Ca^{2+} and synchronous activity in cultured spontaneous beating cardiomyocytes during elevation of the extracellular calcium concentration .

Materials and Methods

The cell cultures were prepared as decribed previously[13]. Intracellular free calcium concentration was estimated, in 3-6 days old cultured cells, from indo-1 fluorescence using the ratio method described by Grynkievicz et al[14]. The cardiac cells grown on cover glass coated with gelatin/collagen were transferred to a chamber on the stage of Zeiss inverted microscope filtered with UV epifluorescence illumination. Indo-1 was excited at 355 nm and the emitted light then split by a dichroic mirror to two photomultipliers with input filter at 405 and 490 nm. The fluorescence ratio 405/490 which is proportional to $[Ca^{2+}]i$ was monitored.

The cellular contraction activity of neonatal rat cardiac myocytes, cultured at the 5th - 8th days of incubation, was analyzed by a video technique previously described by Rich et al1[5]. A culture dish containing adherent cells was attached to the stage of an inverted phase interference microscope. The cells were kept, during the whole experiment, under 37^0C and pH of 7.2 - 7.4. The image of a selected area was passed through the lens to an interlaced video camera at a final magnification of x800. The movement of the cells border, in 4-5 different points, were monitored 400 times/sec. The time variations were converted to voltage, filtered and analyzed by a computer program and recorded simultaneously on Grass polygraph. The type of cellular contraction and the level of synchronization were evaluated.

Results

Our experiments on cell cultured rat cardiomyocytes were divided into two parts: 1/ Fluorescence measurements of [Ca2+]i by indo 1 method (10 experiments 3 cells in each with d-sotalol). 2/ Intercellular synchronization by image analysis (6 experiments with d-sotalol). The results showed that: 1. At days 3-6 of culture, numerous myocytes exhibited spontaneous intracellular Ca^{2+} fluctuations. The average end-diastolic and peak-systolic [Ca^{2+}]i were 100 nM and 320 nM respectively (Fig. 1). Increase in external Ca from 1.8 mM to 3.8 mM decreased spontaneous contractions and increased the diastolic [Ca^{2+}]i from 100 nM to 320 nM (Fig.1). Administration of d-sotalol 10^{-6} M reestablished their spontaneous contraction and reduced [Ca^{2+}]i to its basic level (Fig. 2). The exceleration of the beating rate, observed during the drug induced decrease in Ca is only transient. It decreases very soon to its control rate. 2. At days 6-8 of culture, the majority of the cultured cells exhibited synchronized spontaneous contractions (Fig 3A). Increase of [Ca]o from 1.8 to 3.8 mM in spontaneous synchronized beating myocytes decreased their synchronized activity (Fig.3B) up to total desynchronization with "fibrillating"activity of different cells, more probably due to intercellular electrical uncoupling, followed by termination of the cell movement. Administration of 5x 10^{-6} M d-sotalol restored the synchronized cell activity (Fig.3C) while the "fibrillating"movements disappeared. This effect is most likely due to restoration of the intercellular electrical coupling. Similar effect has been observe following decrease in [Ca^{2+}]o. Pretreatment with either d-sotalol prevented the high [Ca^{2+}]i induced uncoupling and desynchronization.

Discussion

Sotalol is a moderate nonspecific beta adrenergic receptor blocker, as well as potassium channel inhibitor, that dose dependently enables it to prolong action potential duration (APD) and effective refractory period (ERP)[16]. It inhibits time dependent outward delayed rectifier K^+ ionic current and slightly decreases the background K^+ current but not the transient outward current (Ito). It has no effect on the slow Ca^{2+} current and on the fast Na^+ one[11]. The dextroisomer, d-sotalol, has

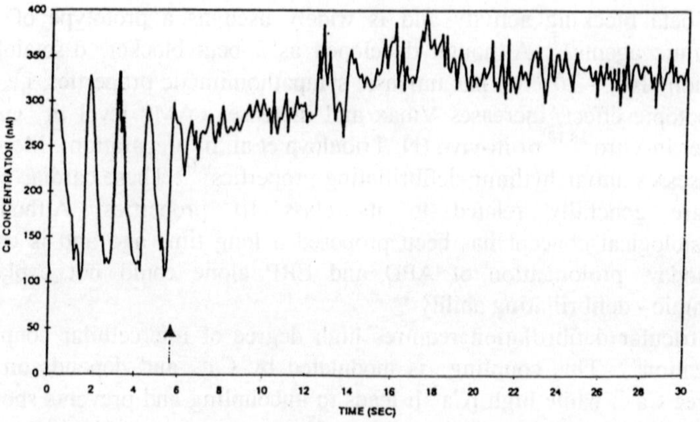

Figure 1.

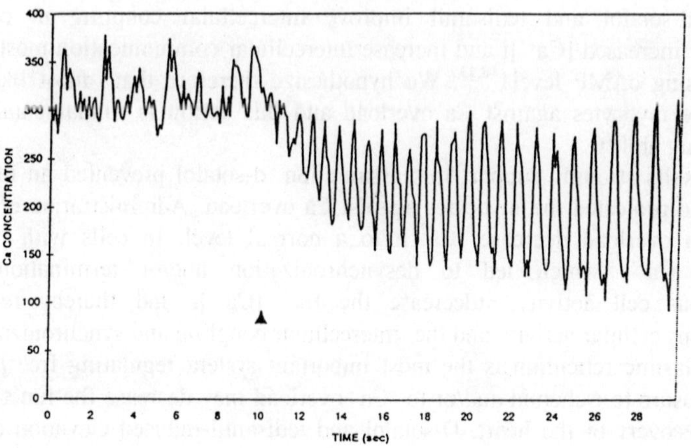

Figure 2.

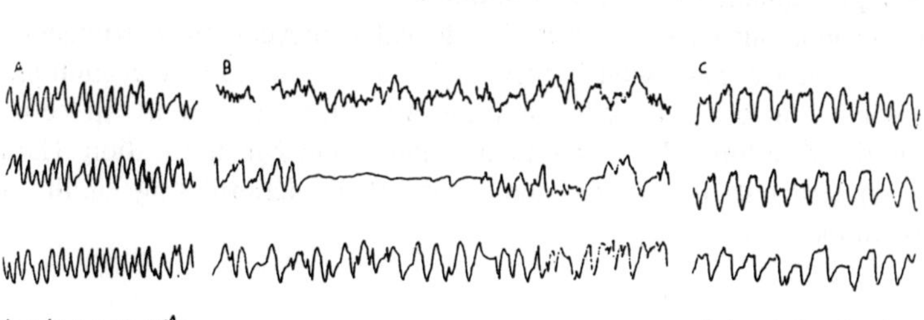

Figure 3.

negligible beta blocking activity and is widely used as a prototype of class III antiarrhythmic agents1[7]. Although developed as a beta blocker, d-sotalol in low concentration (10^{-7} - 10^{-5} M) has intrinsic sympathomimetic properties, i.e. exhibits positive inotopic effect, increases Vmax and increases cAMP level in guinea pig hearts either in-vitro [18,19] or in-vivo (N. Tribulova et.al. in preparation). Moreover ,d-sotalol possesses antiarrhythmic-defibrillating properties[9,10]. These cardiac protective abilities are generally related to its class III properties. Although this electrophysiological concept has been proposed a long time ago and is commonly accepted today, prolongation of APD and ERP alone could not explain their antiarrhythmic - defibrillating ability.

Self ventricular defibrillation requires high degree of intercellular coupling and synchronization[6,8]. This coupling is modulated by Ca^{2+} and depends on the low diastolic free Ca^{2+}, while high $[Ca^{2+}]i$ leads to uncoupling and prevents spontaneous defibrillation. For this reason we hypothesized[8] that any compound which serve as a defibrillating drug, should prevent or decrease Ca overload. Following previous findings d-sotalol and tedisamil improve intercellular coupling in cells with previously increased $[Ca^{2+}]i$ and increase intercellular communication most probably by increasing cAMP levell[18,23]. We hypothesize therefore that most likely they protect the myocytes against Ca overload and this action is fundamental in their defibrilating ability.

Our results strongly support this assumption: d-sotalol prevented an increase in $[Ca^{2+}]i$ and protected the myocytes against Ca overload. Administration of d-sotalol during Ca overload decrease $[Ca^{2+}]i$ to a normal level. In cells with previously increased Ca^{2+}, which led to desynchronization and/or termination of the spontaneous cell activity, itdecrease the free $[Ca^{2+}]i$ and thereby restore the spontaneous cellular activity and the intercellular coupling and synchronization.

Sarcoplasmic reticulum is the most important system regulating free $[Ca^{2+}]i$ [24]. Long exposure to ischemia and/or to Ca overload may decrease the function of SR and the recovery of the heart. D-sotalol and tedisamil-induced elevation of cAMP, could prevent these deteriorating effects and thus to restore intercellular coupling which is a prerequisite for self defibrillation.

In conclusion. Our results showed that d-sotalol prevents the detrimental effect of Ca overload, decreases previously increased $[Ca^{2+}]i$ induced by elevation of external Ca in isolated myocardial cells, prevents asynchronous activity in cell cultured preparation and restored the intercellular coupling and synchronization. These results clearly support our hypothesis and relate their defibrillating ability to their sympathomimetic effects.

References

1. W.H. Bary and H.B. Bridge, Circulation **87**, 1806-1819 (1993).
2. Y. Kihara and J.P.Morgan, Circ. Res. **68**, 1378-1389 (1991).
3. F.Trandroyen A.C. Morris, H.K. Hezler, B. Ziman, L.Pai, J.T. Willerson, L..M. Buja. Circ. Res. **69**,810 - 819 (1991).
4. H. Kimura, Y. Oyamada, H. Ohshika, M. Mori and M. Oyamada, Exper. Cell Res. **220**, 348-356 (1995).
5. S. Kojima, J. Wikman-Cofelt, S.T. Wu & W.W. Parmley, Am. J. Physiol. **266,** Heart Circ.Physiol. 35:,H1473 - H1484 (1994).
6. M.Manoach, D.Varon, M.Neuman, H.Netz, Heart & Vessels **2** Suppl., 56-68, (1997).
7. M. Manoach, and M. Ben-Basat, Int.J. Cardiol. **26**, 129-136 (1990).
8. M. Manoach, & Y. Watanabe, J Cardiovasc. Electrophysiol. **6,** (1995) .
9. P. Dorian and D. Newman, Am. J. Cardiol. **72**, 72A-79A (1993).
10. M.J. Curtis, J. Bassic Clin. Physiol. Pharmacol. **5**, 1-17 (1994).
11. E. Carmeliet, J. Pharmacol. Exp. Ther. **232,**817-825 (1985).
12. I.D. Dukes, L. Cleemann,M. Morad, J. Pharmacol. Exper. Therap. **254,** 560-569 (1990).
13. L. Weinstein, H. Brik, H.H. Rotmanch, and A. SHainberg, J. Cell. Physiol. **148,**124-13 (1991).
14. G. Grynkievitz, M. Poenie,T.Y. Tsien, J. Biol. Chem. **260**,3440-3450, 1985).
15. T.L.Rich, G.A.Langer, M.G.Klassen, Am. J. Physiol. **254**,H937-H 946, (1988).
16. B.N. Sing and E.M. Vaugham-Williams, Br. J. Pharmacol. **39**, 675-687(1970).
17. R. Kato, N. Ikeda, S.M. Yabek, R. Kannan & B.N. Singh, J. Am. Coll. Cardiol. 7, 116-125, (1986).
18. E.I. Miyachi, M. Manoach, H. Uchiyama & Y. Watanabe, Life Sci. **57,**Pl 393-399 (1995).
19. W.W. Parmley, B. Rabinowitz, L. CHuck, G. Bonoris & J.P. Katz, J. Clin. Pharmacol. **12**, 127-135 (1972).
20. K. Baugheer, F. Bode, H.V. Klein, H.J. Trappe, M.R. Franz, P.R.Lichtlen, Eur. Heart J. **15**, 1409-1414 (1994).
21. A.A. Vallace, R.F. Stupienski, E.P. Baskin, A.S.D. Kothstein, J.R. Gehret, S.W. King, D.C. Remy, J.J. Lynch, J. Pharmacol. Exp. Ther. **273**,168-175 (1995).
22. J. Thormann, V. Mitrovic, R. Strasser, H.F. Pitscher, H. Reidel, H. Bahava-rand, M. Schlepper, Z. Kardiol. **82,** 211-221 (1993).
23. H. Uchiyama, M. Manoach, E. Miyachi and Y. Watanabe, Heart Vessels **10,** 185-189 (1995).
24. K.S. Dhalla, H. Rupp, R.E. Beamish and N.S. Dhalla, Cardiovasc. Drug Therapy **10**, 231-238 (1996).

EFFECTS OF VESNARINONE ON THE DELAYED RECTIFIER K+ CURRENT
- EXPERIMENTAL AND SIMULATION STUDY -

J. TOYAMA, MD; K. KAMIYA, MD;
J. CHENG, MD, PhD; J.K. LEE, MD;
the Department of Circulation, Research Institute of Environmental Medicine, Nagoya University, Furo-cho, Chikusa-ku, Nagoya, 464-01, Japan.

R. SUZUKI, BSc; I. KODAMA, MD.
the Department of Humoral Regulation, Research Institute of Environmental Medicine, Nagoya University, Furo-cho, Chikusa-ku, Nagoya, 464-01, Japan.

Vesnarinone, a quinolinone derivative developed as a cardiotonic agent, has complex pharmacological properties but its clinical efficacy is explained partly by the action of I_K block. Therefore, we investigated mode of I_K block by vesnarinone and discussed.**Methods and Results:** I_K of the rabbit ventricular myocyte, in which the rapidly activating component I_{Kr} is predominent, was activated by applying voltage clamp steps from a holding potential to various depolarizing levels up to +50mV. Time courses of both the development of I_K block at depolarization (+10 mV) and its recovery process at hyperpolarization to the physiologic resting potential level (-75 mV) were compared between vesnarinone and E-4031. The I_K block by vesnarinone (3 μmol/L) developed and recovered mono-exponentially with time constants of 400 msec (n=5) and 2.0 sec (n=4), respectively. As for E-4031(0.3 μmol/L), I_K block developed instantaneously and no recovery from the block occurred during hyperpolarization. The frequency-dependence of I_K block was examined by measuring I_K tail currents evoked after a train of depolarizing pulses (for 30 sec at 0.2 to 2 Hz). I_K block by vesnarinone increased with increasing frequency (2 fold at 2 from 0.2 Hz) but that by E-4031 was unchanged. **Conclusion:** Vesnarinone may prolong the repolarization process of human cardiac muscle without reverse frequency-dependence, since the ratio of the rapid to slow component of I_K is as high in the human as the rabbit. Thus, this drug may exert beneficial effects on the decompensated human heart through its I_K blocking action.

Introduction

Vesnarinone, a quinoline derivative developed as a phosphodiesterase (PDE) inhibitor has been reported to improve both morbidity and mortality rates of the patients with chronic congestive heart failure (CHF).[1] However, this drug is effective clinically only at low doses (60 mg/day) below the range at which ventricular contractility and pumping functions are augmented through its PDE inhibitory action. Recent studies on vesnarinone have clarified that this drug has the pharmacological profile of a blocker of the delayed rectifier potassium current (I_K).[2] In particular, the I_K blocking action of vesnarinone is beneficial both for slowing the patient's heart rate which would otherwise be augmented by PDE inhibitory action, and for improving the pumping function of failing hearts, by causing action potential prolongation, similar to that of the methanesulfonanilide derivatives (pure I_K blockers) which inhibit the sinus node activity and augment the contractile force of ventricular muscle. However, the class III antiarrhythmic drugs such as methanesulfonanilide commonly exhibit a "reverse" frequency-dependent prolongation of the action potential duration , limiting its clinical usefulness due to a risk of proarrhythmia.[3]

In this study, we compared the effects of vesnarinone with the selective I_{Kr} blocker E-4031 in rabbit ventricular muscle in which the dominant component of I_K is I_{Kr}.[4] We demonstrate that vesnarinone block I_K in rabbit ventricular muscle in a use-dependent manner.

METHODS

Isolation of Single Ventricular Myocytes: Single ventricular myocytes from rabbit hearts were obtained by an enzymatic dissociation procedure, as described previously.[5] In brief, 2.0 kg the rabbit hearts were rapidly excised, mounted via the aorta to a Langendorff retrograde perfusion apparatus, were initially perfused with calcium-free Tyrode solution until the heart stopped beating, and finally with the same solution containing 0.12 mg/ml collagenase (Yakult, Japan) for 15 min. The isolated cells were stored in the same solution at 4℃ before use. **Electrophysiological Recording:** The single-pipette whole-cell clamp method was used to record currents as reported previously.[6] An aliquot of the cell suspension was placed in the recording chamber on the stage of an inverted microscope (Diaphoto, Nikon Co, Tokyo). Then the cells were superfused with Tyrode solution at 34℃. The pipettes were connected to a patch-clamp amplifier (List-medical, Darmstadt, Germany). When delayed rectifier potassium currents (I_K) were measured, the superfusate was changed to NMG solution (in mmol/L): N-methyl-D-glucamine 149, $MgCl_2$ 5, HEPES 5 and nisoldipine 0.003. **Drugs and Data Analysis:** Vesnarinone (3,4-dihidro-6{4-(3,4-dimethoxybenzoyl)-1-piperazinyl}-2(1H)-quinolinone, OPC-8212) was obtained from Otsuka Pharmaceutical Company. E-4031(N-[4-[[1-[2-(6-methyl-2-pyridinyl)ethyl]-4 -piperidinyl]carbonyl] phenyl]methanesulfonamide dihydrochloride dihydrate) was obtained from Eisai Pharmaceutical Company. They were dissolved in distilled water as stock solutions and diluted in superfusates to the desired final concentrations immediately before each experiment.

All animals were treated in accordance with the principles and procedures outlined by the Committee for Animal Experiment of Nagoya University School of Medicine and the Research Institute of Environmental Medicine.

The curve-fitting program Igor (Wave Metrics, Oregon) was used in data analysis. Data in the text are presented a means ± SE. Statistical analysis in two paired groups was carried out by paired t-test.

Results

Effects on activation of I_K: Dose-dependent effects of vesnarinone on the I_K activation were examined Vesnarinone (3 to 30 μmol/L) depressed dose-dependently both the delayed rectifier outward current (I_K) during the depolarizing pulse and its tail (I_K tail) detected on clamping back to the holding potential. The drug concentration for 50% inhibition of I_K tail following +30 mV depolarization (IC_{50}) was calculated to be 5.5 μmol/L (n=5). The effects of E-4031 on the I_K activation was analysed by the same protocol. E-4031 also depressed I_K tail in a dose-dependent manner and its IC_{50} was 0.9 μmol/L (n=7).

Difference in the development of I_K block was compared between these two drugs. Reduction of I_K tail amplitude (I_K block) by vesnarinone is small (25%) at the conditioning pulse of 0.1 sec but the I_K block is augmented markedly (80%) when the conditioning pulse is prolonged to 1 sec. This implies that vesnarinone blocks I_K through a mechanism of binding to the open state channel.[3] The ratio of I_K tails in the presence and absence of each drug indicates the ratio of the drug-bound fraction to all the available I_K channels. In the presence of vesnarinone, the ratio decreased mono-exponentially (with a time constant 400msec, n=5) with the duration of depolarization, implying a first order reaction which proceeds rather slowly between vesnarinone and its binding site. However, the ratio of I_K tail after E-4031 (0.3 μmol/L) to control remained unchanged even when the depolarizing pulse was lengthened from 0.1 to 3.0 sec. It suggests that the interaction between the I_K channel and E-4031 is either immediate or state-independent. **Effects on deactivation of I_K:** Difference in modulation of the I_K deactivation process was compared compared between vesnarinone and E-4031. The amplitudes of the I_K tail before drug were decreased gradually as the duration of hyperpolarization was lengthened, while those measured after the drug was increased with increase of the duration of hyperpolarization. In the presence of vesnarinone, the ratios were increased mono-exponentially with a time constant of 2.0 sec as the hyperpolarization pulse was prolonged, indicating that recovery from the block of I_K induced by vesnarinone proceeds through a mechanism of unbinding of the drug from the closed state I_K channel when the membrane potential is hyperpolarized to the physiologic resting level. **Frequency dependence of I_K inhibition:** A train of the depolarizing clamp pulses of 200 msec to +10 mV to mimic the configuration of ventricular action potential was applied at a rate from 0.2 to 2.0 Hz. After the train of depolarizing pulses for 30 sec, the I_K tail was measured by applying a test clamp pulse. The amplitude of I_K tail before drug was augmented markedly as the pulse rate was increased from 0.2 to 2 Hz. This indicates that decrease of the resting interval shortens the time for the I_K channel to deactivate, thus leading to a rate-dependent augmentation of the I_K activation. In the presence of vesnarinone, such rate-dependent augmentation of I_K tail disappeared and, on the contrary, the I_K tail amplitude decreased at increasing rates. The measured I_K block by vesnarinone was reduced from 0.84 to 0.50 as the pulse rate increased from 0.2 to 2.0 Hz, and the simulated I_K block was reduced frequency-dependently in the same way as the measured one. In contrast, the I_K block by E-4031 remained unchanged.

Discussion

Carmeliet [4] reported that the unblock of I_K at a physiologic level of the resting potential (-75mV) was practically absent in the presence of either almokalant or dofetilide. Such absence of the unblock at the resting state explains the absence of frequency-dependence, and thus the presence of reverse frequency-dependence is explained by a common feature of the open channel blockers of I_K [3] All the methanesulfonanilide drugs including E-4031 and many class I drugs tested so far share this property. Our data on I_K block are consistent with those reported results. In contrast, vesnarinone blocked I_K frequency-dependently . Such frequency-dependent I_K block was reproduced by our simulation in which our experimental data on the I_K- blocking and -unblocking processes by vesnarinone are assumed to be conducted by the first order reaction between vesnarinone and its specific binding site of the I_K channel. As for E-4031, frequency-dependent I_K block was no recovery from I_K block at the rest period is the reason why this drug blocks I_K frequency-independently. This result supports the hypothesis that E-4031 remains trapped by the closed channel, and explains why the I_K block by this drug is still effective even after a long resting period.

Therefore, in addition to class III antiarrhythmic action, this drug may benefit CHF through themechanisms of opposing the neuro-humorally augmented sinus node activity and improving of the pumping function of failing hearts with a minimal risk of proarrhythmia. [7]

References

1. Feldman AM, Bristow MR, Parmley WW, Carson PE, Pepine CJ, Gilbert EM, Strobeck JE, Hendrix GH, Powers ER, Bain RP, White BG. vesnarinone study group. Effects of

vesnarinone on morbidity and mortality in patients with heart failure. *N Engl J Med.* 1993;329:149-155.

2. Yatani A, Imoto Y, Schwartz A, Brown AM. New positive inotropic agent OPC-8212 modulates single Ca^{2+} channels in ventricular myocytes of guinea pig. *J CardiovascPharmacol.* 1989;13:812-819.

3. Hondeghem LM, Snyders DJ. Class III antiarrhythmic agents have a lot of potential but a long way to go: reduced effectiveness and dangers of reverse use dependent. *Circulation.* 1990;81:686-690.

4. Carmeliet E. Voltage- and time-dependent block of the delayed K^{+} current in cardiac myocytes by dofetilide. *J Pharmacol Exp Ther.* 1992;262:809-817.

5. Toyama J, Sugiura H, Kamiya K, Kodama I, Terasawa M, Hidaka H. Ca^{2+}-calmodulin mediated modulation of the electrical coupling of ventricular myocytes isolated from guinea pig heart. *J Mol Cell Cardiol.* 1994;26:1007-1015.

6. Cheng J, Kamiya K, Kodama I, Toyama J. Differential effects of MS-551 and E-4031 on action potentials and the delayed rectifier K^{+} current in rabbit ventricular myocytes. *Cardiovasc Res.* 1996;31:963-974.

7. Toyama J, Kamiya K, Cheng J, Lee JK, Suzuki R, Kodama I. Ion channel blockers in the treatment of chronic heart failure. *J Cardiovasc Failure.* 1996;2:S243-S249.

A NEW MODEL FOR THE EVALUATION OF POSTHYPOXIC RECOVERY IN GUINEA PIG PAPILLARY MUSCLE

J. E. LØKEBØ, T. RAVINGEROVA[1], J. MUNCH-ELLINGSEN, R. SUNDSET, P. M. TANDE, K. YTREHUS

Department of Medical Physiology, Institute of Medical Biology, University of Tromsø, Tromsø N-9037, Norway; [1]Institute for Heart Research, SAS, 9 Dubravska cesta, Bratislava, 842 33, Slovakia

Brief ischemia or hypoxia has been found to protect the heart against subsequent long-lasting ischemia and to improve contractile dysfunction as well as to reduce the incidence of lethal arrhythmias. This phenomenon termed as preconditioning (PC) has been demonstrated in different species. However, little is known about PC in guinea pigs. Moreover, electrophysiological changes underlying protection have not been studied so far in conjunction with force recovery in a setting of PC. The aim of the study was to establish a new model of PC in a guinea pig papillary muscle, using recovery of contractility after long hypoxic challenge as the main end-point of protection, and to investigate concomitant electrophysiological alterations. In addition, the role of K_{ATP}-channels, potential effectors of PC, was evaluated by application of K_{ATP}-channel blocker 5-hydroxydecanoate (5-HD, 0.5 mM) during recovery in the PC period and subsequent sustained hypoxia. Methods: In guinea pig papillary muscle preparations contracting isometrically (paced at 2 Hz) transmembrane action potentials (AP) and developed force (DF) were recorded by conventional microelectrode technique and a force transducer. In addition, effective refractory periods (ERP) were determined. Hypoxia was induced by superfusion with 100 N_2 ($pO_2 < 5$ kPa) and pacing at 3.3 Hz. In the control group, long hypoxia lasted for 45 min and was followed by 30 min reoxygenation. In the PC group, the muscles were subjected to 5 min hypoxia + 10 min recovery prior to sustained hypoxia/reoxygenation. Results: Long hypoxia induced a similar depression of DF in both, PC and control groups. However, in the PC group loss of contractile activity occurred earlier, and action potential duration (APD) and ERP shortened faster after PC. Upon reoxygenation, these muscles showed significantly better recovery of contractile function (DF 86% of prehypoxic value vs 36% in controls, $p < 0.05$). AP and ERP were completely restored in both, PC and control groups. Treatment with a K_{ATP}-channel blocker attenuated the effects of PC on DF, APD and ERP, but not on resting force (RF) during hypoxia and blocked the recovery of the DF during reoxygenation. Conclusions: Guinea pig papillary muscle can be preconditioned with a brief hypoxic challenge against contractile dysfunction upon long-lasting hypoxia/reoxygenation. During hypoxia, faster shortening of APD and loss of contractility after PC might be beneficial and facilitate preservation of energy. K_{ATP}-channel blockade attenuates protective effect of PC indicating a role of K_{ATP}-channels in the mechanisms of endogenous protection in guinea pigs.

Introduction

Brief episodes of ischemia (hypoxia) have been found to increase tolerance of the heart to a subsequent long-lasting ischemic challenge.[1] This adaptive phenomenon, termed preconditioning, has been found to occur in different animal species (dogs, rabbits, rats) and to include limitation of the infarct size,[2,3] improved postischemic contractile recovery[4] and reduction of severe ventricular arrhythmias in both, open-chest animals and in isolated heart preparations.[5-7]

However, only few reports describe preconditioning in a papillary muscle model[8,9] and little is known about preconditioning in guinea pigs. Moreover, electrophysiological changes underlying protection against arrhythmias still remain unclear and have not been studied in conjunction with force recovery in a setting of preconditioning.

Aims of the study

This study was designed to test whether short hypoxic episodes can provide protection against a long hypoxic challenge in a guinea pig papillary muscle model. Posthypoxic recovery of contractile function has been chosen as the main end-point of protection. A further goal was to evaluate concomitant alterations of electrical activity of the preparation during hypoxia/reoxygenation.

In addition, the role of K_{ATP}-channels as potential effectors of PC, was evaluated by application of K_{ATP}-channel blocker 5-hydroxydecanoate (5-HD, 0.5 mM) during recovery in the PC-periode and subsequent sustained hypoxia (Fig.1).

Methods

Papillary muscles isolated from guinea pig ventricles in a Langendorff perfusion setup were mounted in an organ bath and superfused with modified Tyrode solution containing HEPES buffer (flow rate 5 ml/min). The solution was gassed with 100% O_2 which resulted in pO_2 of ~50 kPa and pH of 7.4 in the organ bath. Temperature in the bath was maintained at 35 °C, and pO_2 was analyzed intermittently.

Muscles were field stimulated at a rate of 2 Hz (2 ms wide rectangular pulses of 1,5 time threshold intensity). Impalement with microelectrode was carried out simultaneously with measurement of developed force via a force tranducer. Transmembrane action potentials were recorded with conventional microelectrode technique. Effective refractory periods (ERP) were determined by a programmed stimulation with a premature pulse applied after a train of 8 basic stimuli until the extra pulse failed to evoke an action potential.

Hypoxia was induced by superfusion with a substrate-free buffer gassed with 100 % N_2 ($pO_2 < 5$ kPa) in an Ar-covered organ bath; pacing rate 3.3 Hz.

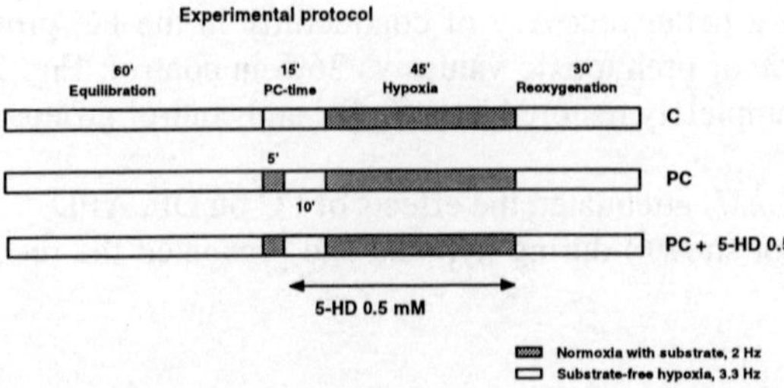

Figure 1: Experimental protocol; 5-hydroxydecanoate (5-HD, 0.5 mM) is given during recovery in preconditioning (PC) period and subsequent sustained hypoxia.

Summary of the results

Short hypoxia and reoxygenation (PC) induced a transient increase and fall in developed force (DF) which was partially recovered (80%) before the onset of long hypoxia, (Fig. 2, left panel). APD (Fig. 2, rigth panel) and ERP (not shown) were initially shortened with a subsequent complete recovery.

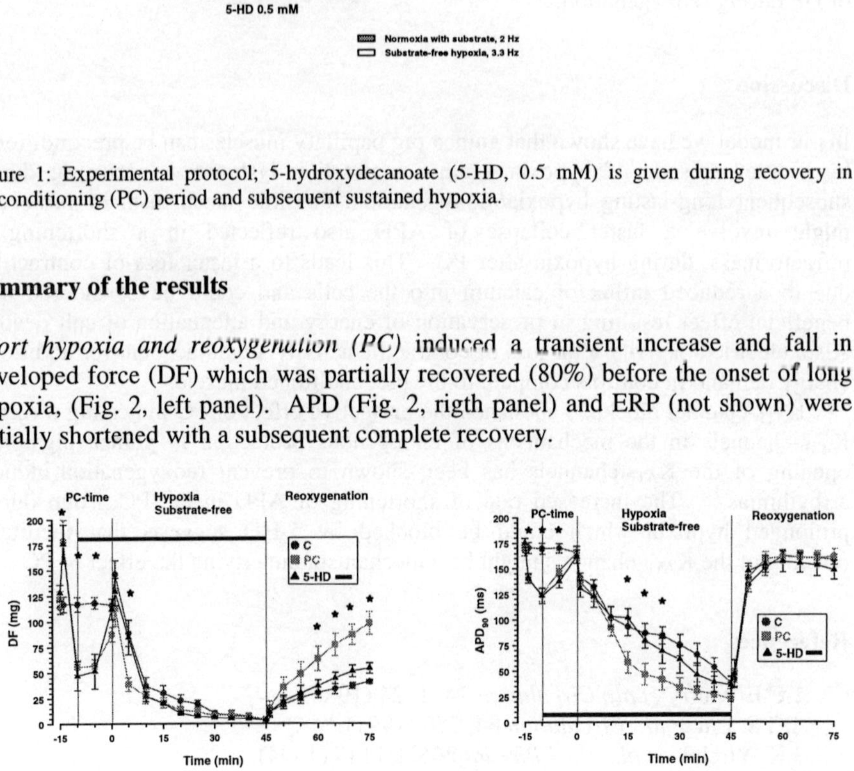

Figure 2: Effects of hypoxic preconditioning (PC) and 5-HD on developed force (DF, left panel) and action potential duration (APD_{90}, right panel) in guinea pig papillary muscles during hypoxia and reoxygenation. Data are means ± SEM of 6 experiments in each group. *$P < 0.05$; PC group vs 5-HD group.

Long hypoxia induced a gradual decline of DF, the rate of which was faster in the PC group (Fig 2 left panel). Increase in resting force (RF) started to develop earlier in the preconditioned muscles, however, the magnitude of RF was as in the control group (not shown). APD and ERP decreased faster and were significantly shorter after PC as compared to the controls (Fig. 2 right panel).

Reoxygenation resulted in a better recovery of contractility in the PC group at the end of the 30 min (DF 86% of prehypoxic values vs 36% in control; Fig. 2 left panel). APD and ERP were completely restored in both, PC and control groups (Fig. 2 right panel).

Treatment with 5-HD (0.5 mM) attenuated the effects of PC on DF, APD (Fig. 2) and ERP, but not on RF (not shown) during hypoxia and prevented the recovery of DF during reoxygenation.

Discussion

In our model we have shown that guinea pig papillary muscles can be preconditioned by a brief episode of hypoxia against contractile dysfunction occurring during subsequent long-lasting hypoxia/reoxygenation. Possible mechanism of protection might involve a faster collapse of APD also reflected in a shortening of refractoriness, during hypoxia after PC. This leads to a faster loss of contractility due to a reduced influx of calcium into the cells and could be considered as a beneficial effect resulting in preservation of energy and attenuation of cell death.[10] Also, electrical activity after loss of contractile activity, could account for additional energy demand in controls compare to the preconditioned muscle.

K_{ATP}-channel blockade abolished the protective effect of PC indicating a role of K_{ATP}-channels in the mechanisms of endogenous protection in guinea pigs. An opening of the K_{ATP}-channels has been shown to prevent reoxygenation-induced arrhythmias.[11] The increased rate of shortening of APD in the PC group during prolonged hypoxia which could be blocked by 5-HD suggests that facilitated opening of the K_{ATP}-channels might be a mechanism underlying the effect of PC.

References

1. C.E. Murry *et al.*, *Circulation* **74**, 1124 (1986).
2. G.S. Liu *et al.*, *Circulation* **84**, 350 (1991).
3. K. Ytrehus *et al., Am J Physiol* **266**, H1145 (1994).
4. M.V. Cohen *et al.*, *Circulation* **84,** 341 (1991).
5. K. Shiki and D.J. Hearse, *Am J Physiol* **253**, H1470 (1987).
6. A. Vegh *et al.*, *Cardiovasc Res* **26**, 487 (1992).
7. T. Ravingerova *et al.*, *Mol Cell Biochem* **147**, 123, (1995).
8. D.M. Walker *et al.*, *Am J Physiol* **266,** H1534, (1994).
9. H.L. Tan *et al.*, *Cardiovasc Res* **27**, 644, (1993).
10. U.K.M. Deckling *et al.*, *Am J Physiol* **269**, H 734 (1995).
11. H. Hayashi *et al.*,*J Cardiovasc Pharmacol* **27**, 816, (1996).

DELAYED PROTECTION OF THE HEART AGAINST ISCHEMIA AND POSTISCHEMIC REPERFUSION (I-R)-INDUCED ARRHYTHMIAS BY 7-OXO-PROSTACYCLIN (PGI_2): MOLECULAR MECHANISMS

A. ZIEGELHÖFFER, T. RAVINGEROVÁ, A. DŽURBA, N. VRBJAR, N. TRIBULOVÁ

Institute for Heart Research, Slovak Academy of Sciences, Dúbravská cesta 9, Bratislava 842 33, Slovak Republic

A stable prostacyclin (PGI_2) analogue 7-oxo-PGI_2 has been shown to exert a delayed and long lasting (2-72h) antiischemic and antiarrhythmic action on the heart. In present study we investigated the protective effect of 7-oxo-PGI_2 on ischemia/reperfusion (I-R)-induced functional, metabolic and morphological perturbations in the rat heart. Special attention was paid to elucidation of molecular mechanisms of the drug action as well as to study of function of the heart sarcolemmal Na,K-ATPase (SL NAK) in respect to arrhythmogenesis. In the untreated group I-R induced 75% of sustained ventricular fibrillation. In animals pretreated with 7-oxo-PGI_2 48 h prior to experiments, incidence of ventricular fibrillation, its duration, as well as arrhythmia score were significantly lower and the recovery of heart function was significantly improved (dP/dt 100% vs. 70% in controls, $p<0.05$). These findings were accompanied with lower lactate accumulation and better preserved ATP contents in hearts during ischemia. Late effect of 7-oxo-PGI_2 was also manifested by a reduced extent of cell damage after I-R, better preserved ultrastructure of cardiomyocytes and by maintenance of the SL integrity as well as prevention of excess Ca^{2+} influx into the cardiac cells. The biochemical base of SL stabilization represented a 7-oxo-PGI_2-induced increase in the amount and activity of SL NAK. This could mitigate the loss of intracellular K^+ and gain of Na^+ and Ca^{2+} in cardiac cells, suppressing thus effectively the incidence, duration and severity of ventricular arrhythmias observed during I-R in the pretreated hearts.

Introduction

Activation of the arachidonic acid pathway as one of the crucial factors of ischemia/reperfusion injury has been extensively studied with rather controversal results. A stable prostacyclin analogue 7-oxo-prostacyclin (PGI_2) has been shown to exert its delayed (2h after administration) and long lasting (until 72h) antiischemic and antiarrhythmic action on the heart in different models and various species[1]. As concerns its mechanism of action, 7-oxo-PGI_2 is comparable with the well known prostacyclin analogue Iloprost[R] and its effect has been ascribed to stabilization of cell membranes. This was manifested by reduction of Na^+ entry and K^+ loss from the myocytes during ischemia.

In the present study we investigated the effect of 7-oxo-PGI_2 on ischemia- and postischemic reperfusion-induced functional, metabolic and morphological derangements in the rat heart with special emphasis on the detrimental effects of Ca^{2+} overload. Our second goal was to clarify the molecular mechanisms involved in functional and structural stabilization of cell membranes, particularly those that are linked with cation homeostasis, and in this respect, to study the function of the heart sarcolemmal Na,K-ATPase.

Material and Methods

All studies have been performed in accordance with the Guide for the Care and Use of Laboratory Animals published by the US National Institute of Health (NIH publication No 85-23, revised 1985.
figure

All experiments were performed in isolated Langendorff-perfused rat hearts. In accordance with the previous findings[1], animals were pretreated with either a single dosage of 7-oxo-PGI_2 (50 μ/kg b.w., i.m.) or saline 48h before the experiment. For the study of myocardial dysfunction, the hearts were subjected to 30 min global ischemia followed by 30 min reperfusion. To induce a non-receptor-mediated calcium oveload, the hearts were subjected to a 3 min Ca^{2+}-free perfusion followed by a 10 min Ca^{2+} repletion. Functional parameters (heart rate, contractility, coronary flow) were monitored. Morphological and metabolic investigations were carried out at the end of the ischemic period and after reperfusion, as well as after Ca^{2+}-depletion and Ca^{2+}-repletion. They included electron microscopy as well as biochemical estimation of high energy phosphates, lactate and pyruvate in the heart tissue[2]. For the study of ventricular arrhythmias, the hearts were subjected to 30 min occlusion of LAD coronary artery and 5 min reperfusion of the occluded area. Arrhythmias occuring upon reperfusion were analysed for incidence and duration as well as for their severity. For the study of Na,K-ATPase, the enzyme activity and its kinetic properties were determined in partially purified sarcolemmal membrane preparations from the hearts of pretreated and control animals[3].

Results

In the 7-oxo-PGI_2-pretreated rats, the recovery of heart function was significantly improved after reperfusion (dP/dt 100% vs. 70% in controls, $p<0.05$) and after Ca^{2+} -overload (dP/dt 60% vs. 0% in controls, $p<0.05$). During ischemia and after Ca^{2+} overload, the tissue contents of ATP and the total pool of adenine nucleotides were better preserved in the hearts of 7-oxo-PGI_2-pretreated rats than in controls (by 20.0 and 23.2 %, $p<0.05$ as well as by 134.3 and 114,2 %, $p<0.01$ respectively).and the lactate content in cardiac tissue during ischemia was lowered by 34.8 % ($p<0.001$) in the pretreated group[2,4]. Protective effect of 7-oxo-PGI_2 was also manifested by a reduced extent of cell damage after ischemia/reperfusion, further by better preservation of myocytes ultrastructure[2,5] as well as by the maintenance of the sarcolemmal membrane integrity. All these prevented an excess Ca^{2+} influx into the cardiac cells[4-5]. Membrane stability has been also found to be enhanced due to a selective stimulation of the sarcolemmal Na,K-ATPase[3]. Both, the amount of enzyme and its activity were significantly increased (by 29.7 and 124.3 % respectively, $p<0.001$) in the pretreated hearts. The V_{max} value of the Na,K-ATPase was also increased by 7 % in the 7-oxo-PGI_2-pretreated hearts. However, this effect was misrepresentingly low since increase in the V_{max} concerned only the smaller newly synthetized portion in the bulk of ATP-ase only[3]. Moreover, the newly synthetized enzyme exhibited a significant decrease in its K_m value (by 43.8 %, $p<0.01$) thus indicating a considerable increase in its affinity to ATP[3]. This finding also idicates these changes in the Na,K-ATPase as a molecular base for effective suppression of the incidence and severity of ventricular arrhythmias which were observed during postischemic reperfusion in the pretreated rat hearts[6].

Discussion

The delayed effects of 7-oxo-PGI_2, protecting the heart against extrasystoles, ventricular fibrillation and cardiac arrest iduced by high doses of ouabain or in ischemia were first described by the group Szekeres et al.[1,7-8]. The compound was shown to provide a preservation of transmembrane transport of cations, particularly Na^+ and K^+. This pointed to Na,K-ATPase, that is believed to be responsible for the outward transport of sodium and inward transport of potassium through myocardial sarcolemma, as a a final link modulated in the chain of events initiated by administration of 7-oxo-PGI_2[3]. In respect to described inhomogeneity in intracellular concentration of sodium[9] as well as to the recognition that precautions taken to prevent the deterioration of Na^+ homeostasis during postischemic reperfusion and the depletion of Ca^{2+}, it could be also assumed that 7-oxo-PGI_2 may protect the heart against calcium paradox[10]. Our results approved the late antiischemic as well as antiarrhytmic effect of 7-oxo-PGI_2 in diverse models of postischemic reperfusion of the rat heart[2,4-6]. The protective effect of the compound against calcium overload of the heart was tested using the model of calcium paradox. Results revealed that depletion of Ca^{2+} lowers the activity of Ca-ATPase, induces a critical depression in the Na,K-ATPase activity and disturbs the integrity of rat heart sarcolemma. Pretreatment of animals with 7-oxo-PGI_2 eliminated the diminution of the Na,K-ATPase activity. The preserved enzyme seemed to be competent to maintain Na^+ concentration in the subsarcolemmal space low enough to prevent an activation of the Na-Ca exchange mechanism. Our results also indicated that in the absence of enhanced Na-Ca exchange, the Ca^{2+} depletion-induced damage to the sarcolemma may be not potent enough to introduce itself an irreversible calcium overload in the rat heart.

Conclusions

Pretreatment of animals with 7-oxo-PGI_2 affords a delayed protection against ischemia/reperfusion injury of the rat heart. Molecular mechanisms of this action involve increased de novo synthesis of Na,K-ATPase molecules. The newly synthetized enzyme is capable to utilize the energy more efficiently since it exhibits increased affinity to ATP. This yields in significant increase in Na,K-ATPase activity of the heart sarcolemma. The latter may be responsible for the better maintenance of intracellular cation homeostasis, prevent intracellular Ca^{2+}-overload and improve the membrane stability of cardiac myocytes.

Well preserved membrane structure and functions may than account for the late antiarrhytmic effect of 7-oxo-PGI_2.

Acknowledgments

The excellent technical assistance of Mr. D. Pancza Msc., Mrs. Marta Hýbelová, Erika Havránková, Zlatica Hradecká and Anna Brichtová is greatfully appreciated.

This project was supported, in part by the Slovak Scientific Grant Agency VEGA, grants No. 1258/96, 1256/96, 1165/96 and the European Communities Grant COST CIPA 92 4009.

References

1. L. Szekeres *et al. Biomed. Biochim. Acta* **47,** 6 (1988).
2. T. Ravingerová *et al. Basic. Res. Cardiol.* **86,** 245 (1991).
3. A. Džurba *et al. Cardioscience* **2,** 105 (1991).
4. T. Ravingerová *et al. Life Sci.* **53,** 1309 (1993).
5. N. Tribulová *et al. Submicrosc. Cytol. Pathol.* **25,** 267 (1993).
6. T. Ravingerová *et al. Cardiovasc. Res.* **27,** 1051 (1993).
7. L. Szekeres et al. *Biomed. Biochim. Acta* **43**, 135 (1987)
8. L. Szekeres et al. .*Pharmacol. Res. Commun.* **20**, Suppl 1, 77 (1988)
9. E. Carmeliet *Cardiovasc. Res.* **26**. 433 (1992)
10. A. Ziegelhöffer et al. *Mol. Cell. Biochem.* **160/161**, 257 (1996)

COOLING EFFECT ON ACTIVATION SEQUENCE OF THE VENTRICULAR EPICARDIUM IN THE RABBIT

D.N. SHMAKOV, J.E. AZAROV, M.P. ROSHCHEVSKY, V.A. VITYAZEV, I.M. ROSHCHEVSKAYA, S.N. HARIN, K.K. MOSTIVENKO

Institute of Physiology of the Komi Science Centre, Ural Division, Russian Academy of Sciences, Syktyvkar, Kommunisticheskaya, 24, Komi, 167610, Russia

E-mail: compcard@online.ru

The changes of the ventricular epicardial activation patterns within the mediastinal temperature range from 38 to 32°C was studied in the adult rabbits. Under heart cooling slight but significant alterations of the ventricular epicardial depolarization sequence were revealed. The total duration of the epicardial activation significantly increased by 3±2 ms while the QRS complex in the II limb lead prolonged by 10±6 ms. These data imply that the major excitation spread slowing occured evidently in the intramural ventricular layers but hardly in the superficial ones. Thus, under moderate hypothermia (32°C) the depolarization delay of the left ventricular epicardial sites was more pronounced than that on the right ventricular surface, and the activation slowing observed in areas of the late depolarization was to a greater extent than that in the area of early excitation.

1 Introduction

Heart cooling widely applied in cardiac surgery causes impulse propagation slowing probably leading to the ventricular arrhythmia. To evaluate the mechanism of the heart electric events occuring under hypothermia it is necessary to study cooling-induced alterations of the ventricular depolarization sequence. The present study continued the investigation of the rabbit's cardiac electric field during the QRS complex already reported from our laboratory[1].

2 Methods

Under mediastinal temperature variations from 38 to 32°C ventricular epicardial depolarization sequences were studied in 14 adult rabbits anaesthetized with sodium thiopental (70-100 mg/kg, i.p.). Unipolar electrograms were simultaneously recorded from 64 epicardial leads evenly distributed on the overall surface of both ventricles. The temperature of mediastinal cavity was varied by the continuous saline perfusion performed with the aid of the thermostat pump. For each epicardial lead site activation time was determined as a minimum of the time-derivative of potential during the QRS-complex. A conventional paired t-test was used for statistical estimation. The differences were considered significant at $p<0.05$. Here the data are presented as M±SD.

3 Results

We found that the mediastinum perfusion procedure itself did not influence significantly the ventricular epicardial depolarization sequence if the thermal conditions were unaltered. In our experiments under mediastinal temperature of 38°C the heart rate was 160-180 bpm, the QRS complex duration in the II limb lead equaled to 29±3 ms and the total duration of the ventricular epicardial activation was 17±3 ms. There were two epicardial depolarization wavefront breakthroughs (Fig.1). One of them was located in the heart apical area in the region of projection of the left ventricular anterior papillary muscle bases. Another one was insignificantly delayed with respect to the first one and observed in the central third of the right ventricular lateral zone. From these centres the excitation wave spread first to a left ventricular lateral surface and then to a ventricular base.

After the mediastinum had been cooled to 32°C the heart rate decelerated to approximately 120 bpm and the depolarization sequence of the ventricular surface changed slightly. The characteristic alteration of the ventricular epicardial activation pattern was excitation time delay. The QRS complex in the II limb lead prolonged by 10±6 ms ($p<0.001$) up to 38±5 ms while the total duration of the epicardial activation significantly ($p<0.001$) increased by 3±2 ms up to 19±3 ms. Throughout the ventricular surface the prolongation of the epicardial depolarizat ion was nonuniform. The cooling-induced activation time delay in various epicardial areas increased ($p<0.05$) in a following order: a lateral right ventricular surface; a right ventricular base and heart apex; left ventricular lateral surface and base. These changes resulted in a depolarization sequence slightly but faithfully different from that under mediastinal temperature of 38°C. In the conditions of cooling the mediastinum to 32°C the excitation wavefront emerged on the epicardium in right ventricular lateral surface (Fig.2). As under normothermic conditions another epicardial breakthrough of the activation wave was found near the heart apex in the left ventricular anterior papillary muscle bases projection region. Depolarization of the lateral right ventricular epicardial zone preceeded insignificantly (1±2 ms) that in the heart apical area. In 5±3 ms ($p<0.001$) after the primary centres of the excitation had appeared on the epicardium the activation wave reached the left ventricular lateral and right ventricular basal surfaces. And 2±2 ms ($p<0.05$) later an epicardium of the left ventricular base was depolarized, i.e., in hypothermic conditions a difference in the activation times between the right and left ventricular basal surfaces appeared.

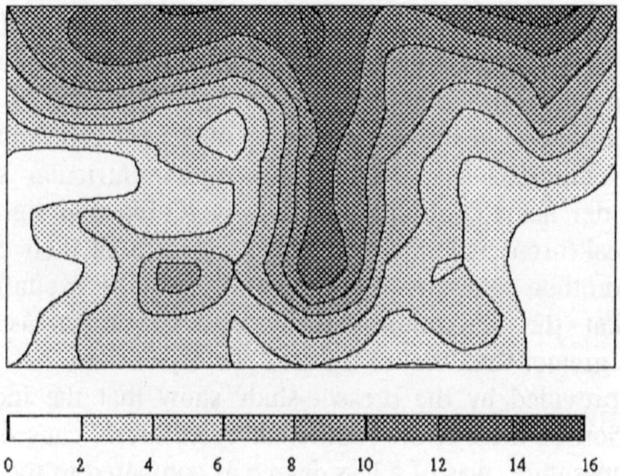

Figure 1: Isochronal map of the depolarization sequence of ventricular epicardium in the rabbit at mediastinal temperature of 38°C.
A top of the map corresponds to the ventricular base and the bottom corresponds to the heart apex. Right and left margins of the map represent the line running from the heart apex to the lateral region of the right ventricular base. The mid portion of the map corresponds the lateral surface of the left ventricle. Time (ms) is measured in respect to the activation epicardial breakthrough.

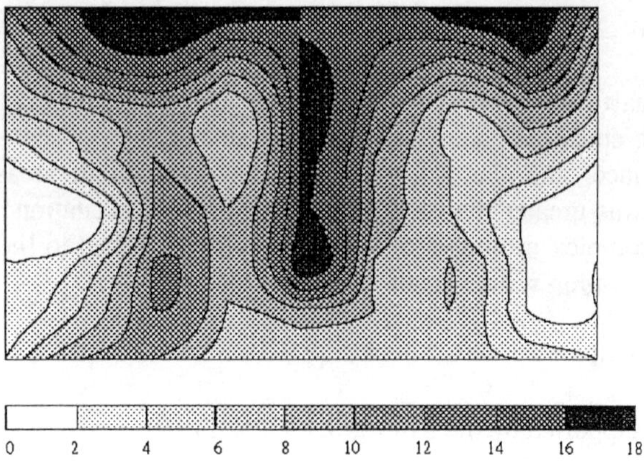

Figure 2: Isochronal map of the depolarization sequence of ventricular epicardium in the rabbit at mediastinal temperature of 32°C.
The data presentation is the same as in figure 1.

4 Discussion

The data obtained indicate that under analysis of the ventricular depolarization order the thermal conditions should be taken into account. There were local peculiarities of the epicardial excitation times changes caused by temperature variations: the prolongation of the depolarization of the left ventricular epicardial sites was more pronounced than that on the right ventricular surface. This resulted in that under heart cooling from 38 to 32°C left and right ventricular activation wave breakthroughs tended to change a priority of their emergence on the epicardium. Another character of the cooling-induced excitation sequence alterations was that the activation slowing observed in areas of the late depolarization was greater than that in the area of early excitation.

The findings provided by the present study show that the increase of the duration of activation of the overall ventricular epicardium, caused by lowering he mediastinal temperature, was of a less degree as compared to the prolongation of the QRS complex period. Pokrovsky et al.[2] found that under heart cooling the impulse propagation slowing occured mainly in the ventricular conductive system. On the basis of our findings, namely the greater prolongation of the left ventricular depolarization, one can speculate that under such moderate hypothermia, as developed in our experiments, he activation spread deceleration should be more pronounced in the left bundle branch than that in the right one.

5 Conclusion

Under rabbit heart cooling from 38 to 32°C the delay of the depolarization of the left ventricular epicardial sites was more pronounced than that on the right ventricular surface, and the activation slowing observed in areas of the late depolarization was greater than that in the area of early excitation. The cooling-induced QRS complex prolongation could be hardly ascribed to the deceleration of epicardial activation wave spread.

Acknowledgements

The study was supported by the RFFI grant 95-04-11910.

References

1. K.Mostivenko, V. Vityasev, B. Kuvetkin in *Electrocardiology'91*, Ed. J.Jagielski, M.Gornicki (World Scientific, Singapore, 1991)
2. V.M Pokrovsky., J.R. Sheykh-Zade, V.V. Vovereydt *Heart under hypothermia* (Leningrad: Nauka, 1984, in Russian)

ALTERATIONS OF VENTRICULAR EPICARDIAL REPOLARIZATION SEQUENCE UNDER MODERATE HEART COOLING IN THE RABBIT

J.E. AZAROV, M.P. ROSHCHEVSKY, D.N. SHMAKOV, V.A. VITYAZEV, N.V. YEVSTIFEEVA

Institute of Physiology of the Komi Science Centre, Ural Division, Russian Academy of Sciences, Syktyvkar, Komi, Russia

E-mail: compcard@online.ru

We examined cooling-induced changes of the recovery sequence throughout a ventricular epicardium in 14 anaesthetized adult rabbits. Under the mediastinal temperature of 38°C apical and lateral left ventricular regions were shown to be repolarized first. The latest recovery occured on a basal surface of both ventricles and in medial areas of the right ventricular free wall. After the mediastinum had been cooled to 32°C the repolarization sequence of the ventricular epicardium was inverted due to nonuniform ($p<0.01$) changes of the recovery properties in various ventricular regions. The greatest cooling-induced activation-recovery interval prolongation was recorded in the heart apical area and the least one was shown to be on the right ventricular basal surface.

1 Introduction

It is well-known that the variations of the lead site temperature influence the action potential duration of the cardiac myocytes[1]. It was suggested that epicardial cooling can cause changes of the ventricular transmural repolarization sequences[2]. However, van Dam and Durrer[3] pointed out that lowering the temperature of the left ventricular surface induced the negative T wave formation which can not be attributed merely to changes of the transmural recovery sequence, but alterations of the repolarization times of the adjacent epicardial sites should be taken into account. It is obscure whether under heart cooling recovery properties should alter within a ventricular surface uniformly or not. In the present study we examined if there were any cooling-induced changes of the recovery sequence throughout a ventricular epicardium.

2 Methods

Experiments were done in 14 rabbits anaesthetized with sodium thiopental (70-100 mg/kg, i.p.). Using an electrode array of 64 electrodes unipolar electrograms were simultaneously recorded from the entire ventricular surface. Activation and recovery times as well as activation-recovery intervals (ARI) were determined according to Wyatt and associates[4] as a minimum of a time derivative of potential during the QRS complex, a maximum of that during the ST-T complex, and a time interval between them, respectively. The temperature within the mediastinum was controled by the continuous perfusion of saline thermostated at 38 and 32°C.

3 Results

Under the mediastinal temperature of 38°C the shortest ARIs were recorded in the heart apical (114±36 ms) and left ventricular lateral (121±35 ms) area. The left ventricular lateral surface had longer ARIs (138±43 ms). The greatest duration of the ARIs was observed on the lateral (155±33 ms) and basal (158±39 ms) right ventricular surface.

In those normothermic conditions (38°C) the repolarization sequence of the rabbit ventricular epicardium was in accordance with the ARI distribution (Fig.1). The surface of the heart apex and lateral left ventricular regions was shown to be repolarized first. The latest recovery occured on a basal surfacc of both vcntricles and in medial areas of the right ventricular free wall.

After the cavity of the mediastinum had been cooled to 32°C the ARI distribution of the ventricular epicardium was inverted. In the right ventricular basal area the shortest ARI (173±43 ms) were observed. On the epicardium of the left ventricular base they were slightly longer (183±39 ms). On the lateral right ventricular surface the ARIs (199±32 ms) were slightly greater than ARIs recorded in the basal area of the left ventricle but significantly longer than those on the right ventricular basal epicardium. The duration of the ARIs registered in the lateral left ventricular area was shown to be essentially greater (226±35 ms). The longest ARIs (243±29 ms) were observed on the surface of the heart apex.

We found that such a cooling-induced inversion of the recovery properties distribution on the ventricular epicardium was caused by a nonuniform ($p<0.01$) increment of the ARI durations in different epicardial areas. The extent of the ARI prolongation increased in the following order: right ventricular base (in this area the cooling-induced alterations of the recovery properties were insignificant); left ventricular base and right ventricular lateral surface; left ventricular lateral surface; heart apex.

Under heart cooling from 38 to 32°C the repolarization sequence of the ventricular epicardium was altered according to ARIs changes. When mediastinal temperature equaled to 32°C the recovery order was inversed as compared to that registered in the normothermic conditions. The earliest epicardial repolarization occured in the right ventricular basal region (Fig.2). Then right ventricular mediolateral area was recovered and at last the repolarization was completed at lateral and particularly apical parts of the left ventricular epicardium. The alteration of the recovery properties was reversible.

4 Discussion

Recently Lux and associates[2] suggested that in tank preparation of isolated canine heart the variations of QRST integral distribution under cooling the

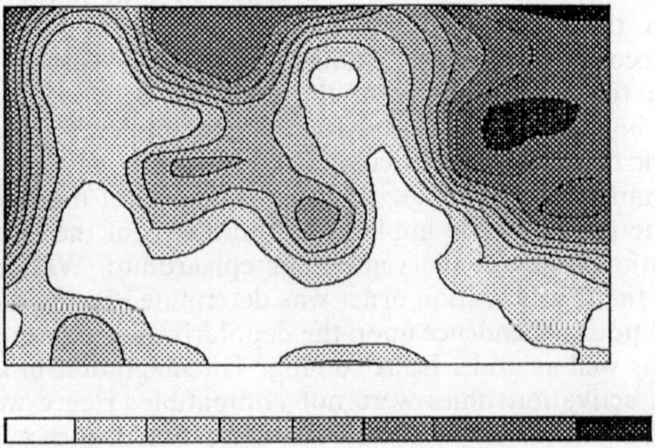

Figure 1: Isochronal map of the repolarization sequence of ventricular epicardium in the rabbit at mediastinal temperature of 38°C.
A top of the map corresponds to the ventricular base and the bottom corresponds to the heart apex. Right and left margins of the map represent the line running from the heart apex to the lateral region of the right ventricular base. The mid portion of the map corresponds the lateral surface of the left ventricle. Time (ms) is measured in respect to the earliest epicardial recovery.

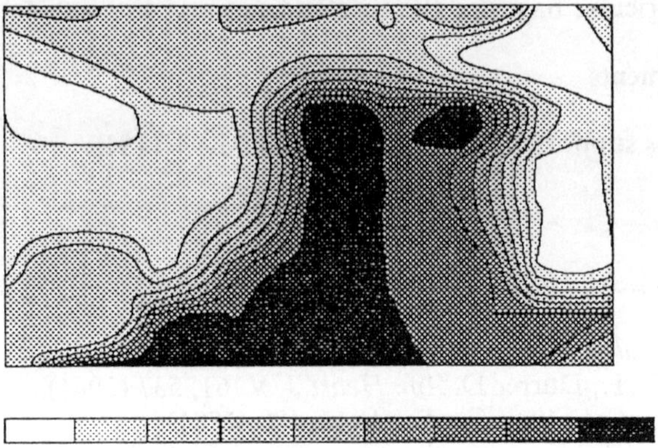

Figure 2: Isochronal map of the repolarization sequence of ventricular epicardium in the rabbit at mediastinal temperature of 32°C.
The data presentation is the same as in figure 1.

irrigating solution are due to prolonged epicardial repolarization as compared to that in the endocardial layers. We observed that under similar thermal conditions in the *in situ* experiments in the rabbit the disparity of the ventricular recovery properties changed within an epicardium. Thus, the differences in the characteristics of the recovery between various epicardial areas should be taken into account for the explanation for the genesis of the cardiac electric field during ventricular repolarization.

The mechanism of the cooling-induced inversion of the recovery sequences revealed in the present study implies the alterations of the recovery properties or the activation times of the ventricular epicardium. We found that under sinus rhythm the repolarization order was determined by the ARI distributions and exhibited poor dependence upon the depolarization sequence under normal temperature as well as under heart cooling. The magnitude of alteration of the recovery and activation times were not compatible. Hence we infer that the inversion of the ventricular epicardial repolarization sequences under lowering the mediastinal temperature to 32°C was mainly due to the recovery properties changes.

5 Conclusion

Under cooling the mediastinum from 38 to 32°C the ventricular epicardial repolarization sequence inversed due to nonuniform alteration of recovery properties: the slightest prolongation of ARIs was found to be in the area of the right ventricular base and the greatest one was observed on the heart apex.

Acknowledgements

The study was supported by the RFFI grant 95-04-11910.

References

1. Woodbury L.A., Hecht H.H., Christopherson A.R. *Am. Physiol.* V. 164, 307 (1951).
2. Lux R.L. *at al. J. Electrocardiol.*- V. 27: Suppl.100 (1994).
3. van Dam R.T., Durrer D. *Am. Heart J.* V. 61, 537 (1961).
4. Wyatt R.F. at al, *Am.J.Cardiol.* V.47, 488 (1981).

PRECONDITIONING WITH NOREPINEPHRINE IN ISOLATED GUINEA PIG CARDIOMYOCYTES

T. RAVINGEROVA, J.-E. LOEKEBOE[1], A. ZIEGELHÖFFER, B. KOIDL[2]

Institute for Heart Research, SAS, 9 Dubravska cesta, Bratislava, 842 33, Slovakia; [1]Department of Medical Physiology, Institute of Medical Biology, University of Tromsoe, Tromsoe N-9037, Norway; [2]Institute of Medical Physics & Biophysics, University of Graz, 21 Harrachgasse, Graz A-8010, Austria

Short ischemia- or norepinephrine (NE)-induced stress preconditions the heart against subsequent ischemic arrhythmias. We investigated whether isolated cardiomyocytes can be protected against arrhythmias by preconditioning (PC) with NE. Ventricular myocytes isolated from guinea pig hearts using collagenase were superfused with Tyrode solution, impaled with patch electrodes to record action potentials (AP) and stimulated (rate 30/min). Regular AP could be monitored for >1h with resting potential (RP) -67($\pm$3) mV. To study arrhythmogenesis, 1 μmol/l NE was added to the buffer. This elicited spontaneous AP generation within 3-5 min (irregular rate ~3/sec) showing no RP, but a maximal diastolic potential of -50 mV and slow diastolic depolarization typical for spontaneous excitations. Spontaneous activity resulting in the irreversible loss of cell excitability within 15 min was blocked by propranolol. To study PC, the preparation was superfused with NE for 5 min and washed out for 50 min, prior to the second superfusion with NE for 15 min. No spontaneous AP were elicited by the second superfusion, which means that the cells were preconditioned. PC was abolished by prazosin, but not by propranolol indicating an involvement of α-, but not β-adrenoceptors. Irregular pacemaker activity of myocytes induced by NE can be interpreted as arrhythmias on the cell level. Prevention of spontaneous AP generation by a prior short application of NE is interpreted as PC of a single cell against arrhythmogenic influence of NE.

Introduction

A new concept of myocardial protection against ischemia termed ischemic preconditioning is based on the exploitation of the heart's own adaptive mechanisms.[1] Brief episodes of ischemia can trigger short-term adaptation leading to a reduction of cell necrosis and life-threatening arrhythmias, during subsequent long-lasting ischemia.[2-4] The exact mechanisms of this protection are not yet fully understood, however, a number of substances released in the myocardium during ischemia have been implicated as triggers of preconditioning. This opens a probability of a pharmacological induction of protection.

Increased sympathetic activity is closely associated with electrophysiological alterations and production of arrhythmias.[5] However, in partially depolarized myocardium arrhythmogenic effects of catecholamines can be attenuated.[6] Moreover, catecholamine-induced short stress has been found to precondition the heart, via stimulation of α-adrenergic receptors, against postischemic myocardial dysfunction,[7] to reduce infarct size[8] and to suppress ischemia- and reperfusion-induced arrhythmias.[9-11] However, the mechanisms of antiarrhythmic protection are still not clear, and the exact role of catecholamines in the effect of preconditioning remains not fully understood.

Aims of the study

To get further insight into the mechanisms of arrhythmogenesis and of antiarrhythmic effect of preconditioning, the present study was designed to test whether arrhythmias and preconditioning can be studied on the level of a single cell. Norepinephrine has been chosen as a tool: 1. to induce arrhythmia and 2. to trigger preconditioning. The second goal was to determine which potential receptors are involved in these effects.

Methods

Ventricular myocytes were isolated from guinea pig hearts using Langendorff perfusion technique with a collagenase solution. Rod-shaped myocytes showing no spontaneous activity at rest were investigated on the stage of an inverted microscope. Cells were continuously superfused with Tyrode solution (rate 2ml/min). Membrane potentials were recorded using the whole-cell patch-clamp technique and a patch-clamp amplifier (Axon Instruments, Foster City, CA, USA). Electrode resistances were 2-3 MΩ. Action potentials (AP) were elicited by intracellular electrical stimulation by rectangular voltage pulses (5ms, rate 30/min). Regular APs with with resting potential (RP) of -67($\pm$3)mV could be monitored for >1h in control experiments.

Drugs used:

Norepinephrine (NE, 1μM) - to induce: spontaneous activity and preconditioning. Propranolol (10μM), Prazosin (2μM) - to study the role of β- and α-adrenoceptors.

Protocols:

1.Control experiment: 15 min stabilization, 70 min superfusion with Tyrode solution;
2.Effect of NE: stabilization, 15 min superfusion with NE;
3.Preconditioning: stabilization, 5 min superfusion with NE followed by 50 min washout, second 15 min superfusion with NE;
4.Preconditioning and Propranolol: stabilization, 5 min superfusion with NE and Propranolol, 50 min washout, second superfusion with NE;

5.Preconditioning and Prazosin: stabilization, 5 min superfusion with NE and Prazosin, 50 min washout, second superfusion with NE.

Summary of the results

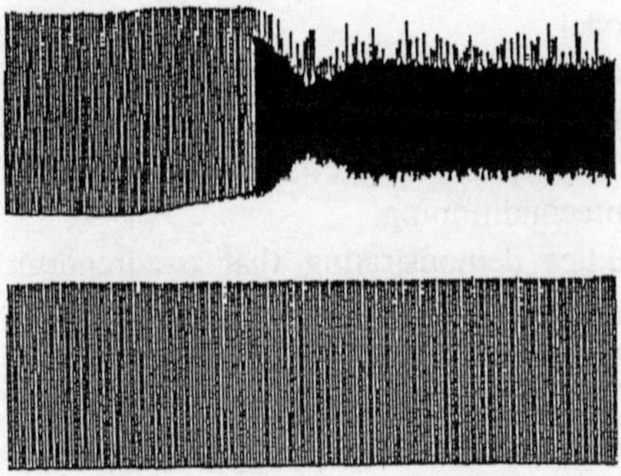

Figure 1: Spontaneous arrhythmic activity induced by superfusion with NE in isolated guinea pig cardiomyocytes. Effect of Propranolol and NE (bottom).

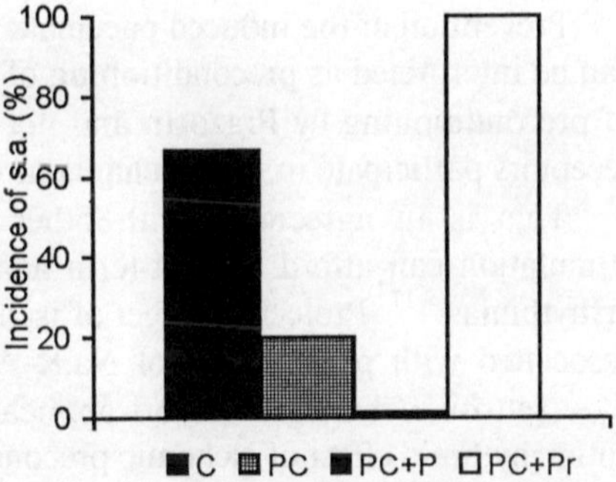

Figure 2: Effect of preconditioning (PC) with NE, and its blockade by Propranolol (P) and Prazosin (Pr) on spontaneous activity in isolated guinea pig cardiomyocytes. n=3-6 cells in each group.

Superfusion with NE induced within 3-5min spontaneous diastolic depolarization and AP generation at an irregular rate of ~3/sec. These APs within the spontaneous bursts showed typical characteristics of spontaneous activity (s. a.): loss of RP, slow diastolic depolarization from the maximal diastolic potential (MDP) of -50mV, a slow upstroke and repolarization to MDP. This arrhythmic activity, which occured in 67% of cells, was not followed by a restoration of normal cell excitability and resulted in a cell death within 15-20min (Fig. 1, top). Propranolol applied together with NE completely blocked spontaneous activity in all cells (Fig. 1, bottom), while Prazosin failed to abolish spontaneous discharge (not shown).

In a setting of preconditioning, 5min superfusion with NE followed by 50min washout, protected 80% of the cells against spontaneous AP generation during the subsequent second superfusion of NE for 15min. S. a. occured only in 1 of 5 preconditioned cells (Fig. 2). Prazosin abolished preconditioning effect in all cells and resulted in nonstable s. a., whereas Propranolol did not block protection afforded by pretreatment with NE (Fig. 2).

Discussion

In this study on isolated ventricular myocytes we demonstrated that administration of NE induced irregular spontaneous AP generation that can be considered as arrhythmic activity on the cell level. Its blockade by Propranolol and a lack of blockade by Prazosin indicates the involvement of β-adrenergic receptors in the mechanisms of arrhythmogenesis in this model.

Prevention of the induced pacemaker activity by a prior short application of NE can be interpreted as preconditioning of a single cell. Inhibition of protective effect of preconditioning by Prazosin and not by Propranolol suggests that α-adrenergic receptors participate in the mechanisms of preconditioning.

This is in agreement with other studies demonstrating that α-adrenergic stimulation can afford a short-term adaptation to a stress and to suppress severe arrhythmias.[9-11] Protective effect of ischemic preconditioning has been found to be associated with preservation of Na,K-ATPase activity and to involve opening of K_{ATP} sensitive channels.[12] Short application of catecholamines mimicks protective antiarrhythmic effect of ischemic preconditioning in isolated rat heart and results in the stimulation of the enzyme activity as well.[9] The latter may contribute to the maintenance of electrical stability of the cell membranes. However, the exact mechanisms of preconditioning cell signaling cascade require further exploration.

Acknowledgements

This work was supported by the Austrian Science Foundation, P11131-MED and SEB 007, as well as by the Protocol of Scientific Cooperation between Austria and Slovakia, project 11 SR 7.

References

1. C.E. Murry *et al., Circulation* **74**, 1124 (1986).
2. G.S. Liu *et al., Circulation* **84**, 350 (1991).
3. A. Vegh *et al., Cardiovasc Res* **26**, 487 (1992).
4. T. Ravingerova *et al., Mol Cell Biochem* **147**, 123 (1995)
5. B.G. Benfey *et al., Br J Pharmacol* **82**, 717 (1984).
6. H.G. Li *et al., Am J Physiol* **265**, H1654 (1993).
7. A. Banerjee *et al., Circ Res* **73**, 656 (1993).
8. Z. Bankwala *et al., Circulation* **90**, 1023 (1994).
9. T. Ravingerova *et al., ANYAS* **793**, 43 (1996).
10. A. Vegh *et al., J Mol Cell Cardiol* **26**, LXXXVII (1995).
11. A. Tosaki *et al., J Pharmacol Exptl Therapeut* **273**, 689 (1995).
12. Y. Morita *et al., J Mol Cell Cardiol* **29**, 1267 (1997).

SUBCELLULAR CHANGES IN THE HEART WITH TRANSIENT OR FATAL VENTRICULAR ARRHYTHMIAS

N. TRIBULOVA, L. OKRUHLICOVA, T. RAVINGEROVA, J. STYK, I. GABAUER, J. SLEZAK

Institute for Heart Research, Slovak Academy of Sciences, Dubravska cesta 9, Bratislava 842 33, Slovak Republic

Coordinated contraction in the heart depends on the rapid, orderly propagation of action potential between cardiomyocytes, a function mediated by sarcolemma and its specialized regions, gap junctions. Accordingly, arrhythmias are likely to arise from disturbances of the active ionic properties of the sarcolemma and abnormal intercellular coupling.We have previously shown that susceptibility of the myocardium to arrhythmias is closely related to electrical heterogeneity and to viability of cardiomyocytes. In this study we attempted to delineate the subcellular alterations of the cardiomyocytes characterizing transient versus sustained ventricular arrhythmias. These were induced, in vivo, in dog hearts by intermitent occlusion of left coronary artery and, in vitro, in the isolated rat heart by perfusion with modified Krebs-Henseleit solution.

Ultrastructural examination revealed moderate subcellular alterations, uniform as well as disturbed patterns of sarcomere units of the myofibrills and no apparent changes in intercellular junctions in the cardiomyocytes of dog and rat hearts affected by transient arrhythmias. On the contrary, fatal ventricular arrhythmias in both species induced heterogenous injury of various degree. Some myocytes were reversibly injured and subcellular alterations resembled these after transient arrhythmias.Besides this, irreversibly injured cardiomyocytes with hypercontracted sarcomeres and contracture of myofibrills as well as disruption of intercellular junctions were detected. The results indicate that arrhythmia-related desynchronisation of contraction is more expressed in the heart with fatal ventricular fibrillation, which is characterized by more pronounced heterogeneity of subcellular changes, probably reflecting higher degree nonuniform anisotropic conduction.

Introduction

Sudden cardiac death in patients who have survived a previous myocardial infarction is often associated with recurrent, sustained ventricular tachycardia though to arise by reentry,[1] thus is attributable to abnormalities in cellular electrophysiology caused by ischemia. The later is closely associated with altered tissue structure. Slow conduction leading to reentry in regions bordering healed infarcts may be due primarily to alterations in specific patterns of myocyte interconnections[2].

Intercellular junctions mediate specific sets of interactions between cells. The fascia adherens and desmosome are adhesive junctions. Communicating junctions, gap junctions, form pathway for direct intercellular signaling as well as low-resistance pathways along which action potentials are propagated. Three types of junctions act in concert to integrate electromechanical function of the myocardium. Thus, intermyocyte coupling and particularly gap junctions, are a principal determinant of intercellular conductance and myocardial conduction velocity[3].

Although cardiac arrhythmias are likely to arise from a combination of disturbances both,the active ionic properties of plasma membrane channels and coupling between cells, abnormal cellular coupling may, under some pathophysiological conditions, be the predominant factor involved[4]. We have previously shown that susceptibility of the myocardium to arrhythmias is closely related to electrical heterogeneity and to reversibility of ultrastructural changes of the cardiomyocytes[5].

In this study we attempted to delineate the subcellular alterations of the cardiac muscle cells characterizing transient versus sustained ventricular arrhythmias. Since pathological changes in tissue structure may markedly alter the electrophysiological properties of the myocardium and thus determine the type of arrhythmia.

Materials and Methods

Male adult Wistar rats were anaesthetized with sodium pentobarbital (50 mg/kg) and heparin (500 U) was given intraperitonealy. After thoracotomy the heart was quickly excised and transfered to Langendorff apparatus. The aorta was cannulated and the heart was perfused at constant pressure 65 mg Hg, temperature 37° C with oxygenated (95% O_2 + 5% CO_2) modified Krebs-Henseleit solution (containing in mmol: NaCl 118, KCl 3.2, $CaCl_2$ 2.5, $MgSO_4$ 1.2, $NaHCO_3$ 25.0, Na_2HPO_4 1.2, glucose 11.0, pH 7.4).

An epicardial electrogram was continuously recorded by means of twoo stainless steel electrodes attached to the apex of the heart and the aortic cannula.The incidence of transient or sustained ventricular fibrillation was monitored. The hearts for electron microscopic investigation were fixed by perfusion with buffered 2,5% gluteraldehyde, the small samples (1mm) from the subepicardial and subendocardial left ventricle were excised and routinely elaborated.

Mongrel male adult dogs were anaesthetized with thiopental Spofa (30mg/kg) and heparinized (3.0 U/kg, i.v.) and maintained on arteficial respiration (95% O_2 + 5% CO_2). After thoracotomy in the 5 intercostal space the left descendent coronary artery branch was occluded and reopened for selected time. An epicardial ECG was continuosly monitored and incidence of arrhythmias was recorded. The small samples from the left ventricle and right atria were excised and fixed by immersion in 2.5% buffered glutaraldehyde for 6 hrs and postfixed with 1% OsO_4. The tissue was further routinely elaboreted for electronmicroscopic examination.

Experimental protocol

1. The rat hearts were perfused with modified Krebs-Henseleit solution and spontaneous ventricular fibrillation was monitored.

5 hearts exibiting transient (< 2 min) ventricular fibrillation and 3 hearts exibiting sustained (> 2 min) ventricular fibrillation were used for electron mocroscopic examination.
2. The dog hearts_were submitted to intermittent short lasting occlusion and reperfusion (3x4 min occlusion + 5 min reperfusion and 40 min occlusion + 60 min reperfusion) and ventricular arrhythmias were monitored.
4 hearts exhibiting transient arrhythmias and 5 hearts exhibiting sustained ventricular fibrillation were used for electron microscopic examination.

Results

1. Ex vivo instrumented rat heart.

A. Transient ventricular fibrillation .
Ultrastructural examination of the cardiomyocytes from the rat heart exibiting transient ventricular fibrillation which was spontaneously terminated revealed moderate subcellular alterations. Mitochondria showed thigtly packed cristae, nonuniform patterns of sarcomeres were present and only rarely slight changes in intercellular connections were found (Fig. 1A).

B. Sustained ventricular fibrillation.
Long lasting ventricular fibrillation induced translocation of specific atrial granules from perinuclear space to the subsarcolemal area. Nonhomogenously injured myocardium was the main feature related to sustained ventricular fibrillation. Besides reversibly changed cardiomyocytes markedly altered myocytes were present. The later revealed contracture of myofibrills, severely damaged mitochondria and lost of integrity of intercellular junctions, including gap junctions. Desynchronisation of contraction was more pronounced (Fig.1B).

2. In vivo instrumented dog heart.
A. Transient arrhythmias.
Intermitent coronary occlusion and reperfusion resulted in high incidence of transient arrhythmias. Ischemic ventricular myocardium revealed moderately edematous mitochondria, nonhomogenous patterns of sarcomeres and slight alterations of intercellular junctions.

B.Sustained ventricular fibrillation.
Nonhomogenous injury was observed. Irreversible subcellular changes were frequently found, they consisted of contraction bands, edematous nuclei and

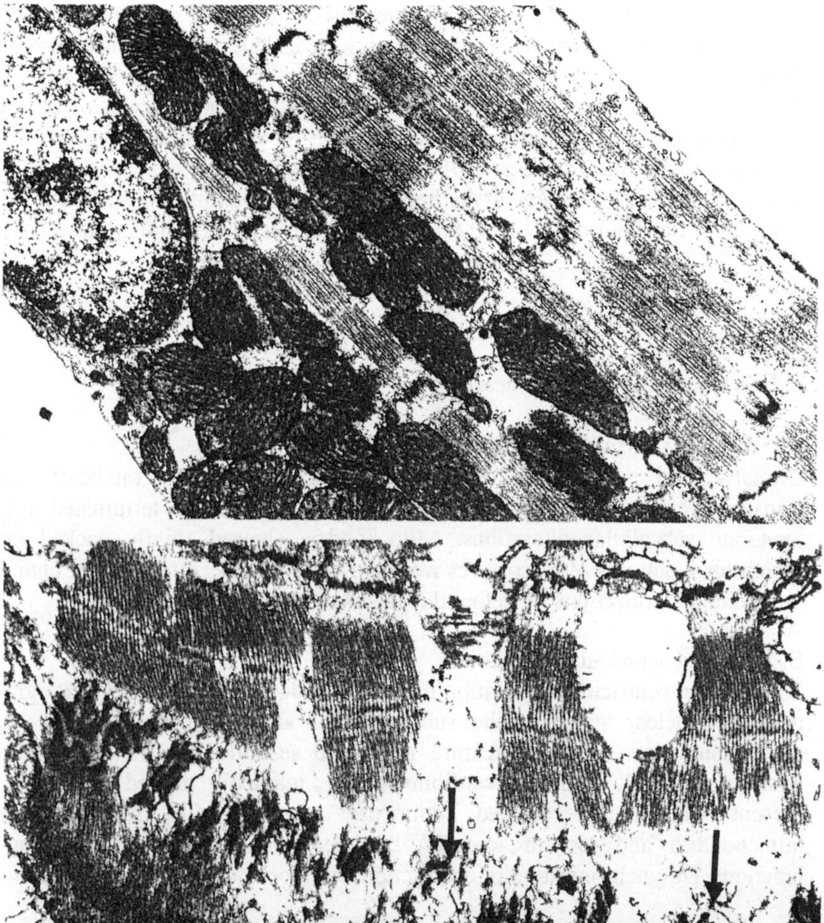

1A

1B

Fig 1A: Transient ventricular fibrillation, rat heart. Electrondense mitochondria with tightly packed cristae and loss of regular sarcomere patterns indicate disturbances in electro-mechanical coupling.

Fig 2A: Subcellular changes of cardiomyocytes from the heart exibiting sustained ventricular fibrillation consist of apparent injury of intercellular connections (arrows) and marked disregulation of contraction.

mitochondria, disruption of myofilaments from fascia adherens junctions, dehiscence of intercellular junctions and loss of integrity of gap junctions. At the perifery of occluded area the majority of cardiomyocytes as well as endocardial Purkinje fibres revealed reversible changes.

Discussion

Arrhythmias and contractile dysfunction are major cause of morbidity and mortality in ischemic heart diseases. Ischemia causes a decrease in myocardial conduction velocity and disturbances in intermyocyte mechanical and electrical coupling and communications[2,5,6] . Thus predisposes the myocardium to reentry, localized usually to the reversibly injured borders of ischemic area[7].

Our results conducted on the dog heart support this assumption and are in accordance with our previous findings [5]. These indicate that transient ventricular arrhythmias are always associated with reversibly altered cardiomyocytes. Although transmision electron microscopy did not reveal the apparent changes in gap junctions , nonuniform patterns of sarcomeres indicate the disturbances in contraction-relaxation proces which can be most likely induced by decreased of intercellular coupling.

Diffrent from transient postischemic arrhythmias which were accompanied with moderate subcellular changes, sustained ventricular fibrillation was manifested with reversible as well as irreversible injury. Severe alterations in intercellular connections, fascia adherens and gap junctions indicate marked disturbance in mechanical and electrical intercellular coupling. Dysfuction of the intercellular communication was more pronounced and resulted in marked desynchronisation of contraction .

To compare the in vivo ischemia/reperfusion induced arrhythmias which can be facilitated by alterations in cardiac autonomic control, such as increase in sympathetic and decrease in parasympathetic tone[8], we used the isolated rat heart perfused with "arrhythmogenic" crystalloid solution. In this model the arrhythmias are facilitated by disturbances in ion homeostasis, particularly associated with elevation of intracellular free Ca [9,10].

Transient ventricular fibrillation in this model was accompanied with moderate ultrastructural changes. Mitochondria with tightly packed cristae resembling "linear densities" occured in Ca overload conditions[11] indicating the increase in [Ca]i. It is known that such elevation can lead to intercellular uncoupling, conduction block [12] and consequently to arrhythmias[9,10]. The indirect evidence of disturbances in electrical coupling was nonhomogeneity in sarcomeric contraction .

Sustained ventricular fibrillation in isolated rat heart resembles those in the dog hearts. The heterogeneity of injury was the main feature of subcellular alterations. Significant desynchronisation of contraction and irreversibly injured cardiomyocytes were apparently evident.

From our results we can conclude that arrhytmia-related desynchronisation of contraction is more expressed in the heart with fatal ventricular fibrillation. This is characterized by more pronounced heterogeneity in subcellular changes probably reflecting higher degree of nonuniform anisotropic conduction.

References

1. M. Manoach, D. Varon and M. Erez, Mol. Cell. Biochem. **147**, 181 (1995).
2. J. E. Saffitz, R. H. Hoyt, R. A. Luke, H. L. Kanter and E. C. Beyer, Trends Cardiovasc. Med. **2**, 56 (1992).
3. N. S. Peters, J. Coromilas, N. J. Severs, A. L. Wit, Circulation **95**, 988 (1997).
4. N. J. Severs, J. Cardiovasc. Electrophysiol. **5**, 462 (1994).
5. T. Ravingerova, N. Tribulova, J. Slezak and M. J. Curtis, J. Mol. Cell. Cardiol. **27**, 1937 (1995).
6. N. J. Severs, R. G. Gourdie, E. Harfst, N. S. Peters and C. R. Green, J. Microscopy **169**, 299 (1992).
7. N. S. Peters, C. R. Green, P. A. Poole-Wilson and N. J. Severs, J. Mol. Cell. Cardiol. **27**, 37 (1995).
8. G.E.Billman, NIPS **7**, 254 (1992).
9. F. T. Thandroyen, A. C. Morris, H. K. Hagler, B. Ziman, L. Pai, J.T.Willerson and L .M. Buja, Circ. Res. **69**, 810 (1991).
10. G. E. Billman, B. McIlroy and J. D. Johnson, FASEB J. **5**, 2586 (1991).
11. N. Tribulova, J. Slezak, T. Ravingerova, J. Submicrosc. Cytol. Pathol. **25**, 267 (1993).
12. M. Manoach, N. Tribulova, I. Imanaga, Heart and Vessels **11**, 445 (1997).

Acknowledgments

The authors are grateful to the Slovak Grant Agency for Science, grant No. 2/999237/93, for partial supporting of this study.

II. Computer Modeling

VENTRICULAR ACTIVATION AS A COMPOSITION OF DETERMINISTIC AND STOCHASTIC PROCESSES

ZS. CSERJÉS, GY. KOZMANN
KFKI Res. Inst. for Materials Science, HAS, 1525 P.O.Box 49., 1525 Budapest, Hungary
E-mail: cserjes@r1.atki.kfki.hu

V. SZATHMÁRY
Inst. of Normal and Pathological Physiology, SAS, Sienkiewiczova 1, 81371 Bratislava, Slovakia
E-mail: szath@unpf.savba.sk

M. TINOVA, M. TYSLER
Inst. of Measurement Science, SAS, Dubravska cesta 9, 84219 Bratislava, Slovakia
E-mail: umermaja@savba.sk

In the paper a generalized interpretation of ventricular activation is given considering it as a composition of deterministic and stochastic processes. The influence of the variability of the intraventricular conduction system on the time instants of characteristic events during ventricular activation is shown by the help of a model experiment. The ability of the linear predictive algorithm, developed earlier for characteristic event detection, was determined for the precise recognition of characteristic event time instant changes due to the above mentioned variability, in the case of normal activation.

1 Introduction

The goal of the model experiments performed was twofold: 1./ to introduce into the numerical heart model a stochastic element in order to show its influence on the time instants of ventricular characteristic events (CEs), like epicardial breakthrough (EB) or collision of waves (CO). 2./ to specify the ability of the linear predictive algorithm (LPA) developed earlier[1] for CE detection, to reveal subtle time instant changes due to the stochastic parameter.

To introduce a stochastic part into the heart model is useful because within a clinically homogeneous group, the ventricular activation process (VAP) has not only deterministic nature, but it is also dependent on some individual parameters which are not measurable in each real case, so we are obliged to handle them as random parameters. Suchlike parameters are e.g. the individual realization of the intraventricular conduction system (sites of activation wave initiations), or the heart geometry.

The LPA for the selection of most informative moments of the activation was based on the assumption that for a given subject the VAP is deterministic in nature. The CEs give the essence of the activation process, in this sense the LPA is a feature extraction method, which might be useful in the interpretation of the heart condition. The performed numerical and biological model studies supported this hypothesis [2,3], but on the other hand the evaluation of the real body surface potential maps showed that the sequence of CEs in a given group had a high variability [4,5,6,7].

To get more information about the influence of a reasonable set of random parameters on the VAP and on the CE sequence, conceptual model investigations were performed.

2 Materials and method

25 different normal activation sequences were generated using a numerical heart model[8] and an inhomogeneous, real shape torso. It was assumed that the cardiac sources of the activation fronts can be approximated by uniform double layers[9].

The model experiment consisted of two main parts:

1./ In the first step a baseline normal activation sequence was defined, then two initiation points were selected in the left ventricle, which were dislocated systematically, at first separately, and then both together. The dislocations were performed into 4 directions: upwards, downwards, left and right on the endocardial surface by 6 model units. The total number of combinations was 25. In each simulation heart cross sections, perpendicular to the main axis of the heart, were defined and activation isochrone maps were drawn in order to determine the CE time instant changes in respect to the baseline case. The CE time instants identified by visual inspection served as reference data for LPA output validation.

2./ In the second part to each heart activation process the corresponding BSPMs were computed in each step of the simulated wave propagation. To check the possible role of the lead system on the LPA output, Oosterom-198 lead, and Lux-192 lead maps were computed. Then the characteristic moments were defined by the LPA from the BSPM sequences. Finally, the CE moments detected by the LPA were compared with the reference data.

3 Results

Time instant data of two CEs are shown in Table 1, as typical examples. The predictive algorithm does reflect properly the CE changes in most of the cases, though by visual inspection all the 25 BSPM series looked quite similar, therefore the detection performance was doubtful. By the use of the Lux-192 lead BSPMs the detection was poorer, than in the case of the Oosterom-198 lead maps, especially regarding the early septal collision.

Using the Oosterom-198 BSPMs the detections are in very good agreement with the references. The result is worse in the case of Lux-192 BSPMs (see Table 2). The difference between the two performances of detection is fairly high concerning CE 1, while the result is more balanced in the case of CE 2.

Table 1: Time instants of two CEs affected by the initiation point changes in 25 cases. (w.i.p.: wave initiation point, 198-Oos.: 198 point Oosterom-type BSPMs, 192-Lux: 192 point Lux-type BSPMs, by refer.: time instants by the references. Time step: 2.5 msec. Zero time instant: the onset of ventricular activation.)

No. of experim.	direction of displacement		CE 1: septal left ventricular collision			CE 2: epicardial breakthrough (left ventricle, posterior)		
	1. w.i.p.	2.w.i.p.	by refer.	by the LPA		by refer.	by the LPA	
				198-Oos.	192-Lux		198-Oos.	192-Lux
1.	-	-	5	5	-	11	11	11
2.	↑	-	5	5	-	11	11	11
3.	↓	-	5	5	-	11	11	11
4.	←	-	4	-	-	11	11	11
5.	→	-	6-7	7	7	11	11	11
6.	-	↑	4-5	4-5	-	12	-	-
7.	-	↓	5	5	-	10-11	11	11
8.	-	←	5	5	-	12	12	-
9.	-	→	5-6	6	-	12	12	-
10.	↑	↑	5	5	-	12	12	12
11.	↑	↓	5	5	5	10-11	11	11
12.	↑	←	5	5	5	12	12	12
13.	↑	→	5-6	5-6	5-6	12	12	12
14.	↓	↑	5	5	-	12	12	12
15.	↓	↓	5	5	-	10 11	11	11
16.	↓	←	5	5	5	12	12	12
17.	↓	→	5-6	5-6	6	12	12	12
18.	←	↑	4	-	-	12	12	12
19.	←	↓	4	5	5	10-11	11	11
20.	←	←	4	5	5	12	12	12
21.	←	→	4	5	5	11-12	11	11
22.	→	↑	7	7	-	12	12	12
23.	→	↓	7	7	7	11	11	11
24.	→	←	7	8	8	12	12	12
25.	→	→	4	4	4	12	12	12

Table 2: Percentage values of correctly detected CE time instants on the basis of Oosterom-198, and Lux-192 lead BSPMs.

No. of CE \ type of the BSPMs	Oosterom-198 BSPMs	Lux-192 BSPMs
CE 1 (CO, LV septal wall)	92%	40%
CE 2 (EB, LV posterior)	95%	88%

4 Discussion

It can be seen in Table 1 that the detection of the early CE (septal collision), has an uncertainty. It is because the surface of the collision is small in itself and its effective size is reduced further by the wavefront roughness due to the numerical approximation technique used to simulate the spherical Huygen's propagation principle in the heart model. In case of the 1st CE, the activation fronts in collision are rough (fjord pattern like), that is why one can only render a probability to the wave collision at these early moments on the reference isochrone patterns. As the wave curvatures decrease in the subsequent moments, the wave surface is getting smoother and the time instants of CEs can be determined without any doubt.

In our view the difference between the two performances of detections was most likely due to the different lead density distributions. While the Oosterom-198 point grid is not equidistant, with a high density in the precordial area[10] , the Lux grid density is uniform over the thoracic surface[11]. The investigated CEs, influence the frontal chest potentials in a higher degree than the back ones, consequently the number of LPA event sitcs in the Oosterom system resulted in a higher score than in the Lux system, yielding finally a higher percentage of correct CE detection.

5 Conclusion

The displacements of wave initiation points on the endocardium changed the time instants of CEs in most cases. The predictive algorithm reflected properly these changes, but the performance of the detection was dependent on the type of BSPM lead arrangement, especially in the early period of the activation. It can be concluded that the LPA is able to detect the electrically small changes ensued not only on the epicardium, but in the myocardium too, if the spatial sampling frequency is high enough.

Acknowledgement

This work was partly supported by the grant of the National Research Found (OTKA - No. T-022605).

References

1. Gy. Kozmann, *et al.*, in *Electrocardiology '83*, eds. I. Ruttkay-Nedecky, P. Macfarlane (Excerpta Medica, Amsterdam, 1984).
2. Zs. Cserjés, *et al., Jpn. Heart J.*, **35**, Suppl. 1994, 93 (1994).
3. Zs. Cserjés, *et al., XXIIIrd Int. Cong. Electrocardiology*, Cleveland, (1996).
4. Gy. Kozmann, *et al.*, in *IEEE EMBS*, Amsterdam (1996).
5. Gy. Kozmann *et al, Circulation*, **79**, 1077, (1989).
6. D. Stilli et al, *J. Electrocardiology*, **21**, 1 (1988).
7. M. Medvegy et al, *Circulation*, **94**, No. 8, Suppl. I-731 (1996).
8. V. Szathmáry *et al, Comp. and Biomed. Res.*, **27**, 27 (1994).
9. M. Tysler, *et al,* in *CIC '93* IEEE Comp. Soc. Press, Washington , (1993).
10. A. van Oosterom, *Comput. J.*, **21**, 253 (1978).
11. R. Lux, C. Smith *et al, IEEE BME*, **25**, 270 (1978).

A SIMULATION STUDY OF TORSADE DE POINTES WITH QT PROLONGATION

OSAMU OKAZAKI, M.D.
International Medical Center of Japan, Tokyo 162
Present address: CVRTI Univ. of Utah, Bldg. 500 Salt Lake City Utah 84112, USA
E-mail: osamu@cvrti.utah.edu

DAMING WEI, Ph.D.*, KENICHI HARUMI, M.D.**
* *Nihon Kohden Co. E-mail: daming_wei@mb2.nkc.co.jp*
***Showa Univ. Fujigaoka Hosp. E-mail:kharumi@ibm.net*

The possible contribution of the conduction delay and QT prolongation in patients with the long QT syndrome was studied by our model in order to clarify the mechanism of polymorphic VT, twisting about a point with the delayed repolarization of M cells and QT prolongation. The simulated condition of the model are anisotropic propagation, premature cycle length-dependent shortening of M cell properties and conduction delay during incomplete recovery. Regions of M cell in anterior and lateral area relatively long refractory period were incorporated according to the evidence of regional prolongation of recovery in long QT syndrome referred to Yan and Antzelevitch. Reentrant excitation fronts around the M cell region initiated a similar series of events, and serial reentry at twisting QRS waveform in torsade de pointes (Tdp). Non-sustained VT was induced by double extra-stimuli under the condition of slower conduction velocity of ventricular muscle than that of in M cells. QT prolongation and the same conduction velocity of M cell and ventricular muscle were required the onset and spontaneous termination of Tdp. Tdp could be induced by double extra-stimuli. BSPM showed a pattern of multipolarity on excitation fronts during VT. On the 3-D images of computer models, the excitation fronts are propagated like reentry from apex to antero-lateral wall around the M cell distribution during Tdp. In this model, these findings suggest the mechanism of Tdp might be caused by the reentry.

Introduction

Torsade de pointes (Tdp) is a type of polymorphic VT in which the QRS complexes underline about the iso-electric baseline, changing their vector within the run. Typical ECG patterns include notched T waves and long QT intervals. The occurrence of Tdp-like behavior including distinctively changing QRS waveform and spontaneous termination of episodes suggests moving site reentry as a physiologically plausible hypothesis of the mechanism of Tdp [1]. Several mechanisms have been proposed to interpret the Tdp, described their possible role in acquired long QT syndrome and Tdp are discussed about M cells [2]. This model included cycle length dependent shortening refractoriness, and the slow conduction variable to incomplete recovery. A possible contribution of conduction delay and QT prolongation for M cell was studied with the anisotropic propagation on the point of induction and spontaneous termination of Tdp. The aim of this study is demonstrated and calculated ECG, BSPM, isochrone maps and 3 dimensional imaging during Tdp in order to clarify the mechanism of the ventricular tachyarrhythmias.

Methods

The anisotropic propagation cells consisted of approximate 50,000 functional cubic units with spatial resolution of 1.5 mm in diameter [3]. The units contained various types of cardiac cells including afria, ventricles, special conduction system and M cell properties with prolonged action potential duration (APD). Each type of the model cell was specified by the electrophysiologic parameters associated with action potential duration, conduction velocity and the sinus pacing frequency. In addition, the absolute refractory period (ARP) and full recovery time (FRT) were included in these parameters. The interval between ARP and FRT was set as relative refractory period (RRP). In the simulation of TdP, we use the prolonged APDof phase 3 repolarization in the area of "M cell". Figure 1 illustrated the horizontal image of M cell distribution [2][4]. They are distributed into the intermediate region of the anterior and lateral ventricular wall, based on the evidence for the existence of M cells in the human heart by Drouin [5]. Figure 2 showed action potential forms of ventricular, M cell and Purkinje fiber. APD90 were set at 265, 342 and 360 msec for ventricular, M cell and Purkinje, respectively. Due to the different duration from endocardial and epicardial action poential, APD adjusted to 12msec per layer reduced. M cells were not included the ventricular gradient adjustment for it's prolonged APD from 20% (296msec) to 50% (342msec). The phenomenon of APD shortening was called "dynamic coefficient" as an important parameter of induction to VT. According to our previous experimental data, APD shortening related to the premature coupling interval were given for ventricular muscle and Purkinje fiber [6]. These data were approximated by linear regression line, dynamic coefficients were set to 9% and 50% for ventricle and Purkinje fiber, respectively. The layer of anisotropic propagated fibers were rotated 90 to 120 degrees from epicardium to endocardium in counterclockwise direction. The conduction velocity ratio for longitudinal to transverse fiber was 3:1. Sinus pacing interval was every 500msec and total simulating time was for 8 sec. Based on anatomical and electrophysiological settings, the surface ECG potentials on a torso model were calculated by boundary element method using Sun-4 / Leia2.

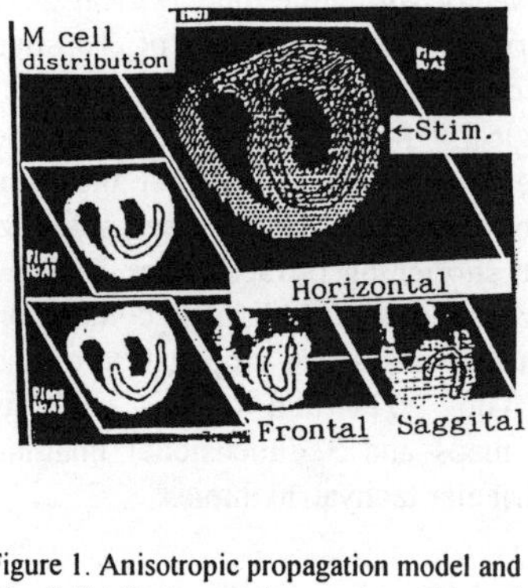

Figure 1. Anisotropic propagation model and M cell distributions at the anterior and lateral region.

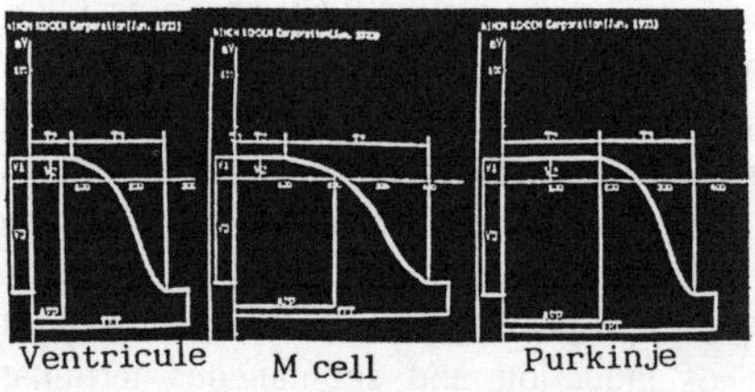

Figure 2. Action Potential Duration (APD) and waveforms of Ventricle (epicardium), M cell and Purkinje

Results

1. Under the same longitudinal conduction velocity of 0.5m/sec for the ventricular fiber and M cell region, Tdp was simulated applying double successive extra-stimuli of 160msec cycle length intervals on the left ventricular epicardium at the delay of 300msec after the sinus pacing excitation. Figure 3-A illustrated polymorphic VT shifting with the direction of QRS vectors. There was a limit to induce Tdp for the longitudinal conduction velocity of 0.52m/sec. When the longitudinal conduction velocity setting was different between the ventricular fiber of 0.47m/sec and M cell region of 0.45m/sec, non-sustained VT was induced as shown in Figure 3-B.

Torsade de pointes　　　　non-sustained VT

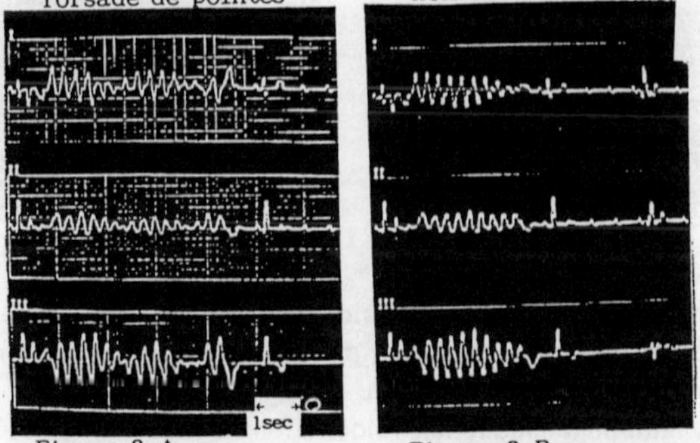

Figure 3-A　　　　Figure 3-B

Figure 3-A : Simulated ECG of Torsade de pointes induced by double extra-stimuli and spontaneous termination of polymorphic VT after refractory period.　Figure 3-B : Non-sustained VT under the different condition of conduction velocity between ventricle and Mcell like properties'

2. QT interval was prolonged with after spontaneous termination of Tdp due to M cell setting and the effect of refractory period. The area of refractoriness recovered from the dispersion on the isochrone maps at the termination of Tdp in Figure 4.

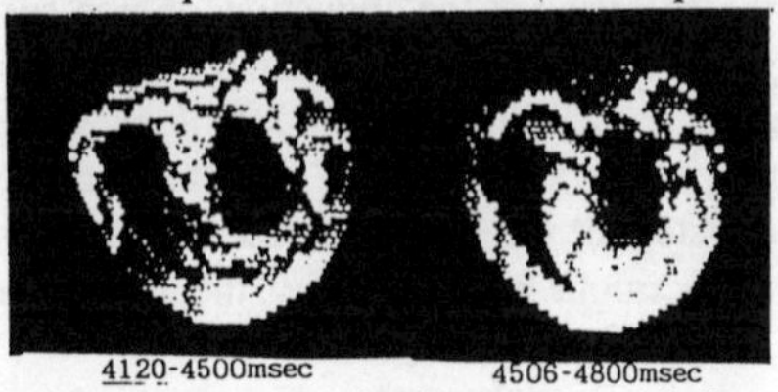

4120-4500msec　　　　4506-4800msec

Figure 4. Isochrone maps at the spontaneous termination. Color step indicated every 3msec interval

3. BSPMs during Tdp and VT showed the pattern of multipolarity at the time of maximum potential in Figure 5-A. Breakthrough site recognized at Tdp after sustaiend VF induced by five extra-stimuli on BSPM as shown in Figure 5-B. Excitation fronts were propagated the reentrant pattern from apex to the ventricle around the distribution of M cell after the refractory area in Figure 6 during Tdp.

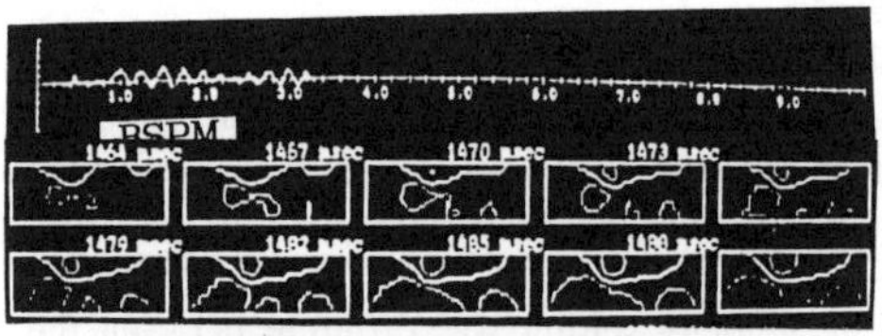

Figure 5-A : BSPMs illustrated the multipolarity during VT and polymorphic VT.

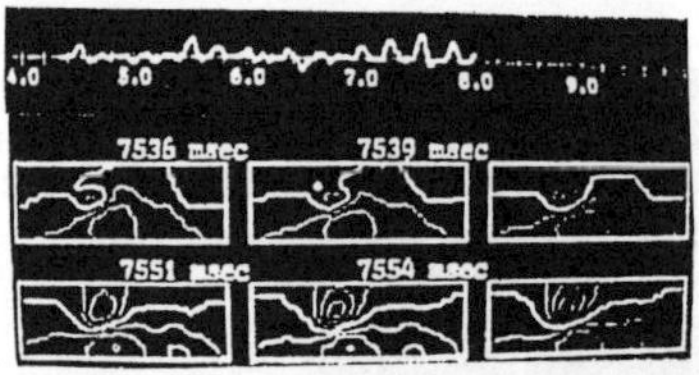

Figure 5-B : Breakthrough site recognized at Tdp after the sustained Vf on BSPM.

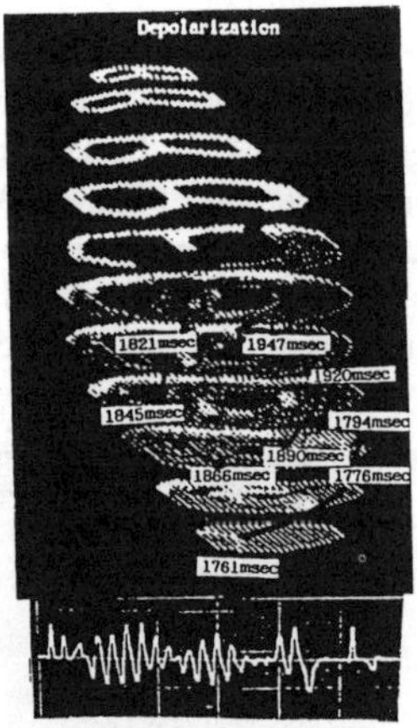

Figure 6. Three dimensional imaging of reentrant propagated excitation fronts

Discussion

Slow conduction is one of important factors of proarrhythmia using anti-arrhythmic agents in patients with reduced cardiac function due to myocardial infarction [7]. We have reported a threshold longitudinal conduction velocity for the induction of VF is from 0.47 to 0.6 m/sec without M cell [8]. For the normal ECG with narrow QRS complex, longitudinal conduction velocity of 0.75 m/sec is required without M cell model. Certainly it is delayed conduction velocity of 0.5m/sec for the longitudinal ventricular fibers. It is required the induction of Tdp as delayed conduction velocity of 0.5 m/sec to the same between the ventricle and M cell like properties. Because of the existence of the area with different conduction velocity caused the reentry for the induction of non-sustained VT. BSPMs indicate the multi-polarization for the dispersion of excitation fronts and isochrone maps illustrate the disparate recovery of excitability. On the 3-D images, the excitation fronts are propagated like reentry from apex to antero-lateral wall around the M cell distribution during Tdp. In this integrated system of the whole heart 3-D anisotropic propagated model, these evidences suggest the Tdp might be caused by the reentry in relation to M cell properties.

References

1. Abildskov JA, Lux RL:Mechanism in Simulated Tdp. J Cardiovasc Electrophysiol, 4:547-560 (1993)

2. Antzelevitch C, Nesterenko VV, Yan GX :Role of M cells in Acquired Long QT syndrome, U waves, and Tdp. J Electrophysiol, 28(suppl):131-138(1995)

3. Wei D, Okazaki O, Harumi K, Harasawa E, Hosaka H:Comparative Simulation of Excitation and BSPM with Isotropic and Anisotropic Computer Heart Models. IEEE 42:343-357(1995)

4. Sicouri S, Antzelevitch C:A Subpopulation of Cells with Unique Electrophysiological Properties in the Deep Subepicardium of the Canine Ventricle, The M Cell. Circ Res 68:1729-1741(1991)

5. Drouin E, Charpentier F, Gauthier C:Evidence for the presence of M cells in the human ventricle. PACE 16:876 (1993)

6. Harumi K, Tsutsumi T, Sato T, Sekiya S: Classification of anti-arrhythmic drugs based on VF threshold. Am J Cardiol 64:10J-14J(1989)

7. Pratt CM, Hallstrom A, Theroux P, Romhilt P, Coromilas J, Myles J: Avoiding interpretive pitfalls when assessing arrhythmia suppression after myocardial infarction: insight from the long term observations of placebo-treated patients in the Cardiac Arrhythmia Pilot Study. JACC 17:1-8(1991)

8. Okazaki O, Wei D, Sekiya S, Tsutsumi T, Mashima S, Harumi K:Conduction velocity as a factor in the induction of VF in an anisotropic computer model. Jap Heart J 35:suppl 267-268(1994)

COMPUTER SIMULATION STUDY OF VECTORCARDIOGRAPHIC MANIFESTATIONS OF HETEROGENEOUS LEFT VENTRICULAR HYPERTROPHY

V. SZATHMÁRY, I. RUTTKAY-NEDECKÝ

Institute of Normal and Pathological Physiology, Slovak Academy of Sciences,
Sienkiewiczova 1, 81371 Bratislava, Slovak Republic
E-mail: szath@unpf.savba.sk

Computer model of propagated activation, with analytically defined ventricular geometry, was used to study the effect of localized asymmetric hypertrophy of the left ventricle on the vectorial representation of its activation. Increase of the wall thickness in parts of the left ventricle affected the magnitude of resultant cardiac vectors differently with respect to its localization. Significant increase of this parameter was found when the lateral and posterior parts of left ventricle were thickened. In the case of interventricular septum, simulated hypertrophy led to a decrease of the magnitude of these vectors. Increase of the wall thickness in the apical part of the left ventricle had minimal effect on cardiac vectors.

1 Introduction

A characteristic feature of hypertrophic cardiomyopathy is most often heterogeneity in the amount of hypertrophy, evident in different regions of the left ventricle, leading to a decrease of its diastolic volume. However, also symmetrical involvement may be found.

The following localizations are usually observed:

Asymmetric:

- septum ("asymmetric septal hypertrophy"),
- septum and anterolateral wall (more the 1/2 of patients),
- posterior portion of the septum, posterobasal free wall.

Symmetric:

- concentric (centripetal) left ventricular hypertrophy with symmetrical thickening of the left ventricle, involving the free wall and the septum equally,
- concentric hypertrophy in the apical left ventricular region (common in Japan)[1].

Since it is practically impossible to induce experimentally such patterns of localized hypertrophy in the left ventricle, computer modeling was used to simulate and study their effects on resultant cardiac vectors.

2 Method

In our computer model of propagated activation[2] the ventricles are determined by parts of ellipsoids. This property of the model allows to change the geometry of ventricles in a simple way. Decrease of the magnitude of two minor axes of the ellipsoid, creating the inner surface of the left ventricle, allows to simulate the concentric (centripetal) increase of the wall thickness, concentric left ventricular hypertrophy. This maneuver accompanied by a parallel shifting of the major axis of the ellipsoid, simulates asymmetric, localized (centripetal) hypertrophy of the left ventricle.

The above described manipulations were performed to simulate asymmetric hypertrophy in the interventricular septum (S), in the anterior (A), posterior (P) and lateral (L) free wall and in the apex (Ap), respectively, as well as in some of their combinations (anteroseptal (AS) and posteroseptal (PS) wall). The thickness of the wall was in these regions increased centripetally to 160% of the reference value. The geometry of the reference model as well as the loci of its initial activation were derived from published data[3,4]. The activation of the ventricle was characterized quantitatively by the spatial time course of the resultant cardiac vector - cardiac vectorgram, and by the time course of the spatial magnitude of these vectors.

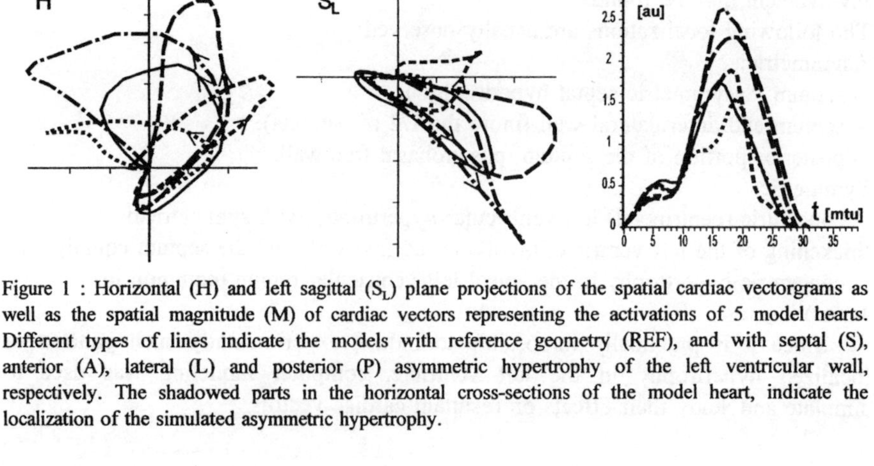

Figure 1 : Horizontal (H) and left sagittal (S_L) plane projections of the spatial cardiac vectorgrams as well as the spatial magnitude (M) of cardiac vectors representing the activations of 5 model hearts. Different types of lines indicate the models with reference geometry (REF), and with septal (S), anterior (A), lateral (L) and posterior (P) asymmetric hypertrophy of the left ventricular wall, respectively. The shadowed parts in the horizontal cross-sections of the model heart, indicate the localization of the simulated asymmetric hypertrophy.

3 Results

The effect of concentric increase of wall thickness in the four major parts of the left ventricle on cardiac vectors is illustrated in Fig.1. Evidently the increase of wall thickness in the lateral and posterior parts of the left ventricle increased significantly the magnitude of resultant cardiac vectors, while the same change in the anterior wall resulted in a slight increase of the magnitude of mid-QRS vectors and in a shifting of the body of the loop to the left. Thickening of the septum led to a decrease of the magnitude of resultant cardiac vectors in the middle part of QRS accompanied by the increase of the posteriorly and to the right oriented forces of the terminal part. In all these simulations the left ventricular mass was increased by 9.5% with regard to the reference.

The cardiac vectorgrams, corresponding to the activations of the model with anteroseptal or posteroseptal asymmetric hypertrophy, are shown in Fig.2. In both cases the left ventricular mass was increased by 16.7% with regard to the reference. Interestingly, in the combination of anterior and septal hypertrophy, the effect of septal hypertrophy prevails in the magnitude-over time curve. The magnitude decreases, but on the orientation of the body of the loop prevails the effect of anterior wall hypertrophy, it is shifted to the left. In the case of

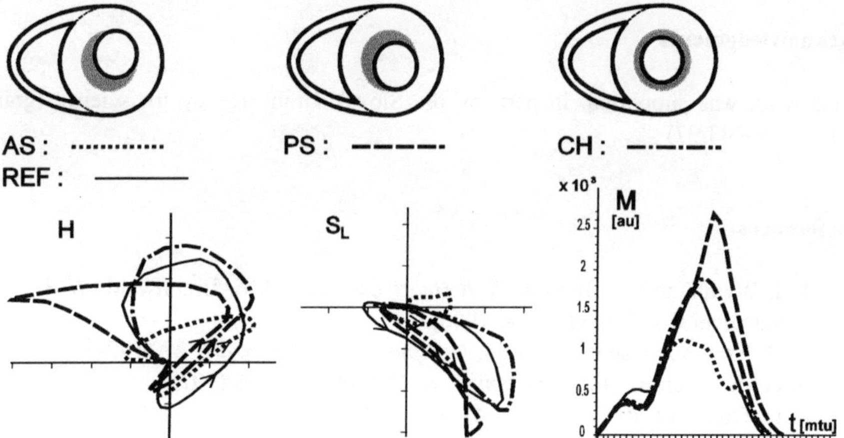

Figure 2 : Horizontal (H) and left sagittal (S_L) plane projections of the spatial cardiac vectorgrams as well as the spatial magnitude (M) of cardiac vectors representing the activations of 3 types of left ventricular hypertrophy. Different types of lines indicate the models with reference geometry (REF), and with anteroseptal (AS), posteroseptal (PS), as well as concentric centripetal hypertrophy (CH) of the left ventricular wall, respectively. The shadowed parts in the horizontal cross-sections of the model heart, indicated the localization of the simulated asymmetric or concentric hypertrophy.

posteroseptal hypertrophy the cardiac vectorgram reflects predominantly the hypertrophy of the posterior wall. In this figure is also evident the difference between cardiac vectorgrams reflecting the activation of the model with symmetric concentric (centripetal) increase of the left ventricular mass and of the above mentioned antero- and posteroseptal hypertrophies. In all cases the mass of the left ventricle was increased by the same amount (16.7%). While symmetric hypertrophy influenced slightly only the initial cardiac vectors, by their shifting to the left and posteriorly, the isolated antero- and posteroseptal hypertrophies led to marked changes, as described above.

Symmetric centripetal thickening of the apical portion of the left ventricle did not affect substantially the shape of the cardiac vector loop.

4 Conclusion

It was the aim of this study to demonstrate the value of computer simulation as an analytical tool for understanding the expected patterns of VCG in different subvarieties of hypertrophic cardiomyopathy with heterogeneous localization of the increased muscle mass.

Acknowledgments

This work was supported, in part, by the Slovak Grant agency for science (grant VEGA 2/4043/97)

References

1. J. Wynne and E. Braunwald in *Heart Disease,* ed. E. Braunwald (W.B. Saunders Co., Philadelphia, 1980).
2. V. Szathmáry and R. Osvald, *Comput. Biomed. Res.* **27**, 27 (1994).
3. G.M. Hutchins *et al, The Am. J. of Cardiol.* **41**, 646 (1978).
4. D. Durrer *et al, Circulation* **41**, 899 (1970).

INVERSE LOCALIZATION OF PREEXCITATION SITES USING "JUMPING DIPOLE"

M. TIŇOVÁ, M. TYŠLER, M. TURZOVÁ, J. ŠVEHLÍKOVÁ
Institute of Measurement Science, Slovak Academy of Sciences,
Dúbravská cesta 9, 842 19 Bratislava, Slovak Republic
E-mail: umermaja@savba.sk

In the study, a set of activation sequences was simulated using the cellular automata model of ventricles with analytically defined shape. Each activation was initiated in a single starting point on AV ring, to represent the preexcitation in case of WPW syndrome. Corresponding body surface potential maps (BSPMs) were simulated on the realistic inhomogeneous torso using the uniform double layer as an equivalent cardiac generator. Computed maps served as an input for the inverse localization procedure. For the inverse solution, volume of the ventricles was divided into 39 segments (18 of them on AV ring). Linear single dipole inverse solution was computed repeatedly for dipoles placed in the centers of all segments for all time steps. The relative residual error of surface potential was evaluated for the whole period of preexcitation (the first 25 ms). Preexcitation was localized into the segment with the lowest error. The method has been tested on data simulated from 16 activation sequences (8 of them iniciated at subepicardium and 8 iniciated at subendocardium). The method performs very well in presence of noise with normal distribution (up to $\sigma = 20\ \mu V$) but is sensitive to the shifts of the position of the cardiac generator.

1 Introduction

Several noninvasive techniques have been tested for the pre-operative localization of the single site of preexcitation in case of WPW syndrome. They were either based on knowledge of experts evaluating the measured body surface potential maps (BSPMs) [1] or inverse computation of parameters of cardiac generator, like multiple dipole [2] or moving dipole [3], from BSPMs. Presented approach was named "jumping dipole", since the cardiac generator was represented by a single dipole placed in predefined limited number of possible locations - centers of the ventricular segments. Amplitude and orientation of the dipole was computed during the whole period of preexcitation and for each possible dipole location. The location with the lowest root mean square of the relative error of the inverse solution was identified as the center of the ventricular segment containing the site of accessory pathway.

2 Method

For simulation of BSPMs a cellular automata model of the activation propagation [4] have been used. Altogether 16 locations of preexcitation were simulated.

In 8 cases the accessory pathway was situated on the subendocardial part of Atrio-Ventricular Ring (AVR), in 8 cases preexcitation was initiated on the subepicardial part of AVR. The BSPMs were computed for the first 25 ms of preexcitation using the uniform dipole layer representation of the cardiac generator, inhomogeneous torso (including lungs and ventricular cavities) as a volume conductor and a boundary element method.

For the inverse computation a volume of ventricles was divided into 39 segments (18 of them on the AVR). The localization procedure consisted of 2 steps. First, for each preexcitation an inverse solution was computed 39 times, having a single dipole always placed in the center of one of the segments. Second, initial point of the preexcitation was localized into the segment where the inverse solution (first step) was computed with the lowest error for the whole period of 25 ms. 4 factors which may influence the inverse localization were simulated: 1) neglection of inhomogeneities (lungs and cavities) within the torso, 2) limited knowledge of the position of the heart - 5 shifts and rotations with mean displacement of centers of segments of the cardiac generator within 1 cm were simulated, 3) number of leads for BSPM measurement - 3 cases were studied - the use of 198 leads (full torso), 63 leads system according to Savard and 24 leads according to Barr, 4) presence of noise in input data, i.e. BSPMs: additional normally distributed noise with value of standard deviation σ equal to 10, 15 and 20 μV was modelled. For each σ and each location of preexcitation 5 realizations were computed.

The resulting dipole was expressed in local coordinate system predefined for each ventricular segment. The local coordinate system consisted of 3 orthogonal coordinates $(\vec{n}, \vec{th}, \vec{tv})$ defined as follows: $\vec{n}$ was in direction from endocardium to epicardium, normal to the epicardial surface of ventricle, $\vec{th}$ was the circumflex tangential and $\vec{tv}$ was in direction from base to apex, tangential to the epicardial surface of ventricle. Compare to global coordinate system $(\vec{x}, \vec{y}, \vec{z})$, the local coordinates were invariant to the heart rotations.

3 Results

The mean dimensions of the segments on the AVR were: length 15.4 mm, hight 26 mm and width 6 mm. With the exact knowledge of the heart position, full number of 198 surface potential leads and considering the presence of lungs filled with air and cavities filled with blood, the simulated accessory pathway was localized into the correct segment in 12 cases, the neighbouring segment in 3 cases and the localization procedure was not successful in 1 out of 16 cases.

The results obtained for homogeneous and inhomogeneous volume conductors and different number of leads are shown in Table 1. All of the following

Table 1: Results obtained for inverse localization using different number of leads and inhomogeneous or homogeneous torso for 16 simulated types of preexcitation.

		Localization (in # of cases)		
		Correct	1st neigh.	Out
	error	7.7 mm	15.4 mm	> 15.4 mm
198 leads	**torso inhomogeneous**	**12**	**3**	**1**
	torso homogeneous	8	3	5
63 leads	torso inhomogeneous	11	4	1
	torso homogeneous	7	7	2
24 leads	torso inhomogeneous	7	8	1
	torso homogeneous	4	9	3

Table 2: Results obtained for 63 lead system according to Savard in %.

	Localization (in %)		
	Correct	1st neigh.	Out
error	7.7 mm	15.4 mm	> 15.4 mm
inhomogen. torso (16 cases)	68.75	25.00	6.25
shift 1cm (16 x 5 cases)	31.25	36.25	32.50
noise 10μV (16 x 5 cases)	52.5	40.00	7.50
noise 15μV (16 x 5 cases)	53.75	38.75	7.50
noise 20μV (16 x 5 cases)	52.50	40.00	7.50
shift 1cm + noise 10μV (16 x 5 cases x 5 cases)	28.50	36.00	35.50

presented results were computed considering torso as an inhomogeneous volume conductor.

In all simulated cases, the localization procedure worked better for the 198 lead BSPMs , than for 63 leads Savard system. 63 leads system performed better than 24 leads system according to Barr. In Table 2, the results obtained for 63 leads system are shown. Accuracy of localization was evaluated for 16 locations of preexcitation with the precise knowledge of cardiac generator within an inhomogeneous torso, for 5 cases of 1 cm shifts and rotation with mean displacement of centers of segment of cardiac generator about 1cm for each location of preexcitation (totally 80 cases), for 5 realizations of additional noise for each location of preexcitation (totally 80 cases) for each σ. The last row shows the results when inaccurate position of the cardiac generator together with the additional noise 10μV was taken into account (totally 400 cases). The results are shown in % of all simulated cases.

Detailed analysis of the results revealed, that the method localized better the initial points placed on the left ventricular wall than those placed on the right ventricular wall. The accessory pathways placed on subepicardium were localized with lower error than the pathways on the endocardium.

4 Discussion and Conclusions

The "jumping dipole" method appeared to be very robust and the results remained stabile even when additional normally distributed noise up to $\sigma = 20\mu V$ was present in input data. The localization procedure was much more sensitive to misplacements of the segmental dipoles that modelled the inaccurate knowledge of the precise position of the cardiac generator. Introduction of the *local* instead of *global* coordinate system can be used in future for distinction between endocardial and epicardial preexcitation. In a former case the normal component of the segmental dipole $\vec{n}$ is positive, while in the latter case it has negative values during the period of preexcitation. The method might be improved if an individual time period of preexcitation would be chosen for each location of preexcitation according to[1] instead of constant 25 ms, as used in the study.

Acknowledgments

The work was supported by grant 2/1216/94 from the Grant Agency for Science of the Slovak Republic and by The Open Society Found.

References

1. J. Liebman, J.A. Zeno, B. Olshansky, A.S. Geha and et al., *Circulation* **83**, 886 (1991).
2. M. Tyšler, M. Tiňová, M. Turzová and P. Kneppo, *Jap. Heart Journal, Suppl.1*, 95 (1994).
3. R. Gulrajani and et al., *Journal of Electrocardiology* **17**, 271 (1984).
4. V. Szathmary and R. Osvald, *Computers and biomed. Research* **27**, 27 (1994).

MODELS FOR SIMPLIFIED MAPPING OF HEART ELECTROPHYSIOLOGICAL STATES

M. G. DANILOUCHKINE
Eindhoven University of Technology,
P.O.Box 513, 5600 MB Eindhoven, the Netherlands

L. I.TITOMIR
Institute for Problems of Information Transmission,
Russian Academy of Sciences
Ermolovoy 19, Moscow 101447, Russia

Abstract

Simplified models of the heart electric generators for the ventricular depolarization and repolarization are proposed for mapping of the electrophysiological states of myocardium on the basis of noninvasive measurements of the heart dipole moment (HDM) obtained by three orthogonal leads.

1 Introduction

Nowadays the orthogonal lead systems such as Frank leads etc. are of frequent use for data acquisition in computerized electrocardiography. These systems allow one to obtain the signals which are proportional to the components of the HDM during cardiac cycle. For the purposes of diagnostical interpretation, the initially measured data are represented as separate time–dependent curves or as VCG loops. However, the parameters extracted by using these methods are usually represented in rather an abstract form. The noninvasive identification of cardiac excitation process using the HDM can be facilitated by means of an intelligible–pictorial representation of the acquired data, with the electrophysiological characteristics and states of the myocardium being more explicitly depicted and related to the heart anatomy. This calls for development of models, or cardiac equivalent generators described by the parameters which can be interpreted electrophysiologically. Two such models intended for a simplified visual interpretation of the orthogonal electrocardiographic signals are presented in this paper.

2 Methods

2.1 Model of Cardioelectric Generator for Depolarization.

During the depolarization, the electric generator of the myocardium is approximated with sufficient accuracy by a uniform double layer coinciding with the depolarization front and having moment proportional to the amplitude of the transmembrane action potential (TAP). In particular, we represent the ventricular depolarization process at each time instant in the form of single summary double layer bounded by a circle lying on the image sphere, which surrounds the heart and has the center coinciding with the center of the heart (this sphere may be interpreted as a spherical quasiepicardium in the framework of a thin-wall heart model [1]). Further simplification is based on the assumption that the maximum magnitude D_m of HDM is achieved at the instant when the radius of double layer edge ρ becomes equal to the image sphere radius R_{ep}. The position of the circle is determined by the orientation angles θ, ψ of the instantaneous HDM $\bar{D}(t)$, and its radius with respect to the image sphere radius $r = \rho / R_{ep}$ is determined by the instantaneous magnitude of the HDM with respect to its maximum magnitude. The parameters r, θ, ψ of the generator can be determined from noninvasive measurements of the HDM components D_x, D_y, D_z at a particular time instant t from the system of equations

$$D_x = D_m r^2 \sin\theta \cos\psi, \quad D_y = D_m r^2 \sin\theta \sin\psi, \quad D_z = D_m r^2 \cos\theta. \tag{1}$$

The heart wall regions possessing three basic electrophysiological states are projected onto the image sphere. These are the state of resting or polarized myocardium (*Res*); the state of wall activation, where a depolarization front is traversing the wall (*Act*); the state of completely depolarized myocardium after propagation of the depolarization front (*Dep*). At the beginning of the ventricular depolarization the wall is assumed to be in the polarized state. At each subsequent time instant, the activation state is defined by belonging of a given point to the circular depolarization front. The point possesses the completely excited state if it has been in the activation state before the present instant. The distributions of the aforementioned states for sequential time instants make up the instantaneous maps of heart depolarization.

Maps of integral kind can also be computed. In particular, these are the isochrone maps representing the time delay of activation arrival or departure and the activation duration map representing the time during which the activation state is retained.

2.2 Model of Cardioelectric Generator for Repolarization.

During the ventricular repolarization, the electric generator is essentially distributed all over the ventricles, its intensity being proportional to the TAP gradient. It is supposed that the region of generator existence is restricted by two concentric spheres with the radii approximating, respectively, the epicardial and endocardial surfaces of the ventricles, R_{ep} and R_{en} ($R_{ep} > R_{en}$). On the assumption of uniform spatial distribution of this generator, we have proved that for the spherical model considered, the summary generator is described by the strictly dipolar terms of multipole expansion with the following dipole components in the coordinate system with the z axis coinciding with the HDM vector [2]:

$$D_x = 0, \qquad D_y = 0, \qquad D_z = \frac{4\pi}{3}(R_{ep}^3 - R_{en}^3) J_V, \tag{2}$$

where J_V is the intensity (volume dipole moment density) of the generator.

Using the aforementioned approach to normalization of the HDM with respect to the epicardium radius and an exponential approximation of the mean time course of the repolarization process[3], we obtain the following expression for the instantaneous distribution of the myocardium cell polarization levels on the image sphere:

$$U(\theta, \psi, t) = \frac{1}{1 + e^{-c(t-t_m)}} - \frac{3}{4} \frac{D(t)\cos\alpha}{D_m} \left(1 - \frac{R_{en}^3}{R_{ep}^3}\right)^{-1}, \quad (3)$$

where c is a constant characterizing the slope of average variation of the TAP in the repolarization phase, t_m is the time of achieving the maximal magnitude of the HDM during the repolarization phase, and α is the angle between the HDM vector and the radius vector of the considered point θ, ψ. The first term of the right side describes the mean temporal course of ventricular recovery. The second term is an additive component with the spatial distribution coinciding with the potential distribution of a dipole proportional to the magnitude of the HDM at a given time instant t. The distributions of U for sequential time instants make up the instantaneous maps of heart repolarization.

The ventricular gradient map representing the distribution of the time difference τ of TAP length with respect to the longest one, can be computed by the formula

$$\tau(\theta, \psi) = -\frac{3}{4} \cos\alpha \left(1 - \frac{R_{en}^3}{R_{ep}^3}\right)^{-1} \int\limits_{QRST} \frac{D(t)}{D_m} dt. \quad (4)$$

The map of τ is assigned to the integral maps of heart repolarization.

The topographic representation of orthogonal electrocardiographic signals on the basis of the models described, was implemented by the computer application software "DECARTO" (Dipolar electrocardiotopography) and tested on a group of healthy and diseased persons.

3 Results and Conclusions

Examples of instantaneous and integral maps, sometimes referred to as decartograms, for depolarization and repolarization phases for the heart cycle of a normal subject are presented in the figure 1. Experimental studies on various groups of patients have shown that the topographic characteristics supplement significant diagnostic information to the commonly used electrocardiographic curves. In many cases, straightforward visual recognition of the heart pathologic states such as myocardial infarction, hypertrophy, conduction blocks etc., is possible.

The models described above correspond, as to their simplicity, to the limited initial information delivered by the orthogonal electrocardiogram. While being extremely simplified, this approach nevertheless provides a new useful means for visual diagnostic interpretation of the electrocardiographic data.

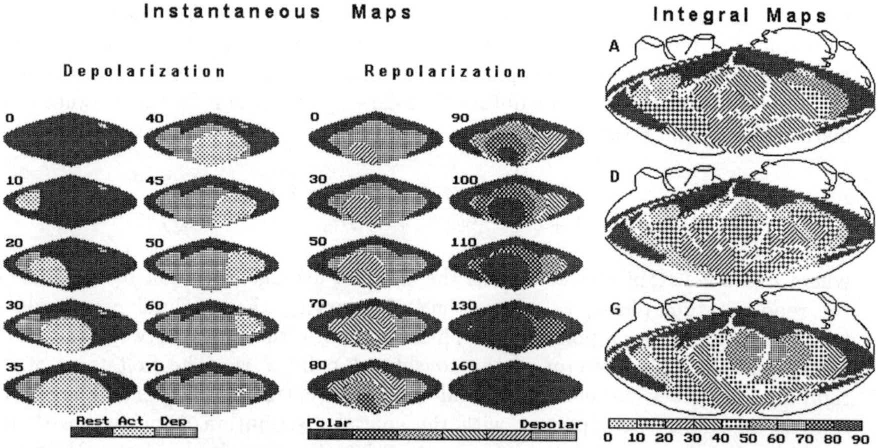

Figure 1: Instantaneous and integral decartograms for a normal subject. Time instants are indicated in milliseconds on the left top corner of each instantaneous map from the onset of the depolarization and repolarization phases. The integral maps of activation arrival, activation duration, and ventricular gradient are denoted by A, D, and G.

References

1. L.I.Titomir and I.Ruttkay–Nedecký in *Analysis of Orthogonal Electrocardiogram* (Nauka, Moscow, 1990, in Russian).
2. M.G.Danilouchkine,*Proc. IPPI Y. Inv. Conf.*,**XXVI**, 17 (1994).
3. B.Wohlfart,*Europ. Heart J.***8**, 409 (1987).

BIOPHYSICAL APPROACH TO THE COMPARATIVE ELECTROCARDIOLOGY

O.V. BAUM, O.D. KOTCHETKOVA, L.A. POPOV, V.I. VOLOSHIN
RAS Institute of Theoretical & Experimental Biophysics, Pushchino, Russia.

The application of quantitative methods based on biophysical models of cardiac equivalent generators to theoretical and experimental tasks of comparative electrocardiology is considered.

One of the main problems of the modern comparative electrocardiology consists in how anatomo-physiological and electrophysiological parameters of the heart (parameters that are characteristic for various classified groups of animals) are related with the spatio-temporal structure of cardioelectric fields generated by the heart[1]. However, while the comparative systematization of the heart parameters is rather well developed (its geometry, transmembrane action potential, speed of the excitation propagation and other characteristics of the excitable myocardium), the interpretation of particularities and distinctions of the registered electrical fields are performed in qualitative and descriptive manner. It is rather difficult to compare these distinctions physiologically, as well as physically. True distinctions of the electrical fields created by the activities of the hearts of various animals are sometimes masked by the influence of the specific extracardial factors, especially, by the influence of the boundary conditions.

The combination of experimental studies and the development of models of the ECG genesis seems to be the most reasonable way to solve this problem. The general idea — using already known electrocardiological methods — is to disengage oneself from such factors as the trunk shape and heart orientation within it and to consider cardiac electric field (CEF) on some standard surfaces of two types: (i) quasi-epicardium one closely enveloping the heart and (ii) quasi-torso surface. Such a surface, being a sphere of a certain radius, is normalized with respect to the maximal heart size. It is desirable that the spherical coordinate system and the own heart coordinate system were correlated. Such a standardization provides obvious advantages. For instance, the body surface potential mapping (BSPM) restricts to the SSPM (standard surface potential mapping). This facilitates real comparative studies and makes them more objective. It should be stressed that the majority of CEF researchers that worked with the isolated heart installed the measuring electrodes precisely on the spherical surface[2].

The development of the above idea is not to "rewrite" the CEF part of the comparative electrocardiology *ab initio* using the "cut-and-measure" method for all the systematic animal groups, but to use the modelling method of direct and inverse problems in the comparative electrocardiology together with the concept of equivalent electrical heart generator (EEHG) well known in the theoretical electrocardiology[3]. This approach is applicable both to theoretical and experimental researches. In a physiological experiment the transfer to SSPM is executed in three stages. First, as usually, the BSPMs are created by means of synchronous multichannel recording. In addition, geometrical trunk parameters are measured. Then in accordance with the known theorems of the theoretical electrocardiology the current parameters of EEHG of multipole type are calculated[4]. These parameters are the intrinsic characteristics of the source, i.e. they change only when transferred to another coordinate system. Finally, the obtained multipole components are used to calculate the potential distribution on the chosen standard surface at the appropriate time moments. The truncation of the multipole series used to define the EEHG parameters is determined by the precision and discreteness of the measurements.

As regarding the theoretical research using the simulation methods of direct problems, attention should be paid to the biophysical models of electric activities of the heart and genesis of its CEF, which parameters describe the heart work in terms of modern electrophysiology permitting physical interpretation[5]. A computer system for simulation of the cardiac electric activity of the heart which may be applied for large scale investigation in cardioelectrodynamics has been developed in our laboratory on the basis of the previously performed investigations. Two models make out the conceptual basis of the system: the 3-D model of myocardium activation with account of specialized conducting His-Purkinje system and CEF genesis model[6] — double electrical layer on the boundary surfaces of electrically active myocardium and boundaries of jump-like changes of its properties. Both models are imbedded into one shell and represent a software package for IBM-compatible PC. The main parameters of the heart electrical activity model are: the geometry of the heart and His-Purkinje system, excitation propagation velocities in different parts of the heart, location of pacemakers, shapes of the generated transmembrane action potentials (TAP), biophysical and some other parameters of the myocardium and intact heart. Taking one of the existing models from the "Patient" data-base or creating a new model on the basis of parameters stored in the "Archive" data-base it is possible to view and edit the model by section in any of the three planes: frontal, horizontal and sagittal. The system allows the choice and correction of the TAP forms distribution regime on the epi- and endocardium surfaces. It defines ultimately the form of the repolarization part of electocardiosignals (e.g. ST-T interval on ECG). The 3-D excitation media model is represented by a space non-dimensional matrix with tightly packed elements which are differentiated into clusters "Myocardium", "His", "Purkinje", "Empty" and make up the "HEART" body on the matrix. One of the system units in accordance with the initial data, biophysical parameters of the model, location and function of the pacemaker elements defines a set of elements, which belong to the excitation wave front for the consequent time moments, and activation time instances — for elements of "HEART" body boundaries. The chosen model parameters and the obtained picture of excitation propagation in the simulated heart correspond to the obtained solution for the direct problem — the calculated ECG curves for the systems of 12 standard and 3 orthogonal leads, as well as VCG loops QRS and T, carried out in three planes (Fig. 1).

One of the possible application of the model is its special modification for the CEF problems in comparative electrocardiology[7]: elucidation of regularities of waves changes in cardiocycle with onthogenetic and phylogenetic heart morphology complication, test of hypotheses concerning distinctive characteristics impact of the conducting system upon the sequence of the ventricle activation, simulation of the indirect influences of ecological changes through the parameters of TAP upon the ECG form. There is a unified model which is adequate to the up-to-date knowledge in the field of CEF biophysics. So it seems natural to formulate all tasks in terms of the model. The parameter values of the model are changed.

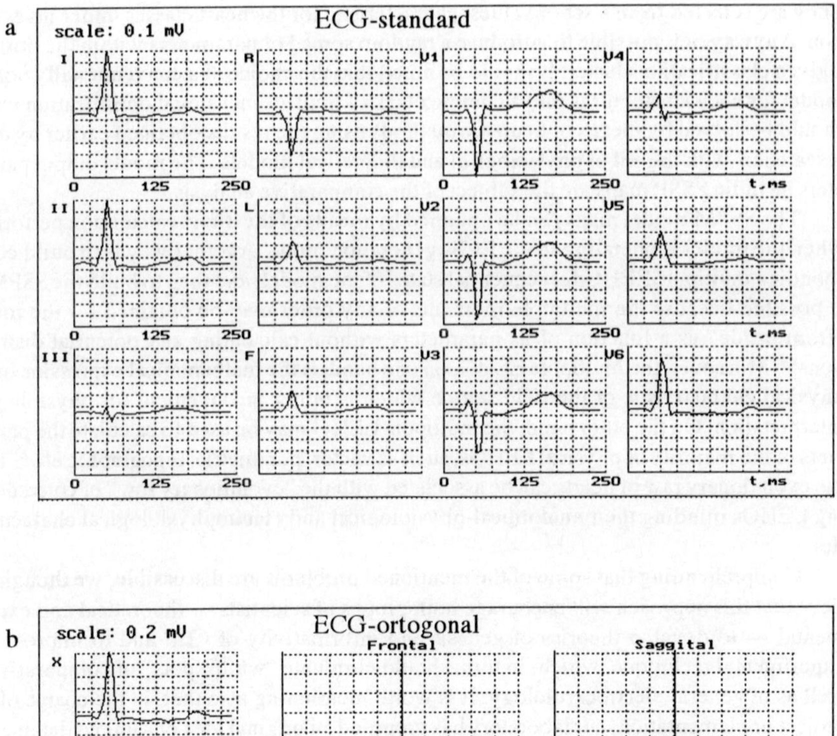

Figure 1. Simulated ECGs corresponding to some shosen parameters of the cardiac electrical activity model: a — ECG in the standard lead system, b — orthogonal ECG and VCG loops QRS and T in XY, XZ, YZ planes.

They are selected from a set of values, characteristic for the heart classes under investigation. Anyway, it is possible to introduce a random spread of parameters within the limits of a given classification cluster. It should be noted that the choice of a conventionally normal model for each cluster turns into a complex task of multi-dimensional optimization which should be solved by means of heuristic methods using the results obtained earlier by other researchers with the aid of physiological and theoretical models. The model output parameters including SSP maps are the subject of the comparative analysis.

The SSPM model maps can be obtained by means of the direct calculation performed when the model is operating in the ECSs generation mode. Another way is to build corresponding multipole EEHG for sequential states of the model, and then to build the SSPM. It is possible because the multipole moments of any order may be obtained for the model "from inside" as a function of its parameters without calculating any potential distributions[8,9]. Moreover, the multipole EEHG, on one hand, is the mathematical expression of the physical characteristic of the field source which is rather inconvenient for physiological interpretation. On the other hand, the multipole EEHG may be used to calculate the parameters of the majority of physical EEHGs, such as vector, parametric, topographic etc.[4]. Thus the evolutionary raw of hearts can be associated with the "evolutionary row" of corresponding EEHGs minding their anatomical-physiological and electrophysiological characteristics.

Comprehending that some of the mentioned problems are discussible, we though believe that this approach will encourage both groups of scientists — theoretical and experimental — to develop theories of genesis and informativity of CEF and to improve the experimental technique, which, in turn, should eliminate "white spots" of comparative as well as of general electrocardiology. It is worth mentioning also that, in the coarse of the project implementation, our laboratory has proposed an original idea of a united database of model and experimental electrocardiosignals.

This work is supported by RFBR grants No. 96-04-48789 and No. 96-01-01080.

References

1. M.P.Roshchevskiy. Evolutional Electrocardiology (Nauka, Leningrad, 1972).
2. O.V.Baum et al. In Cardiac Electric Field (Satell. Symp. 17th Int. Congr. Electrocardiol.). Abstracts, 21, (SAV, Bratislava, 1990).
3. The Theoretical Basis of Electrocardiology, eds. C.V.Nelson and D.B.Geselowitz (Clarendon Press, Oxford, 1976).
4. L.I.Titomir and P.Kneppo. Bioelectric and Biomagnetic Fields. Theory and Applications in Electrocardiology (CRC Press, Boca Raton etc., 1994).
5. O.V.Baum in Biophysics of the Complex System, ed. G.M.Frank, 119 (Nauka, Moscow, 1977).
6. O.V.Baum and E.D.Dubrovin, Biofizika, **16**, 898 (1971).
7. O.V.Baum and L.I.Orlova in Comparative Electrocardiology, ed. M.P.Roshchevskiy, 185, (Nauka, Leningrad, 1981). In Russian.
8. D.B.Geselowitz, Proc. IRE, **48**, 75 (1960).
9. L.I.Orlova and O.V.Baum in Electrocardiology'83, eds. I.Ruttkay-Nedecky and P.Macfarlane, 122 (Excerpta Medica, Amsterdam etc., 1984).

FORWARD SOLUTION BASED ON EXPERIMENTAL DATA MEASURED IN ANIMALS WITH DIFFERENT MYOCARDIAL ACTIVATION PATTERNS

N.V. YEVSTIFEEVA, I.M. ROSHCHEVSKAYA, N.A. ANTONOVA, V.A.VITYAZEV, D.N. SHMAKOV, M.P. ROSHCHEVSKY

Institute of Physiology, Ural Department of Russian Academy of Sciences, Kommunisticheskaya, 24, 167610, Syktyvkar, Komi Republic, Russia

E-mail: compcard@online.ru

The reflection of depolarization wavefronts of various configuration in ventricular myocardium onto the heart and body surfaces and the reflection of epicardial potential distributions onto the body surface was studied by means of forward problem solution by the use of three mathematical models based on experimental data. The first model («interpolation») allows to reconstruct the depolarization sequence of the whole ventricles' myocardium on the base of extracellular cardiac potentials recorded from several cross-sections of the ventricles. The other two models are the models of forward problem solution. One of them permits simulation of epicardial and body surface potentials on the base of 3D configurations of real excitation wavefronts in the heart ventricles reconstructed by the use of the «interpolation» model. Another forward model allows to calculate body surface potentials from real epicardial ones.

1 Introduction

Solution of the forward problem of electrocardiology by the use of mathematical models is an important tool for investigation of cardiolelecric field formation.

The peculiarity of the present study is that the forward models used were based on experimentally measured electrical heart parameters and real geometrical characteristics of the animals. Besides we have used a comparative-physiological approach: forward problem was solved for the sheep and the dog - animals differed both in heart and torso geometry as well as in ventricles' depolarization patterns.

2 Methods

Cardioelectric potentials were recorded by the use of the 64-channel computer system on body surface, ventricles' epicardium and within ventricular myocardium in 6 dogs ("successive" type of myocardial activation) and 6 sheep ("flash" type of myocardial activation).

For every examined animal realistic heart and torso surfaces as well as the real 3D depolarization wavefronts in the heart ventricles were reconstructed. The wavefronts of excitation were reconstructed as isochrone surfaces of depolarization by means of the «interpolation» mathematical model[1]. This model allows to reconstruct 3D patterns of excitation wave spread through the heart ventricles on the base of extracellular potentials recodered from several ventricles' cross-sections.

Epicardial and torso potentials were simulated as potentials of uniform double electric layers coinciding with real wavefronts of excitation in the heart ventricles. Besides the body surface potentials were calculated from the measured epicardil ones by means of a model connecting potential distributions over heart and torso surfaces through transfer coefficients depending on torso and heart geometry. Simulated potentials were in a good agreement with experimental data.

3 Results

In the frame of the model represented by double electrical layers coinciding with real wavefronts of excitation we investigated the reflection of depolarization wavefronts of various configuration in ventricular myocardium onto the heart and body surfaces at the initial and final stages of ventricles' depolarization[2].

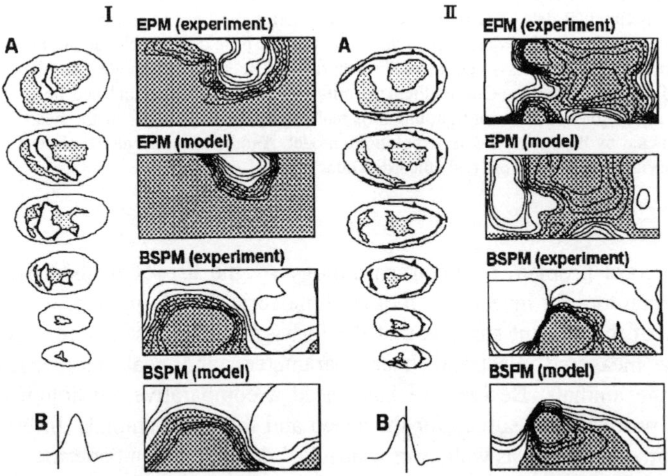

Figure 1: Cardioelectric potentials of a dog at the initial (I) and final (II) periods of ventricles' depolarization, real and simulated as potentials of uniform double layers coinciding with real wavefronts of activation.

A - localization of excitation wavefronts (bold lines) on the cross-sections of heart ventricles (the direction of wavefronts propagation is depicted by arrows, ventricular cavities are shaded). B - forelegs lead ECG with a time marker. EPM - epicardial potential map, BSPM - body surface potential map (positive potential areas are shaded). The left half of the maps corresponds to the ventral, the right half - to the dorsal surface of torso or ventricles' epicardium. The interval between isopotential lines is 1 mV for EPMs and 0.1 mV for BSPMs (I), 5 mV for EPMs and 0.5 mV for BSPMs (II).

The model allowed to distinguish the contribution of electrical activity of different layers of heart ventricles to the cardioelectric field in dependence on the myocardial activation pattern. It was shown that during the initial period of ventricular depolarization the cardioelectric potentials both in the dogs and in the sheep are determined by the electrical activity of subendocardial layers (fig. 1, I and 2, I). At the final stages of depolarization the cardioelectric field in the dogs is formed due to the activity of myocardial and subepicardial layers (fig. 1, II), while in the sheep - due to the activity of intramural, subepicardial and subendocardial

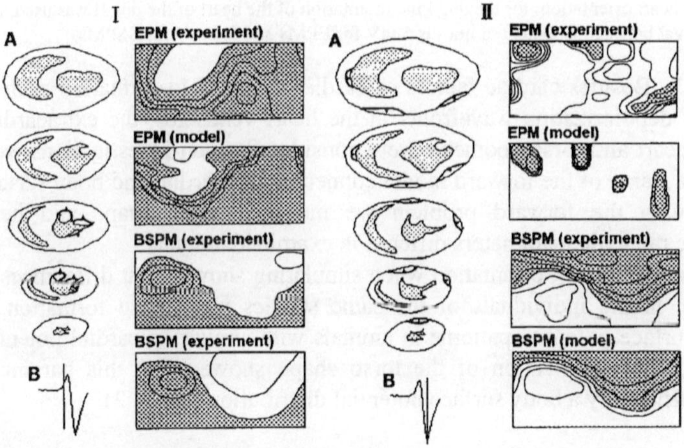

Figure 2: Cardioelectric potentials of a sheep at the initial (I) and final (II) periods of ventricles' depolarization, real and simulated as potentials of uniform double layers coinciding with real wavefronts of depolarization.

Conventional signs are the same as on fig. 1. The interval between isopotential lines is 0.5 mV for EPMs and 0.1 mV for BSPMs (I), 1 mV for EPMs and 0.2 mV BSPMs (II).

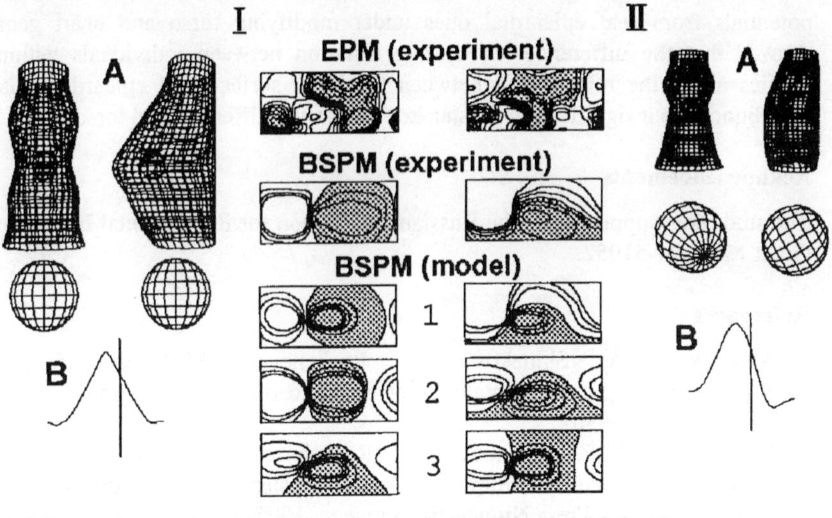

Figure 3: Influence of heart orientation and torso shape on body surface potentials in a dog.

I and II - animals with various heart and torso geometry. A - heart and torso surfaces reconstructed on the basis of measurements. B - forelegs lead ECG with a time marker. BSPM (model) - torso potential distributions simulated from real epicardial potentials. (1) - potentials simulated under real heart and torso geometry. (2) - potentials simulated under a real heart orientation but a changed torso shape: for the dog I the torso shape of the dog II was used, and vice versa. (3) - potentials simulated under a real torso shape but a changed heart orientation: for the dog I the orientation of the heart of the dog II was used, and vice versa. The interval between isopotential lines is 5 mV for EPMs and 0.5 mV for BSPMs.

layers (fig. 2, II). Besides cardiac factors of cardioelectric field formation such as configuration of depolarization wavefronts in the heart ventricles, the extracardiac factors such as heart and torso geometry were considered. Such investigations were carried out in the frame of the forward model connecting epicardial and body surface potentials[3]. Solving the forward problem we modified torso shape and heart orientation in the range the parameters differed in examined animals.

Modification of the heart orientation when simulating showed that differences in heart orientation in the individuals of the same species may cause formation of different body surface potential patterns in animals with similar epicardial potential patterns (fig. 3, 3). Modification of the torso shape showed that this parameter doesn't affect sufficiently a body surface potential distribution (fig. 3, 2).

4 Conclusion

The forward problem solution on the base of real chronotopographic characteristics of the heart ventricles' depolarization process allowed to distinguish the contribution of the electrical activity of different ventricular layers to the cardioelectric field in dependence on the myocardial activation pattern. Simulations of body surface potentials from real epicardial ones under modifying torso and heart geometry showed that the differences in heart orientation between individuals within one species affect the relationship between the body surface and epicardial potential distributions to a significantly greater extent than the differences in torso shape.

Acknowledgements

The study was supported by the Russian Foundation for Fundamental Investigations, Grant № 96-04-51052.

References

1. Antonova N.A., Shmakov D.N., Roshchevsky M.P. in *Advances in Electrocardiology*, Ed. Antaloczy et al. (Excerpta Medica, Amsterdam, New York, Oxford, 1990).
2. Roshchevsky M.P., Shmakov D.N., Roshchevskaya I.M. et al. in *Building Bridges in Electrocardiology*, Ed. A. van Oosterom, T.F. Oostendorp, G.J.H. Uijen (University Press Nijmegen, Nijmegen, 1995).
3. Shmakov D.N., Roshchevsky M.P., Roshchevskaya I.M. et al. in *Abstr. XXIIIth Intern. Congr. on Electrocardiology* (Cleveland, Ohio, USA, 1996).

THERMAL REGIMES OF HEART, MYOCARDIUM REPOLARIZATION AND ST-T GENESIS. A MODEL STUDY

O.V.BAUM

RAS Institute of Theoretical & Experimental Biophysics, Pushchino, Russia.

The effect of heat processes on the distribution of transmembrane action potential durations in the ventricle wall has been studied in connection with the ST-T interval genesis by means of mathematical modelling methods.

The repolarization part of the ventricle complex, i.e. the ST-T interval, is the most variable, and at the same time, the most informative characteristic of the cardiac cycle as it carries indirect information about the metabolic processes in myocardium, about electrolytic balance changes, etc.

Distribution of the transmembrane action potential (TAP) durations existing in the working heart gave the rise to the concept of the ventricle gradient G in electrocardiology[1]. In its scalar interpretation G_I is an integral of $ECG_I(t)$ taken in limits of QRST segment for the discussed ECG lead I. The difference in temperature on the epi- and endocardium surfaces is one of the causes (and may be the main one) of the G_I origin in normal conditions.

Indeed, the duration of TAP phases is the temperature-sensitive characteristic of the excitable myocardium and therefore depends on the temperature field in the cardiac muscle. The presence of some transmural temperature difference $\Delta t°$ has been noted in many experimental works, which though disagree with value estimations and $\Delta t°$ sign assessments. Several problems are still disputable, for instance those related the informativity of isointegral QRST maps and ST-T interval form changes that are observed under the sharp change of the ambient or intracavital temperature in invasive electrophysiological experiments[2]. Therefore the biophysically based theoretical investigation of the ST-T genesis should include the development and investigation of myocardium electric activity models as well as models suitable for the calculation of heart thermal conditions.

In the biophysical models of ECG genesis, which are represented by the double electrical layer on the boundary surfaces of the electrically active myocardium, for the ST-T changes simulation it is necessary, as a minimum, to know the durations of TAPs generated on these surfaces[3] and dependent upon the above mentioned temperature field, which, in turn, is defined by the heat because of metabolic energy, transmural convection due to the blood perfusion, thermophysical properties of myocardium, and by boundary conditions[4]. Such conditions are defined by the possible heart work regimes in natural or experimental conditions: *in situ*, in the air, and in the extensive conductive medium.

For the calculation of the transmural temperature profile θ (x) of the ventricle wall with the thickness L, temperature extremum position x_{extr}, epicardium temperature θ_L, heat fluxes on endo- and epicardium it is required to work out and solve a suitable heat conduction equation for a ventricle wall model in the case of distributed heat sources **q** and transmural convection **m**, where **q** is the heat due to metabolic energy and **m** is proportional to the blood perfusion value in the ventricle wall ($[q] = wt \cdot cm^{-3}$, $[m] = wt \cdot cm^{-3} \cdot deg^{-1}$).

Taking into account the possible assumptions and expected errors as well as being guided by the aim to obtain estimating analytical solution useful to investigate the impact tendencies of q and m changes upon $\theta(x)$ for the heart working in the air and in the extensive liquid medium a rather simple stationary heat conduction equation has been chosen:

$$\frac{d^2\theta}{dx^2}+\frac{q}{\lambda}-\frac{m}{\lambda}\theta=0 \tag{1}$$

with boundary conditions:

$$\theta\Big|_{x=0}=0,\quad -\lambda\frac{d\theta}{dx}\Big|_{x=L}=\alpha(\theta_1-\theta_{extr}), \tag{2}$$

where λ is the heat conduction constant, α is the free heat convection coefficient, $\theta(x)=T^{\circ}(x)-T^{\circ}_B$, T°_B is the blood temperature, θ_{ext} is the excessive external temperature.

Analytical solutions of the above equation for each heat regime of the heart work have been obtained in the form of curve families with the parameters represented by relative levels of heat production and convection, wall thickness and boundary conditions. In particular, for the $\theta(x)$ function the solution of equation (1) is:

$$\theta(x)=\frac{\frac{q}{m}\left[\left(\alpha-\sqrt{\lambda m}\right)e^{-\sqrt{\frac{m}{\lambda}}\cdot L}-\alpha\right]+\alpha\theta_{extr}}{\alpha\cdot sh\left(\sqrt{\frac{m}{\lambda}}\cdot L\right)+\sqrt{\lambda m}\cdot ch\left(\sqrt{\frac{m}{\lambda}}\cdot L\right)}\cdot sh\left(\sqrt{\frac{m}{\lambda}}\cdot x\right)+\frac{q}{m}\left(1-e^{-\sqrt{\frac{m}{\lambda}}\cdot x}\right). \tag{3}$$

Figure 1 shows as an example the $\theta(x)$ curves for normal values of q and m (0.02 wt · cm^{-3} and 0.045 wt · cm^{-3} · deg^{-1} accordingly) when modelling the heart work in the air (a) and in the liquid medium (b); the figure also shows two stationary temperature profiles of the ventricle walls under the transmural temperature difference $\Delta t^{\circ}=+2^{\circ}C$ (c) and $-2^{\circ}C$ (d) accordingly in the case of the liquid external medium.

Figure 2 shows the excessive epicardium temperature q_L dependent on the wall thickness L when modelling the heart under the perfusion in the air in normal conditions (a) and under the decreasing of the coronary blood flow by four times (b). It should be noted that under some θ_{ext} values the epicardium temperature may be less (for a thin wall) or more than T°_B under other equal conditions.

Thus, the researchers investigating the repolarization processes in the cardiac muscle in laboratory conditions on a myocardium specimen or an isolated heart working in the air or in the liquid medium, should take into consideration the boundary conditions of the experiment when trying to extend the obtained electrophysiological knowledge for the visceral level *in situ*.

The estimating results obtained show also the need for the further development of joint thermal and electric models of the heart in direct problems of cardioelectrodynamics. Such joint models will provide for TAP distributions adequate to the simulated heat regime of the

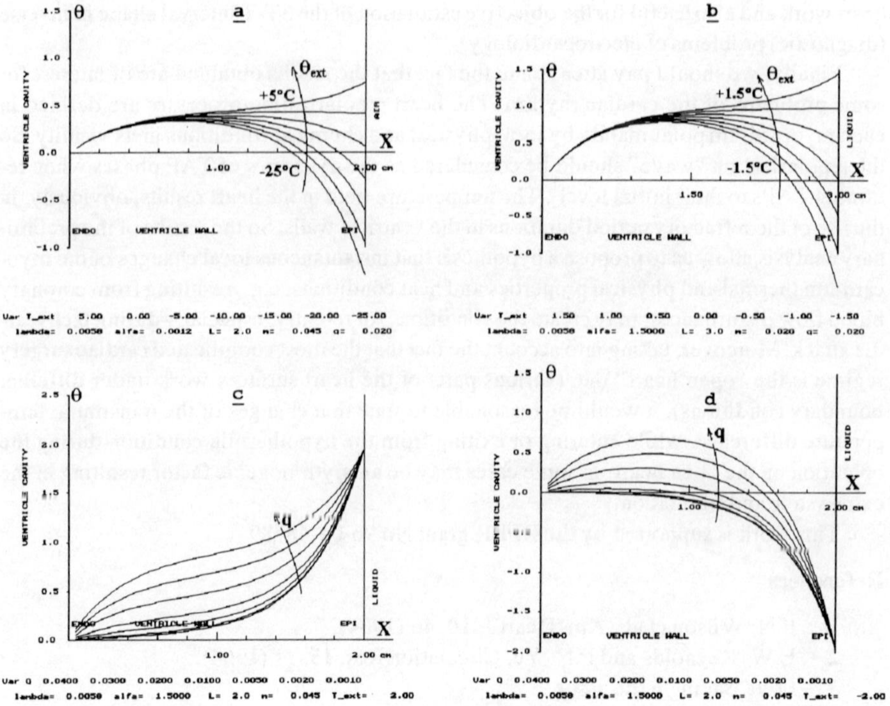

Figure 1

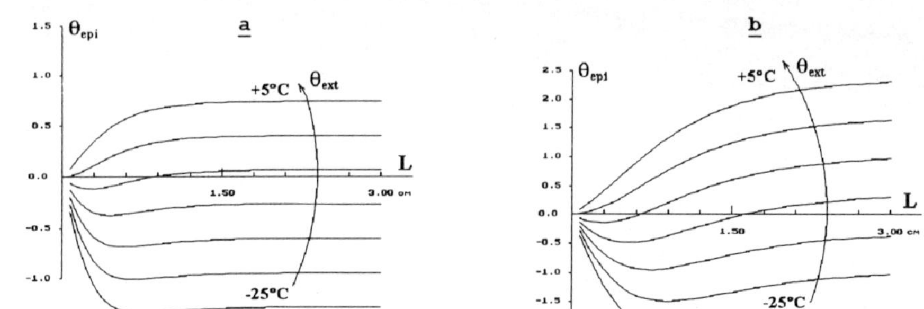

Figure 2

heart work and also useful for the objective estimation of the ST-T interval shape in inverse (diagnostic) problems of electrocardiology.

Finally, we should pay attention to the fact that the results obtained are of interest for some problems of the cardiac rhythm. The heart repolarization processes are defined in each myocardium point mainly by local physical and chemical conditions in its vicinity. So the repolarization "wave" should be considered as the dynamics of TAP phases when returning TAPs to their initial level[5]. The temperature field in the heart results, obviously, in the rise of the refractory period durations in the ventricle walls. So the results of the preliminary analysis allow us to propose a hypothesis that instantaneous local changes of the myocardium thermal and physical properties and heat conditions, e.g., resulting from coronary blood flow disturbances, may create the conditions for re-entry, especially during tachycardia attack. Moreover, taking into account the fact that the most complicated cardiac surgery regime is the "open heart" one (various parts of the heart surfaces work under different boundary conditions), it would be reasonable to state that changes of the transmural temperature difference, while entering or exiting from the hypothermia condition during the operation on the open heart, in some cases may be an arythmogenic factor resulting in the extrasystole and fibrillation.

This work is supported by the RFBR grant No 96-04-48789.

References

1. F.N. Wilson et al., Am. Heart J. **10**, 46 (1934).
2. E.W. Reynolds and P.N. Yu, Circulation Res. **15**, 11 (1964).
3. O.V. Baum in this issue.
4. E. Barta et al., Int. J. Heat Mass Transfer **28**, 663 (1985).
5. O.V. Baum in Electrocardiology'83, eds. I. Ruttkay-Nedecky and P. Macfarlane, 88(Excerpta Medica, Amsterdam etc., 1984).

III. Heart Rate Regulation and Rhythm Disturbances

HEART RATE CONTROL AND HEMODYNAMICS DURING SLEEP IN CAD PATIENTS WITH SLEEP APNEA SYNDROME

G.VARONECKAS, R.DAUKŠYS, A.MARTINKĖNAS, D.ŽEMAITYTĖ
Institute Psychophysiology and Rehabilitation, Vydûno Str 4,
Palanga 5720, Lithuania
E-mail: giedvar@ktl.mii.lt

Modification of autonomic HR control and hemodynamics during individual sleep stages was analysed in CAD patients with and without sleep apnea syndrome (SAS). CAD patients with SAS, as compared with patients without SAS, during sleep have reduced hemodynamics and autonomic heart rate control, especially sympathetic one, and lower level of hemodynamics. An increased contribution of relative impact of humoral control was found during episodes of apnea.

Introduction

Obstructive sleep apnea is a serious, potentially life-treathening condition in cardiac patients [1]. Earlier we found that approximately one half of coronary artery disease (CAD) patients displayed an episodes of apnea during different sleep stages, and periodic breathing was associated to heart rate (HR) oscillations with a period of 30 seconds accompanied by vasoconstriction and an increase in HR frequency and variability [2]. From the other hand, those modifications followed by the changes in autonomic control of cardiovascular system as well as in hemodynamics might be a risk factor for occurrence of cardiac abnormalities during sleep in CAD patients.

The goal was an investigation of modification of autonomic HR control and hemodynamics during individual sleep stages in CAD patients with and without sleep apnea syndrome (SAS).

Contingent and Methods

The contingent was 184 CAD patients (52.9±1.24 yr.), including 18 patients (55.1±4.86 yr.) with SAS. Patients with SAS, as compared with patients without SAS, were characterised by overweight (Broka index more 20%), disturbed cerebral blood flow, lower workload at symptom-limited exercise, and more frequent presence ($p<.1$) of heart failure and previous myocardial infarction.

Recordings of EOG, EEG, and EMG as well as RR intervals and stroke volume (SV), measured by impedance cardiography, were performed throughout the night sleep. Sleep stages were identified visually according to conventional criteria [3]. Computerised analysis of HR, hemodynamics, and HR power spectrum was done. Three major oscillatory components of HR power spectrum were used as a noninvasive instrument, reflecting HR control: (i) very low frequency component (VLFC), associated with thermal-metabolic regulation; (ii) low frequency component (LFC), reflecting predominantly sympathetic control; (iii) high frequency component (HFC), reflecting parasympathetic one [4].

Sleep apnea syndrome was characterised by more than 30 apnea episodes of no less than 10 seconds duration during 8 hours of sleep.

Results and Discussion

An example of HR power spectrum during normal breathing and apnea episode is presented in Figure 1. The HR power spectrum during apnea episodes is characterised by clear-cut diminution of HFC and LFC, representing a reduction of parasympathetic and sympathetic input into HR regulation. The pick in the zone of frequency of 30 seconds is very characteristic for HR oscillations during apnea episodes.

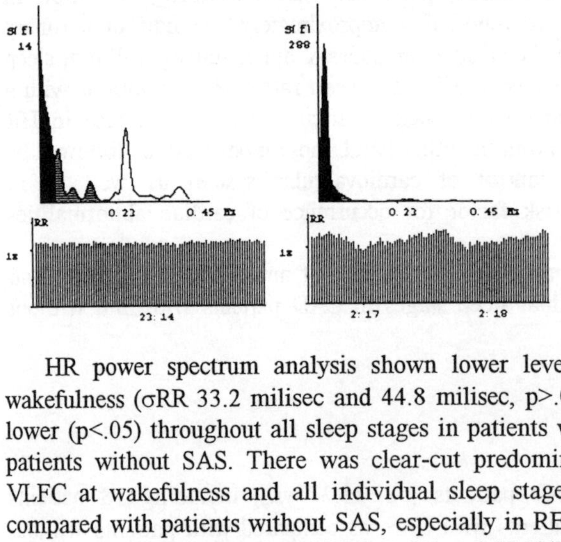

Figure 1. An examples of heart rate power spectrum (top) and rhythmogram (bottom) during normal breathing (left side) and apnea episodes (right side).

HR power spectrum analysis shown lower level of HR variability during wakefulness (σRR 33.2 milisec and 44.8 milisec, p>.05), which was significantly lower (p<.05) throughout all sleep stages in patients with SAS, as compared with patients without SAS. There was clear-cut predominance of relative impact of VLFC at wakefulness and all individual sleep stages in patients with SAS, as compared with patients without SAS, especially in REM sleep (79.6% and 66.6%, respectively) due to diminished LFC (9.5% and 17.8%) and HFC (8.1% and 12.8%) (Figure 2).

HR and hemodynamics during apnea episodes, as compared with normal breathing, in patients with SAS have shown significantly increased impact of VLFC (77.4%, and 68.7%, respectively during apnea episodes and normal breathing) and reduced LFC (11.3%, and 16.3%, respectively) during stage II, which becomes more expressed during stage III (LFC 9.4% and 17.8%, respectively). Those differences disappeared in REM sleep when VLFC dominates

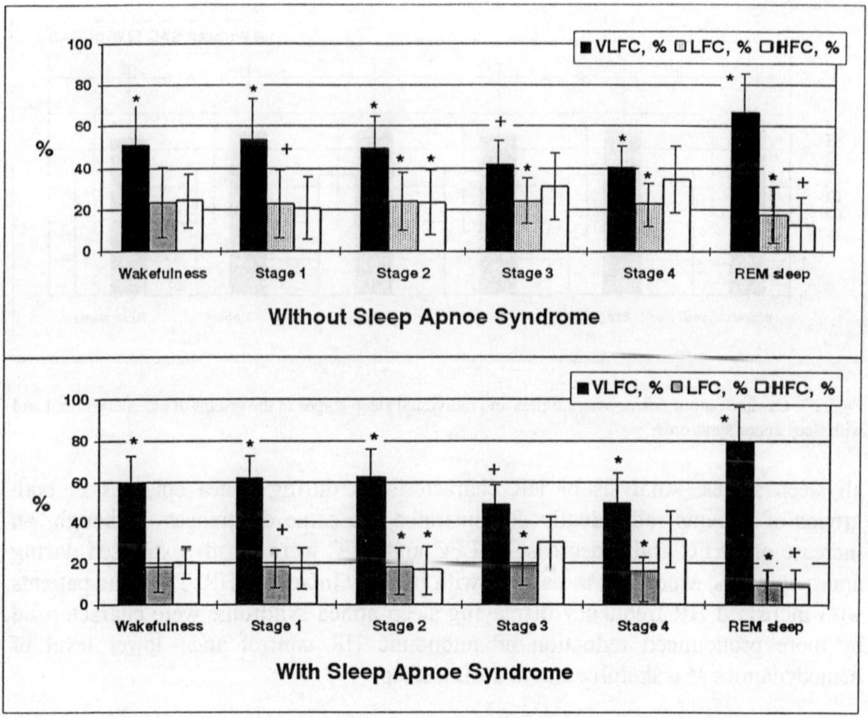

Figure 2. Characteristics of HR power spectrum analysis in the groups of patients without and with sleep apnea syndrome

in both situations, during apnea episodes and normal breathing (82.6% for both groups).

HR and hemodynamics during normal breathing over sleep in patients with SAS, as compared to patients without SAS, demonstrated lower level of SV and CO at wakefulness (57.4 ml and 1.17 l/min and 82.7 ml and 2.45 l/min, respectively) and all sleep stages (Figure 3).

Although the group of patients displaying SAS was non-homogeneous, being composed from two groups: 1) patients with baseline bradycardia, and 2) patients with initially increased HR frequency. Both groups demonstrated reduced HR modifications over sleep stages during normal breathing: changes of RR interval during individual sleep stages did not exceed 5% and 7%, respectively in patients with increased HR and patients with bradycardia. Patients with initially increased HR, as compared with bradycardia patients, at wakefulness were characterised by lower level of CO 2.60 l/min and 4.22 l/min, respectively), HR variability, with more increased relative impact of VLFC (72.8% and 59.7%, respectively) and decreased HFC (12.9% and 29.3%, respectively). The same was characteristic for

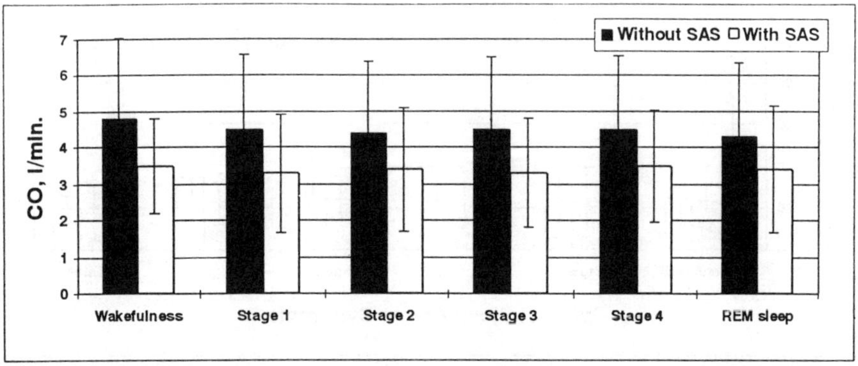

Figure 3. Cardiac output during wakefulness and individual sleep stages in the groups of patients without and with sleep apnea syndrome.

all sleep stages. Analysis of HR characteristics during apnea episodes in both groups of patients individually demonstrated the same differences. Although, an increase of VLFC and a decrease of LFC and HFC were mostly expressed during apnea episodes, especially in patients with initially increased HR. Thus, the patients with increased HR frequency displaying sleep apnea syndrome were characterised by more pronounced reduction of autonomic HR control and lower level of hemodynamics at wakefulness and during sleep.

Conclusion

CAD patients with SAS at wakefulness and during sleep have reduced hemodynamics and autonomic HR control, especially sympathetic one, with increased contribution of relative impact of humoral control. This effect is more pronounced during apnea episodes, as compared with normal breathing of the same patient. It might be a predisposing factor for cardiac abnormalities during sleep, especially in cardiac patients.

References

1. Mooe T. et al. *Chest* Vol. 109, 659-663 (1996).
2. Žemaitytė D., Varoneckas G., Sokolov E. *Psychophysiology*. Vol. 21, 290-298 (1984).
3. A. Rechtschaffen and A. Kales (1968).
4. Žemaitytė D. et al. *Int. J. Psychophysiology* Vol. 4, 129-141 (1986).
5. Varoneckas G. *Sleep Research* Vol. 24A, 418 (1995).

BAROREFLEX SENSITIVITY AND HEART RATE VARIABILITY

D.ŽEMAITYTĖ, G.VARONECKAS, V.DILKAITĖ, A.MARTINKĖNAS
Institute Psychophysiology and Rehabilitation, Vydûno Str 4,
Palanga 5720, Lithuania
E-mail: giedvar@ktl.mii.lt

Correlation between of baroreflex sensitivity (BRS) and heart rate (HR) variability including HR response to active orthostasis was studied in healthy subjects and CAD patients. Maximal HR frequency at active orthostasis, but not response to it, was found mostly related to BRS. Thus, BRS and maximal HR response to active orthostasis might bee seen as independent markers of negative prognosis in coronary artery disease patients.

Introduction

Heart rate (HR) variability was seen as a marker of negative prognosis for patients after myocardial infarction [1, 5, 7]. Baroreflex sensitivity (BRS) as well as HR variability was demonstrated as being most significant marker of sudden death [2, 3, 4, 6]. Although correlation between of HR variability and BRS have been found not very high. Maximal HR response to active orthostatic test (AOT) have been shown being more informative, than HR variability characteristics, as prognostic index for coronary artery disease (CAD) patients [7].

The goal of the study was an analysis of relationship between of BRS and HR variability, including HR responses to AOT and bicycle ergometry, in healthy subjects and CAD patients.

Contingent and Methods

The contingent was 30 adult subjects: 13 healthy subjects (age 37.7 yrs) and 17 CAD patients (age 55.2 yrs). Among CAD patients six patients demonstrated evidence of congestive heart failure, seven patients - hypertension.

Autonomic HR control have been evaluated using HR frequency and variability at rest, maximal HR response to AOT and parasympathetic-sympathetic interaction according HR power spectrum analysis into three major oscillatory components: very low (VLFC), low (LFC) and high (HFC) frequency components. Bicycle ergometry was performed in addition. BRS was measured during phenylephrine infusion. Analysis of HR, stroke volume and systolic blood pressure by Korotkoff method was performed using computerised system on each infusion stage: (i) physiological saline; (ii) phenylephrine 0.4 μg/kg/min; (iii) phenylephrine 0.8 μg/kg/min; and (iv) physiological saline. Phenylephrine infusion was discontinued if systolic blood pressure raised more tan 30 mmHg or cardiac abnormalities manifested. BRS was assessed from linear regression slope of RR interval (in msec) versus increment in systolic blood pressure (in mmHg). Linear regression analysis was performed on each infusion stage data or during all stages of test. The slopes were calculated using linear regression analysis according:

$$RR = a + b \cdot BPsys, \text{ where } a = \overline{RR} - b \cdot \overline{BPsys} \text{ and } b = r\frac{\sigma_{RR}}{\sigma_{BPs}}.$$

Cardiac output (CO) and total peripheral resistance (TPR) were calculated from stroke volume and arterial blood pressure. HR and hemodynamics characteristics were analysed using computerised system [8].

Mean values of BRS or slope, HR and hemodynamic parameters during AOT and bicycle ergometry for healthy subjects and CAD patients have been compared using Students criteria, correlative analysis between of BRS level and investigated data have been performed. Spaerman R correlation between presence of CAD and all investigated parameters have been performed as well.

Results

Basic recordings at rest before test in supine position have not demonstrated any significant difference of average values of HR frequency (RR interval) and hemodynamics (SV, CO, TPR) between the groups of healthy subjects and CAD patients. CAD patients, as compared with healthy subjects, demonstrated statistically lower level of HR variability (σRR=18 ms and σRR=27 ms, correspondingly in CAD pts and healthy Ss) and respiratory arrhythmia (RA=30 ms and RA=53 ms, correspondingly), reflecting decreased tonic HR control. Analysis of HR power spectrum shown significant difference between both groups for all three relative oscillatory components of HR power spectrum: very low frequency component (VLFC) was higher in CAD pts group (56% and 40%, correspondingly in CAD pts and healthy Ss) indicating a prevalence of humoral HR control; low frequency component (LFC) (17% and 30%, correspondingly) and high frequency component (HFC) (27% and 30%, correspondingly) were higher in healthy subjects indicating a prevalence of reflex HR control. Maximal HR response to AOT (ΔRR_B=22% and ΔRR_B=32%, correspondingly in CAD pts and healthy Ss), maximal HR frequency at AOT (RR_B=728 ms and RR_B=615 ms, correspondingly), difference of RR interval at maximal HR decrease and increase during transitory period while standing at AOT (ΔRR_C=140 ms and (ΔRR_C=262 ms, correspondingly), HR frequency at symptom limited work load (RR_W=467 ms and RR_W=396 ms, correspondingly) have been significantly lower in CAD patients.

BRS values were higher in healthy subjects (8,6 ms/mmHg), as compared with CAD patients (3,8 ms/mmHg). Baseline arterial BP was higher in CAD patients (142 mmHg), as compared with healthy subjects (114 mmHg). An increase of BP during phenylephrine test was higher in CAD patients (39 mmHg), as compared with healthy subjects (28 mmHg). A gain of RR interval was more significant in healthy subjects (258 ms) than in CAD patients (147 ms). An example of BRS in healthy subject and CAD patient is demonstrated in Figure 1.

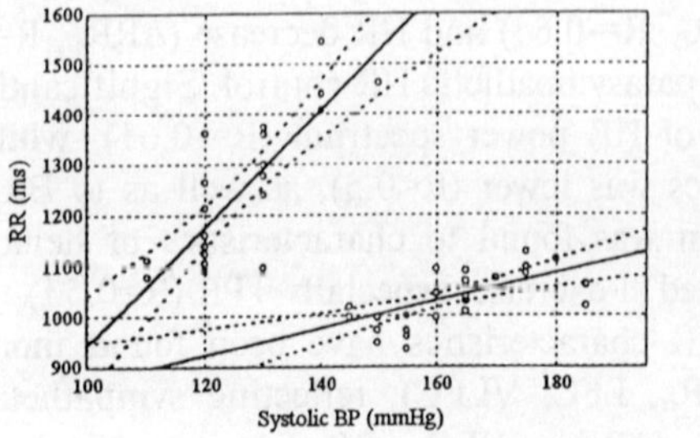

Figure 1. Baroreflex sensitivity: healthy subject (left) (BRS=11.66 ms/mmHg; r=.82) and CAD patient with mild congestive heart failure (right) (BRS=2.71 ms/mmHg; r=.62).

BRS level have shown strong negative linear correlation to maximal HR frequency at AOT (RR_B, R=-0.68). The most strong correlation was found between of BRS and HR characteristics. Moderate positive correlation was found between of BRS and LFC (r=0.52) or BRS and ratio LFC/HFC, (r=0.52) and mild negative correlation was found between of BRS and VLFC (r=-0.43).

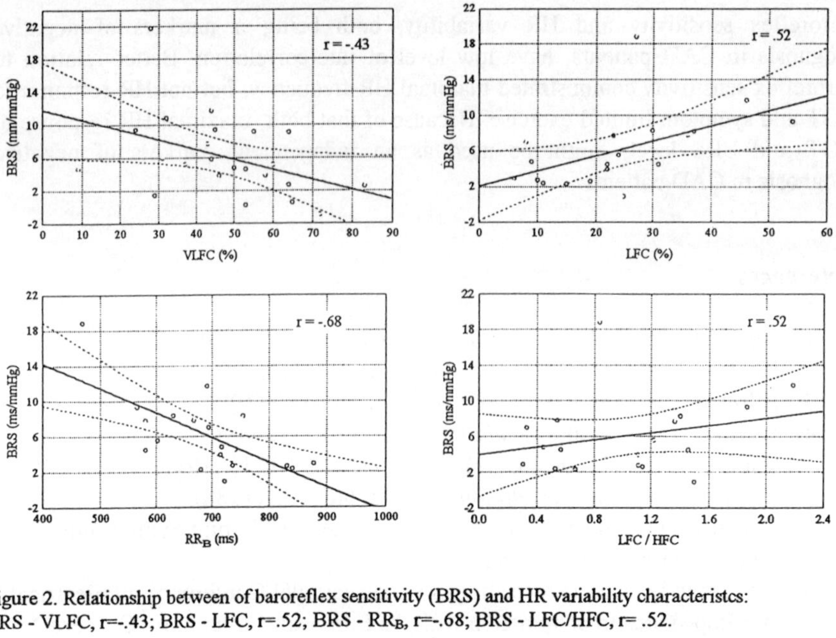

Figure 2. Relationship between of baroreflex sensitivity (BRS) and HR variability characteristcs:
BRS - VLFC, r=-.43; BRS - LFC, r=.52; BRS - RR_B, r=-.68; BRS - LFC/HFC, r= .52.

Spaerman R correlation between of evidence of CAD and HR variability parameters have shown quite strong relationship to HR responses during AOT and bicycle ergometry. Positive correlation was found to maximal HR frequency during tests (to RR_W, R=0.67; to RR_B, R=0.56), reflecting level of reduction of sympathetic HR control for CAD patients. Although relationship was negative to maximal HR responses during both, HR increase (ΔRR_B, R=-0.64) and HR decrease (ΔRR_C, R=-0.60) during AOT, reflecting the level of parasympathetic HR control. Significantly negative correlation was found to LFC of HR power spectrum (R=-0.61), while correlation to the other HR characteristics was lower (R<0.5), as well as to BRS (R=-0.47). The same level of correlation was found to characteristics of hemodynamics at rest. They become more related at exercise, especially TPR (R=0.53).

Correlation between of BRS and HR characteristics have been found more expressed through parameters (RR_W, RR_B, LFC, VLFC), reflecting sympathetic gain, but not trough characteristics (ΔRR_B, HFC, RR_C etc.), reflecting parasympathetic one. The latter might be seen as independent characteristics of cardiovascular reserve in CAD patients, related mostly to central parasympathetic control level.

Conclusion

Baroreflex sensitivity and HR variability, both being a markers of negative prognosis in CAD patients, have low level of intercorrelation. Better relation to baroreflex sensitivity demonstrated maximal HR frequency, but not HR response to AOT and symptom limited exercise. Because of that both, maximal HR response to AOT and BRS level, might be used as an independent markers of negative prognosis in CAD patients.

References

1. Bigger J.T. et al, *J. Am. Cardiol.* Vol. 61, 208-215 (1988).
2. Bigger J.T. et al, *Circulation.* Vol. 85, 164 (1992).
3. Billman G.E. et al, *Circulation.* Vol. 66, 874-880 (1982).
4. La Rovere M.T. et al, *Circulation.* Vol. 78, 816 (1988).
5. Lombardi F. et al, *Am J. Cardiol.* Vol. 60, 1239-1245 (1987).
6. Schwartz P.J. et al, *Circulation.* Vol. 78, 969-973 (1988).
7. Žemaitytė D. and Brožaitienė J. (Third USA-USSR Joint Symposium. Sudden Cardiac Death, 1984).
8. Žemaitytė D. et al. (Proceedings IX International Conference on Electrical Bio-Impedance In conjunction with the European Community Concerted Action on Impedance Tomography, Heidelberg, 1995).

AUTONOMIC HEART RATE CONTROL MODIFICATIONS IN RELATION TO LOCALISATION OF PATHOLOGICAL PROCESS IN CORONARY ARTERY DISEASE PATIENTS

G.ŽILIUKAS, D.ŽEMAITYTĖ, G.VARONECKAS
Institute Psychophysiology and Rehabilitation, Vydûno Str 4, Palanga 5720, Lithuania
E-mail: giedvar@ktl.mii.lt

Differences of modification of autonomic HR control in CAD pts depending on localisation of coronary arteries involved in to pathologic process were studied. Reduced HR variability, particularly of maximal HR response to AOT, was found in patients with disturbed coronary blood flow, supplying anterior wall of left heart ventricle but not posterior one in both cases, after MI and without it.

Introduction

Experimental and clinical studies demonstrated relationship of autonomic heart rate (HR) control modifications, especially negative impact of increased activity of sympathetic control and protective role parasympathetic one to negative prognoses in coronary artery disease [4, 8, 9]. Because of that HR variability analysis in coronary artery disease patients (CAD pts) was seen as having diagnostic and prognostic value [1, 3, 5, 13, 15]. There was demonstrated clear cut differences of modification of autonomic HR control due to myocardial infarction (MI) in relation to its localisation [10, 11, 12, 17]. HR variability might be related to localisation of coronary arteries, involved into pathological process, even in cases without MI. The reason for such expectations were differences in innervation of anterior and posteriorinferior wall's of left ventricle of the heart [7, 14].

The goal of the study was an investigation of modifications of autonomic HR control and hemodynamics in relation to localisation of MI and stenosis of coronary arteries in CAD patients.

Methods and Contingent

Contingent was 409 CAD patients. One hundred fifty five patients were after MI. Congestive heart failure (CHF) was evident in 65 patients. Patients after MI were grouped: (i) 78 patients with anteroseptal; and (ii) 76 patients with posteriorinferior localisation of myocardial lesion without evidence of CHF and myocardial ischemia. Patients without MI with isolated myocardial ischemia were grouped: (i) 21 patient with anteroseptal; and (ii) 50 patients with posteriorinferior localisation of myocardial lesion and without CHF). One hundred nineteen CAD patients without

MI undergone coronary angiography: isolated stenosis of LAD was found in 22 patients, in RCA - 17 patients, multiple stenosis with dominant in LAD or main left coronary artery - 53 patients, and with dominant stenosis in RCA - 27 patients. Thus, prevalent stenosis of LAD have been found in 75 patients, while RCA - in 44 CAD patients.

Computerised testing of cardiovascular function have been performed, including active orthostatic test (AOT) and bicycle ergometry until submaximal HR frequency or symptoms, limiting exercise. HR variability and HR frequency responses to tests, as well as hemodynamics (measured by impedance cardiography) were analysed. Power spectrum analysis of HR was performed, evaluating total HR variability (σRR) and an impact of three main frequency components: very low frequency (VLFC), low frequency (LFC), and high frequency (HLC) components.

Results

Comparison of data from CAD patients with different localisation of MI, as well as, with different localisation of myocardial ischemia or coronary artery stenosis, obtained by coronary arteriography, demonstrated some differences in autonomic HR control and hemodynamics (fig. 1). Anterior localisation of MI, as compared to those with inferior posterior one, shown significant reduction of HR variability (σRR 32 ms and 45 ms, correspondingly) and especially HFC (14 ms and 27 ms), maximal HR response to AOT (ΔRR_B 25% and 28%), if CHF was absent. The same tendencies have been found in CAD patients with isolated myocardial ischemia of anteroseptal and posteriorinferior localisation: reduced HR variability (σRR 36 ms and 47 ms, correspondingly), HFC (16 ms and 22 ms) and tendency of reduction of maximal HR response to AOT (27 % and 28 %), followed by increased TPR (3165 $dyn \cdot s \cdot cm^{-5}$ and 2291 $dyn \cdot s \cdot cm^{-5}$). Those differences have been attenuated in the patients with evidence of CHF due to additional impact of the latter: reduction of HR variability (σRR 22 ms), maximal HR response to AOT (ΔRR_B 23%), and an increase of TPR.

Principally the same differences have been found in CAD patients after coronary angiography. Reduction of HR variability (σRR 20,3±1,4 ms; RA 31,1±2,5 ms), especially of maximal HR response to AOT (ΔRR_B 19,7±0,8%) have been shown in patients with LAD stenosis, while patients with RCA stenosis, even in a cases of multiple involvement, have no significant impact on autonomic HR control (σRR 26,3±2,1 ms; RA 44,0±4,6 ms; ΔRR_B 27,5±0,9%)- it remains nearly normal. Thus, predominance of LAD involvement was related to increasing prevalence of sympathetic and humoral HR control, while parasympathetic control prevalence in CAD patients with RCA dominating involvement. The differences of hemodynamics level are following the same direction.

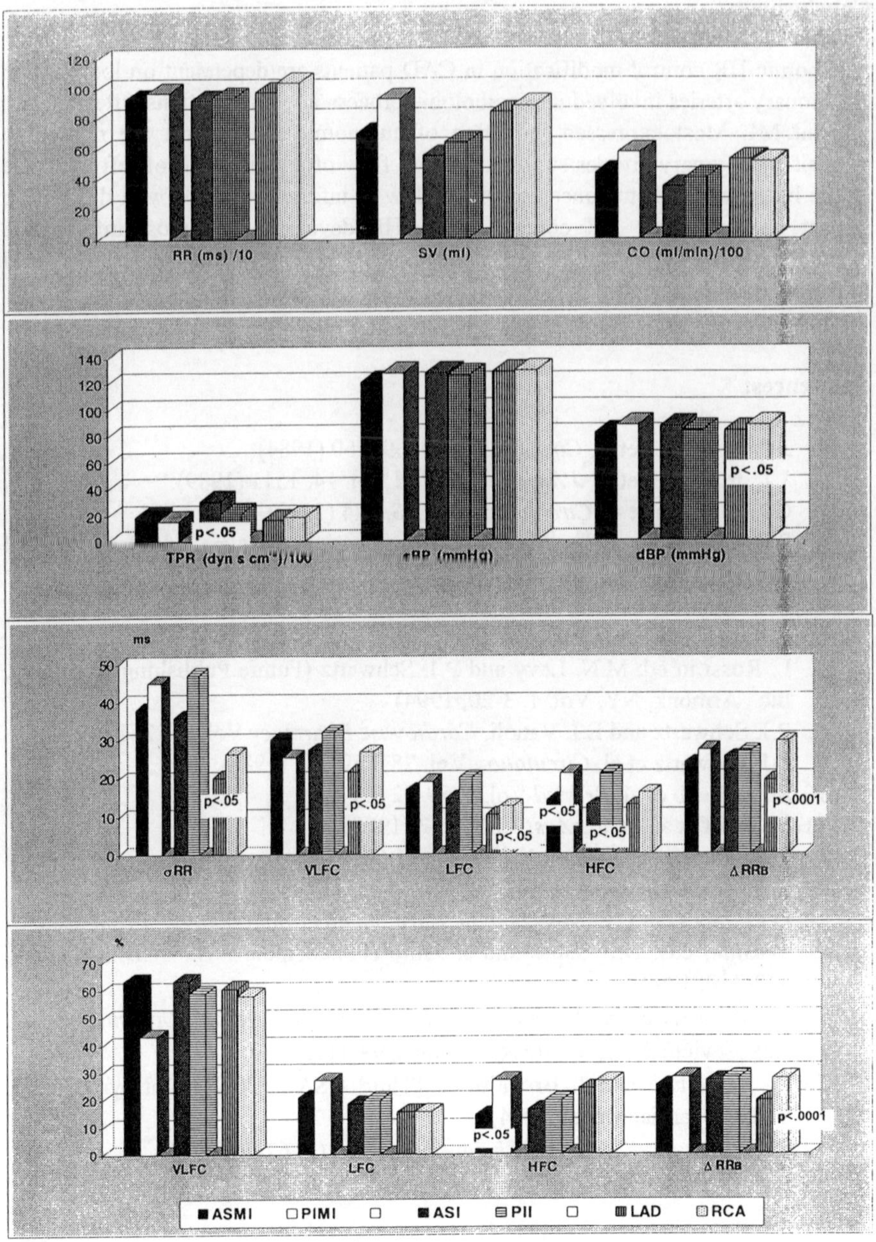

Figure 1. Autonomic HR control and hemodynamics moduliation due to different (anterior and postero-inferior) localization of pathology in CAD pts: (1) after myocardial infarction; (2) with myocardial ischemia; (3) after angiography (with predominance of LAD and RCA stenoses).

Conclusions

Autonomic HR control modification in CAD patients are dependant on localisation of coronary arteries involved into pathologic process in both situations, after MI and without MI. Most expressed reduction of autonomic HR control are related to stenosis of coronary arteries supplying blood flow of anterior wall of left ventricle of the heart, while disturbances of blood flow at inferior-posterior wall did not an impact on autonomic HR control until CHF develops. The most informative characteristic of HR was maximal HR response to AOT, reflecting mainly the level of parasympathetic control.

References:

1. J.T. Jr. Bigger et al, *Circulation* Vol. 69, 250 (1984).
2. J.T. Jr. Bigger et al, *J Am Coll Cordial* Vol. 14, 1511 (1989).
3. G.E. Billman et al, *Circulation* Vol. 66, 874 (1982).
4. P.B. Corr et al, in *The Heart and Cardiovascular System,* eds H.A. Fozzard et al (Raven Press, New York, NY, Vol. II, 1343-1403, 1986).
5. F. Lombardi et al, *Am J Cardiol* Vol. 60, 1239-1245 (1987).
6. B. Lown and R.L. Verrier, *N Engl J Med* Vol. 294, 1165 (1976).
7. L. Rossi in ed. M.N. Levy and P.J. Schwartz (Future Publishing Company, Inc., Armonk, NY, Vol. 1, 3-20, 1994)
8. P.J. Schwartz and E.J. Vanoli, *Cardiovasc Pharmacy* Vol. 3, 1251 (1981).
9. P.J. Schwartz et al, *Circulation* Vol. 78, 969-973 (1988).
10. S.W. Webb et al, *Br Med* Vol. 3, 89-92 (1972).
11. M. Wolf et al, *Med J Aust* Vol. 2, 52 (1978).
12. D.P. Zipes et al, *Circulation* Vol. 76, 1 (1987).
13. D.P. Zipes, *Circulation* Vol. 82, 1093-1105 (1990).
14. D.P. Zipes and T. Miyazaki in *Cardiac Electrophysiology: From Cell to Bedside*, eds. D.P. Zipes and J. Jalife (Philadelphia P.A., W.B. Saunders, 312-330, 1990).
15. D. Žemaitytė in *Normal and Pathological Cardiac Rhythm*, ed. A. Lukoševičiūtė and V. Meška (Vilnius, 99-111, 1970).
16. D. Žemaitytė and J. Brožaitiene (Third USA - USSR joint symposium. Sudden Cardiac Death, 1984).
17. D. Žemaitytė, *Fiziologija Cheloveka* Vol. 17 (1) 62-70 (1991).

COMPARISON OF DISCRIMINATIVE ABILITY OF SIGNAL AVERAGED AND SINGLE BEAT CARDIAC MICROPOTENTIALS IN SUBJECTS WITH/WITHOUT MYOCARDIAL ELECTRICAL INSTABILITY

Z. DRŠKA

Expert Laboratory of the Inspector of Air Forces and Air Defense of the Army of the Czech Republic, Mladoboleslavská 197 06, Prague, CR

P. ŠŤOVÍČEK

2nd Dept. of General Medicine, 1st Faculty of Medicine, Charles University, U nemocnice 2, 128 08, Prague, CR

P. TILŠER

1st Dept. of Cardiovascular Investigations, University Hospital, Hradec Kralové

Signal-averaged late potentials (SA LP) were compared with single-beat late potentials (SB LP) in order to verify the base of differences in statistical characteristics for both approaches using the logistic regression of standard micropotentials parameters. The simultaneously measured matrix of eighty surface ECGs and three orthogonal VCG electrocardiograms from single systole were processed by Singular Value Decomposition allowing necessary noise reduction. 38 subjects with CAD were studied. Subgroups were 28 subject (19 males) with history of Q-MI without positive positive ventricular stimulation (PVS) and 10 pts with positive PVS. SA LP detected by standard method of evaluation leads to the sensitivity = 85.71, specificity = 41.17 and total predictive accuracy (TPA)= 65.79. Logistic regression of these SA LP parameters leads to the sensitivity = 85.71, specificity = 63.64 and TPA = 81.58. Using the logistic regression to evaluate SB cardiac micropotentials parameters, the sensitivity = 85.71, specificity = 72.73 and TPA = 86.84 were found. We concluded that the discriminative ability of cardiac micropotentials depends significantly on the method of evaluation. Evaluation of parameters of SB LP and SA LP by logistic regression appears significantly more successful then generally used comparison of signal averaged cardiac micropotentials with their individual borderline values. The "single beat" procedure appears also substantially less sensitive to the random errors of parameters values because of elimination of their comparison with borderline limit.

1 Introduction

Signal-averaged late potentials (SA LP) have been shown to exhibit predictive ability for ventricular arrhythmias [1-3]. Their significance is limited by relatively low specificity [4]. Specificity reached by Single-Beat Late Potentials (SBLP) extracted from one systole by original procedure described in previous papers [5-9] exhibited significantly higher value in comparison with specificity obtained evaluating the cardiac micropotentials using the standard rules. These findings leads to the present study based on the comparison of discriminative ability of signal-averaged late potentials (SA LP) and single-beat late potentials (SBLP) in subjects with negative or positive programmed ventricular electrical stimulation. The main objective of this study is to verify the base of differences in statistical characteristics between the method of SA LP (a) using the generally known rules (i.e., for example Simpson rules) or (b) using the logistic regression of standard micropotentials parameters to detect the late potentials. This is valid for both SA and SB cardiac micropotentials.

2 Material and methods

The simultaneously measured matrix of eighty surface ECGs and three orthogonal VCG electrocardiograms from single systole were processed by Singular Value Decomposition (SVD) allowing necessary noise reduction [10]. The QRS onset and offset were detected manually on the computer screen. All ECG measurements were carried out by multichannel system Cardiag 128.2 (METE Ltd, CR).

The noise reduction has been achieved by elimination of higher order orthogonal components from data reconstruction in the final step of SVD procedure. This was performed by elimination of members of orthogonal expansion having the order number in orthogonal expansion sequence higher then twenty.

Subsequent signal processing and evaluation were performed analogous to that standard extraction procedure. After described preprocessing, vectorcardiographic orthogonal ECGs are transformed to the spatial amplitude, and then they are filtered using the bidirectional high-pass Butterworth filter at frequency 40 Hz. Signal discretization frequency being equal to 500 Hz, the Nyquist value is equal to 250 Hz. From these data the module and RMS of potential at individual time instants were calculated.

Data evaluation consisted of determination of standard micropotential parameters as filtered QRS duration (TQRS), low amplitude signal within the final part of the QRS (LAS) and RMS within the last 40 ms of the QRS interval (RMS40).

Resulting data were analyzed by stepwise logistic regression (system of statistical procedures SOLO). SA LP were evaluated by Simson's method. Classification results were expressed in terms of specificity, sensitivity and total predictive accuracy.

Programmed ventricular stimulation was carried out using standard protocol with up to three extrastimuli at pacing drive 100, 120, 140 and 180 min^{-1}. The positive diagnostic result of programmed stimulation was given if a sustained monomorphic ventricular tachycardia was provoked. Application of antiarrhythmic drugs was stopped before five-fold half time of respective drug.

Data of 38 subjects with CAD and mean age of 54 yrs (38 to 72 yrs). were studied The subgroup of pts without positive programmed ventricular stimulation (PVS) consisted of 28 subject (19 males) with history of QMI, second subgroup consist of 10 pts with positive PVS.

3 Results

Classification results are summarized in Table 1.

Table 1: Summary table of classification. SA LP = Signal averaged late potentials, SA LP LR = Signal averaged late potentials parameters evaluated by logistic regression, SB LP = Single beat late potentials evaluated by logistic regression, TPA = Total predictive accuracy.

	SA LP	SA LP LR	SB LP
SENSITIVITY	85.71	85.71	89.29
SPECIFICITY	41.17	63.64	72.73
TPA	65.79	81.58	86.84

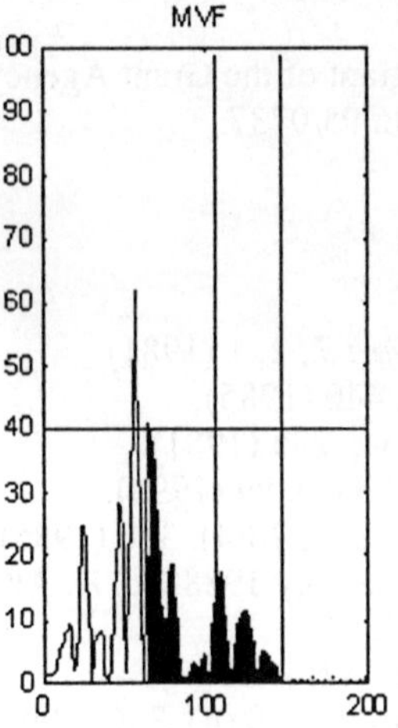

Fig. 1: An example of characteristic single beat late potentials of subject with positive programmed ventricular stimulation. The scale on the vertical axis is equal to 100 uV, the scale on the horizontal axis is equal to 200 msec. Vertical lines represent end point of the total

filtered QRS interval and last 40 msec of the QRS. Black area corresponds to the low amplitude signal in terminal part of the QRS interval.

4 Discussion

Using the principle components expansion was proved, for example by Horan and coworkers [11], that ECGs from body surface could be reconstructed with sufficient accuracy using the 15 orthogonal components. For higher frequency compartments of ECG signal (as are late potentials) can be demonstrated that even this set of components can be insufficient. Therefore, first twenty singular value decomposition components were adopted for final signal reconstruction.

Present study testify for the statement that the discriminative ability of cardiac micropotentials depends significantly on the method of evaluation. Evaluation of parameters of SB LP and SA LP by function resulting from the logistic regression (or discriminative analysis) appears significantly more successful than generally used comparison of signal averaged cardiac micropotentials with their individual borderline value. The "single beat" procedure appears also substantially less sensitive to the random errors of parameters because of elimination of their comparison with borderline limit.

Acknowledgments

This study was supported by grant of the Grant Agency of the Czech Republic No. 406/95/0737

References

1. G. Breithardt et al., *Eur. Heart J.,* **2,** 1 (1981).
2. N. El-Sherif et al. *PACE,* **8,** 440 (1985).
3. M.B. Simson, *Circulation,* **64,** 235 (1981).
4. J.S. Steinberg et al., *JACC,* **23** (1), 99 (1996).
5. Z. Drska et al., *J. Electrocardiol.,* **28**(4), 340 (1985).
6. Z. Drska et al. in Electrocardiology 1988, ed. H. Abel (Elsevier Excerpta Medica, Amsterdam, 1989), 361.
7. Z. Drska, et al., Physiol. Res. **42,** 7 (1993).
8. Z. Drska et al., J. Electrocardiol. **28** (4), 340 (1995).
9. Z. Drska et al., in Proc. of XXIIIrd Internat. Congress onElectrocardiology, (Cleveland, Ohio USA 1996), 16.
10. G.J.H. Uijen, (Drukkerij Brokkenstein Nijmegen 1991), 207.
11. L.G. Horan et al., *Circulat. Res.*, **2,** 131 (1964).

COMPARISON OF THE TIME-FREQUENCY MAPPING OF THE SIGNAL AVERAGED ECG SIGNAL USING FFT ALGORITHM AND WIGNER DISTRIBUTION.

HUBKA P., BERNADIC M., HULIN I.

Institute of Pathological Physiology, School of Medicine, Comenius University, Sasinkova 4, 811 08 Bratislava, Slovak Republic

The aim of this study was to examine the usefulness of the spectrograms of signal averaged ECG (SA ECG) signals based on Wigner distribution (WD) algorithm in comparison with standard Fast Fourier Transform (FFT) algorithm. The advantages of WD as a non-stationary signal processing method are described. Time-frequency maps of the 20 healthy men and 20 healthy dogs have been composed by both techniques. Spectrograms based on WD have showed more distinguished frequency peaks, especially for higher frequencies (> 30 Hz). For this reason WD could be considered as a very useful technique for identification of late potentials as well as the low amplitude and high frequency signals in whole cardiac cycle.

The majority of standard electrocardiographic techniques uses algorithm based on Fourier Transform (FT) for frequency domain analysis. On the other hand it is well known that FT is suited for stationary signals and electrocardiographic signal do not belong to this group. This is the reason why the spectrum of electrocardiogram (ECG) resulting from FT is only an estimation of real spectrum. It was necessary to find algorithms for acquiring more precise spectral estimation.

Firstly, it was the short time fast Fourier transform (STFFT). This algorithm have taken into account the non-stationary character of ECG signal. This is the most simple method for construction of spectro-temporal mapping. Spectro-temporal mapping allows us to see dynamic changes of spectrum with time, but limitations have still remained. The choosing of the length of analyzing time period and the need of windowing appears to be the basic limitations of this method. Other method which could give us the possibly more precise image of dynamic changes in ECG spectrum during the whole QRS duration was gliding window FFT (GWFFT). GWFFT compute area ratios obtained from STFFT. This could help us to find where is the highest contribution of higher frequencies.

The limitations of these methods could potentially lead to misinterpretations of their results. These confusing results have confirmed the opinion that frequency domain analysis is not reliable method. We think that using more precise algorithms for decomposition of signal into its frequency components could change this opinion.

One of these methods is Wigner distribution (WD). WD, in contrast to STFFT which is resolution limited either in frequency or time (caused by the windowing function), and suffers from smearing and sidelobe leakage, offers more precise resolution in both the frequency and time domains. Comparison of the spectro-temporal mapping resulting from STFFT and WD have showed differences especially for higher frequency ranges (20-100 Hz). Comparison was made also for GWFFT and the area ratios based on WD. The peaks of area ratios based on GWFFT have no corresponding peaks in curves of area ratios based on WD.

We can conclude that we have to find which offers the most precise image of time frequency interpretation of ECG signal. On the other hand the spectral distributions are not the only signal processing techniques which could lead to misinterpretation of the ECG signal. For example, averaging itself could artificially produce components which have no biological basis. Therefore we propose the exact knowledge of each cycle included to averaging beside the signal averaged ECG analysis. Comparison between the spectra of adjacent cardiac cycles and composing of heart spectra variability could bring the other point of view.

References

1. T A C M Claasen and W F G Mecklenbraeuker, The Wigner Distribution - A Tool for Time-Frequency Signal Analysis, *Philips J. Res.* **35**, 217-250, 1980.
2. W Martin, P Flandrin, Wigner-Ville Spectral Analysis of non-stationary processes, *IEEE ASSP* **33**, 1985
3. I Hulin, P Slavkovsky, R Hatala, H Petrasova, V Cik, J Murin, Glinding Window Fast Fourier Analysis - A new method for discovering the contribution of Higher Frequencies in Signal-averaged ECG, *Can J. Cardiol.* **9**, 789-796, 1993.
4. P Lander, E J Berbari, Principles and signal processing of the High-resolution Electrocardiogram, *Prog. Cardiovasc. Dis* **35**, 169-188, 1992.
5. G Breithardt, M E Cain, N El-Sherif, N C Flowers, V Hombach, M Janse, M B Simson, G Steinbeck, Standards for Analysis of Ventricular Late Potentials Using High-Resolution Or Signal-Averaged Electrocardiography: A Statement by A Task Force Committee of The European Society of Cardiology, The American Heart Association, And The American College of Cardiology, *JACC* **17**, 999-1006, 1991

COMPARATIVE STUDY ON ANTIARRHYTHMIC EFFECTS OF A NEW CLASS IC DRUG, PILSICAINIDE AND DISOPYRAMIDE ON PATIENTS WITH PAROXYSMAL ATRIAL FIBRILLATION

N. IKEDA, MD;
Chunichi Hospital, 3-6-38, Marunouchi, Naka-ku, Nagoya, Japan
J. TOYAMA, MD;
Research Institute of Environmental Medicine, Nagoya University, Furo-cho, Chikusa-ku, Nagoya, Japan
M. OHNO, MD;
Japanese Red Cross Nagoya First Hospital, 3-35, Michishita-cho, Nakamura-ku, Nagoya, Japan
K. YAMADA, MD.
Meitetsu Hospital, 2-26-11, Sakoh, Nishi-ku, Nagoya, Japan

Efficacy and safety of a new class Ic antiarrhythmic drug, pilsicainide were compared with those of disopyramide in patients with paroxysmal atrial fibrillation (PAf) in a multicenter open randomized trial. Pilsicainide had a significantly higher suppressive effects than disopyramide, although its side effects due to anticholinergic action were significantly less than those of disopyramide, suggesting that class Ic drug, like pilsicainide may be more profitable in the treatment of PAf than class Ia drug.

Introduction

Pilsicainide,N-(2,6-dimethylphenyl)-8-pyrrolizidinylacetamide hydrochloride hemihydrate, (see Fig.1), is a new class Ic antiarrhythmic drug developed in Japan. [1] It has been demonstrated that this drug has potent antiarrhythmic effects on supraventricular as well as ventricular tachyarrhythmias. [2,3] However, its clinical usefulness has not been comparatively studied with other antiarrhythmic agents. In the present study , efficacy and safety of pilsicainide on PAf were compared with those of class Ia drug, disopyramide, in a multicenter open randomized trial.

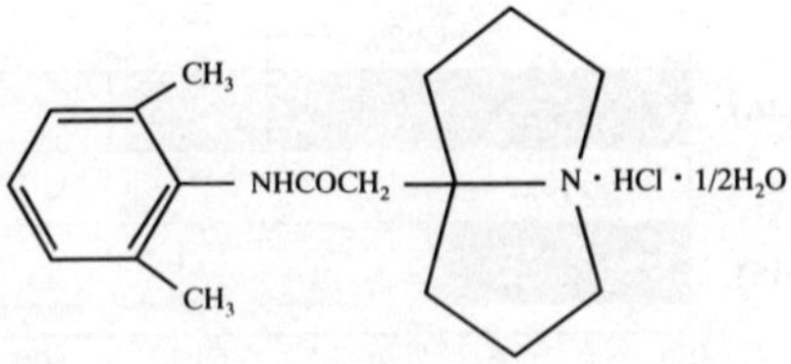

Figure 1: Chemical structure of pilsicainide.

Methods

Ninety-two patients with symptomatic PAf were divided into pilsicainide group (n=46), and disopyramide group (n=46) by open randomized method. PAf was confirmed by conventional ECG monitoring at the attack or by Holter ECG. The subjects had at least more than once of PAf attack in a month of control period. The effects of each drug on the frequency and the duration of PAf, in addition to accompanying symptoms such as palpitation, dyspnea, and chest discomfort were evaluated at both 4 weeks and 12 weeks after starting the treatment. The efficacy was defined as the total percentage of the patients who showed marked or moderate effectiveness evaluated by each doctor considering objective (frequency and duration of PAf) and subjective symptoms. Safety of each drug was defined as the percentage of the patients with no or minor side effects.

Each drug was administered orally at daily doses of 100-150 mg for pilsicainide, and 200-300 mg for disopyramide, respectively. The side effects of each drug were also observed at the same time schedule. Statistical analysis was performed by using Chi-test.

Results

The results on the efficacy of each drug are shown in Fig. 2. Drug efficacy at 4 weeks was not different between pilsicainide and disopyramide (52.5% vs 32.5%, NS) but it became significant (85.7% vs 46.3%, p=0.043) at 12 weeks.

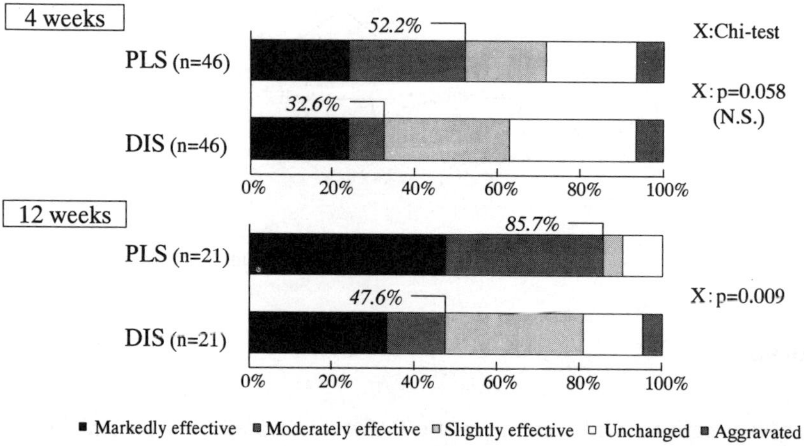

Figure 2: Efficacy of pilsicainide and disopyramide evaluated at 4 and 12 weeks.
Figure of each column shows total percentage of patients with marked and moderate efficacy.
PLS, pilsicainide; DIS, disopyramide

Safety of pilsicainide also was higher than disopyramide at 4 weeks (91.3% vs 78.3%, p=0.009), but it became insignificant (95.5 vs 85.7%,) at 12 weeks. In pilsicainide group, one patients with hypertrophic cardiomyopathy (HCM), experienced an attack of ventricular tachycardia, which was converted to sinus rhythm by withdrawing the drug. Symptomatic side effects of each drug are shown in Table 1. Among these, symptoms considered to be due to anticholinergic action, such as dysuria, urinary retention, dry mouth were significantly less (4%) for pilsicainide than that of disopyramide group (24%) (Table 2). None of the patients had to stop the treatment because of abnormal changes in blood examination.

Table 1: Side effects of pilsicainide and disopyramide.

PLS		DIS	
10/46 (22%)		14/46 (30%)	
P=0.270 (N.S.)			
	No. of Events		No. of Events
1) Dysuria	2	1) Dysuria	7
2) QT prolongation	1	2) Dry mouth	2
3) VT	1	3) Urinary retention	2
4) AV Block (First degree)	1	4) QT prolongation	1
5) CRBBB	1	5) VT	1
6) Bradycardia	1	6) Tinnitus	1
7) Sinus arrest	1	7) Headache	1
8) Urticaria	1	8) Abdominal discomfort	1
9) Anorexia	1	9) Anorexia	1
10) Dizziness	1	10) Sleepiness	1
		11) Dizziness	1

PLS, pilsicainide; DIS, disopyramide; VT, ventricular tachycardia;

CRBBB, complete right bundle branch block.

Table 2: Anticholinergic side effects.

PLS		DIS	
2/46(4%)		11/46 (24%)	
P=0.005			
	No. of Events		No. of Events
1) Dysuria	2	1) Dysuria	7
		2) Dry mouth	2
		3) Urinary retention	2

PLS, pilsicainide; DIS, disopyramide.

Discussion

In the present study, it was clarified that efficacy of pilsicainide on PAf tended to be higher at 4 weeks than that of disopyramide (without statistical significance) , but it became significant at 12 weeks. These discrepant results may be explained as follows: if " Atrial fibrillation begets atrial fibrillation" is approved, vice versa may be also true: then such vice versa mechanism may makes the drug efficacy more prominent as the drug treatment is prolonged. The mechanism of such concept remains to be clarified, but it may be related to alterations of the repolarization process of the atrial muscle mediated through the altered potassium expression during atrial fibrillation. [4] Thus, it is considered that suppression of PAf itself reduces PAf in a time-dependent manner. It also has been reported that pilsicainide is useful for rapid conversion of atrial fibrillation (Af) by single oral dose, demonstrating high efficacy on terminating Af. [5]

Considering the side effects, pilsicainide had a significantly higher safety at 4 weeks, but there was no significant difference at 12 weeks. The reason for this is considered to be due to the decrease in number of the patients at 12 weeks. Percentage of the patients who complained dysuria, urinary retention, or dry mouth was significantly lower in pilsicainide group than disopyramide group. These side effects are due to anticholinergic action, indicating that pilsicainide has little such action. However, in pilsicainide group, severe side effects such as ventricular tachycardia was observed in on case. This patients had hypertrophic cardiomyopathy. In the case of HCM with PAf, QRS duration at tachycardiac PAf may be prolonged rate-dependently because pilsicainide has a potent depressive effect on atrial as well as ventricular impulse conduction. Therefore, in patients with HCM accompanying PAf, treatment with class Ic drug should be done with great care.

In conclusion, pilsicainide has been proved to be more profitable for the treatment of PAf than class Ia drug in cases without HCM.

References

1. T. Hattori et al., J. Cardiovasc. Pharmacol. 8, 998, (1986).
2. H. Niitani et al., Jap. J. Clin. Pharmacol. Ther. 20, 719, (1989).
3. H. Niitani et al., Jap. J. Clin. Pharmacol. Ther. 23, 557, (1992)
4. MC. Wijffels et al., Circulation 92, 1954, (1995).
5. H. Atarashi et al., Am. J. Cardiol. 78, 694, (1996).

HIGH RESOLUTION ECG IN DOGS - GLIDING WINDOW FAST FOURIER TRANSFORM ANALYSIS AND WIGNER'S TRANSFORMATION

M. BERNADIC, P. HUBKA, B. MLADOSIEVICOVA, J. HOLZEROVA, L. ZLATOS, I. SULKOVA, H. PETRASOVA, I. HULIN

Institut of Pathophysiology, School of Medicine, Comenius University, Sasinkova 4, 851 01 Bratislava, Slovakia

E-mail: bernadic@fmed.uniba.sk

R. HATALA

Slovak Heart Institut, Pod Krasnou horkou 1, 833 48 Bratislava, Slovakia

The main aim of our work is to define "etalon" of averaged values of time and frequency domain analysis ECG for healthy dogs, to describe the onset and the termination of activation regarding the "steepness" of QRS-on ans QRS-off and to describe the composition of frequency spectrum of ECG signal during the ventricular activation by Wigner transformation in healthy dogs. This detailed study is very important from two aspects: the dogs are very often used as experimental animal for modelling arrhythmias and MI, and there are no standards for experimental animals, up till now.

1. Introduction

High resolution ECG (HR ECG) is usefull mostly for identification of electrical instability risk in patients after myocardial infarction (MI) (1). Prolonged, fractionated ECG's are detectable after MI and are a marker of arrhythmia-prone state. QRS late potentials (LP) detected on the body surface with signal-averaged ECG (SA ECG) are thought to arise from the diseased tissue that generates prolonged ventricular electrograms and as such are also a marker for arrhythmias (2). The high-frequency contribution is also intensively investigated in ECG signal (3,4). Further possibilities of HR ECG are tested in some experimental studies (5,6).

The main aim of our work is to define "etalon" of averaged values of time and frequency domain analysis ECG for healthy dogs, to describe the onset and the termination of activation regarding the "steepness" of QRS-on ans QRS-off and to describe the composition of frequency spectrum of ECG signal during the ventricular activation by Wigner transformation in healthy dogs. This detailed study is very important from two aspects: the dogs are very often used as experimental animal for modelling arrhythmias and MI, and there are no standards for experimental animals, up till now. It is not necessary to emphasize that in the essential arrhytmogenic studies experimental animals have been used.

necessary to emphasize that in the essential arrhytmogenic studies experimental animals have been used.

2. Material and methods

In order to form an etalon of the time domain analysis of ECG signal mean values a group of 25 healthy dogs (body weight 12-15 kg) was examined. Ethical norms established for animal experiments were respected consistently during the whole examination.

Standard ECG was recorded in dogs in leight total anaesthesia (i.v. Pentobarbital Sp., 25 mg/kg b.w.). The recording was performed in dogs in right side position. The Ag-loops as a permanent subcutaneous electrodes were used in all dogs.

2.1. High-resolution electrocardiogaphy

We used the Arrhythmia Research Technology model 1200 EPX device to record simultaneous orthogonal X,Y and Z leads. The signal from each lead was AD converted at a 16 bits accuracy with a sampling rate of 4000 Hz. Ectopic or noisy beats were eliminated. At least 100 beats were averaged with mean noise level (1,0 μV). After signal-averaging, the data were stored in a file with a sampling rate of 1000 Hz and transferred to a computer.

2.2. Time domain analysis

The data were filtered using a bidirectional digital filter (25, 40, and 80 to 250 Hz). Three leads X,Y,Z were combined in a root-mean-square vector termed the filtered QRS. The earliest onset and latest offset of the QRS were determined from unfiltered leads by a computer algorithm. The parameters studied included: the filtered QRS (ms), the terminal of QRS under 30 μV (ms), and the RMS amplitude of the terminal 20 ms (μV). All parameters were calculated at 25, 4O and 80 to 250 Hz.

2.3. Frequency domain analysis

2.3.1. Gliding window fast Fourier transform analysis (GW FFTA)
The analysis of frequency spectrum of activation was performed by GW FFTA (40 ms) (7). The X,Y,Z leads and a composite one were constructed from the values of area ratio.

2.3.2. Wigner's transformation
The algorithm for Wigner's transformation calculation was used for description

of the whole frequency spectrum of the heart activation. Wigner's distribution describes the spectrum of the given signal taking into consideration its unstable character. The method results in spectro-temporal mapping, by means of which we can acquire a review of the dynamics of changes in the contribution of individual frequencies during ventricular activation.

3. Results

The average values of time domain analysis of a group of healthy dogs are shown in the table 1. In recording evaluation the shorter duration of QRS complex in dogs in comparison with human QRS has been taken into consideration.

Table 1. The average values of time domain analysis SA ECG at 25 healthy dogs (±SEM)

item	24-250 Hz	40-250 Hz	80-250 Hz
standQRS (µV)	726.29±63.97	462.51±36.42	166.55±14.69
fQRS (µV)	694.66 39.86	441.80 35.99	157.46 13.65
total QRS (ms)	62.41 1.32	60.87 1.50	57.91 1.67
RMS<30 µV (ms)	15.33 1.06	17.91 0.98	20.20 1.01
LAS20 ms (µV)	40.37 10.84	40.64 10.96	23.27 6.78

In frequency domain analysis we used GW FFTA of the whole heart activation. Results are formed from the values of area ratios for contribution of frequencies of 0-5O Hz/0-120 Hz. There are curves of all dogs drawn in one figure. The peak on the curve expresses the higher contribution of higher frequencies, or the decrease in lower frequencies. The picture of a complete spectrum of frequencies was obtained by Wigner transformation. Inside the ventricular complex the spectrum is the largest, as well as the presence of high frequencies is clearly visible.

4. Conclusions

There is not right to use human's criteria for indentification of late ventricular potentials in experiments with dogs. Our approach to determination of mean values etalon in healthy dogs is in agreement with the approach of Spear et al (8). The voltage of the terminal part of ECG in duration of 40 ms is consider to be one of the criteria of LVP in human medicine. Because of very short

Figure 1. GW FFTA - curves of all investigated dogs.

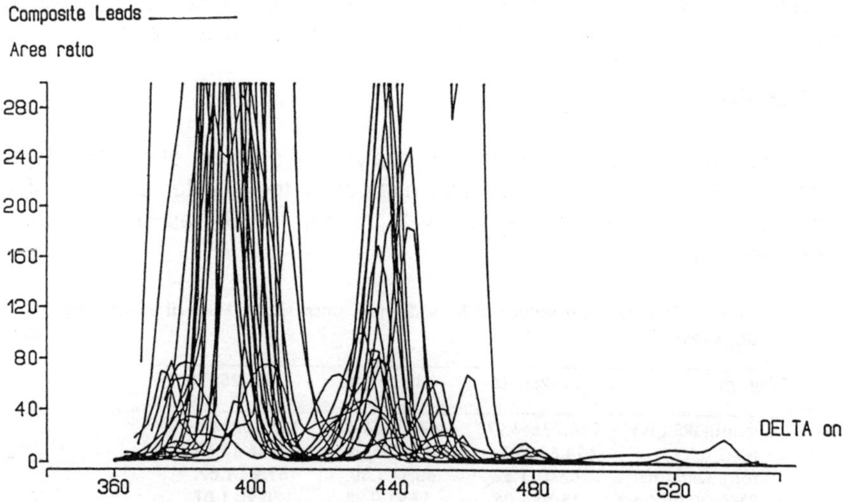

ventricular complex duration in dogs is this parameter not usable. The investigation using GW FFTA informs on the changes in higher and lower frequencies ratio during the whole activation of the heart. Generally, the etalons may be used for investigation of arrhythmogenesis in experiments in dogs. For the LVP identification, SA ECG was used till now in all experimental investigations. In dogs with experimental MI the frequency domain analysis by FFTA has been examined. Unanbiguous results were not obtained. In frequency analysis by Wigner transformation we stated that the frequency spectrum is during activation almost uniform. In all 25 dogs is the higher frequencies accumulation situated in the 2nd third of QRS complex. We assume that these high frequencies are caused by the activation transmision from the conducting system of the myocardium.

References

1. G. Breithardt et al.: J Am Coll Cardiol 1991,17:999-1006.
2. R.A. Freedman et al.: Circulation 1991,84:2,871-883.
3. S. Yakubo et al.: J Electrocardiol 1995,28 Suppl:234-238.
4. G. Steinbeck et al.: Coronary Artery Disease 1991,2:27-32.
5. M.B. Simson et al.: Am J Physiol 1981,241:3,H363-369.
6. S. Yoh et al.: Pacing Clin Electrophysiol 1990,13:4,469-479.
7. I. Hulin et al.: Can J Cardiol 1993:9;(9); 789-796.

FIRST EXPERIENCES WITH RADIOFREQUENCY CATHETER ABLATION

A. PINTÉR, Á. SZÉKELY, S. KAYSER, I. PRÉDA
Cardiovascular Center, Haynal Imre University of Health Sciences, 35 Szabolcs street, Budapest, Hungary, H-1135

K. ZÁMOLYI
Department of Cardiology, Bajcsy-Zsilinszky Hospital, 89-91 Maglódi street, Budapest, Hungary, H-1106

Z. CSANÁDI
2nd Dept. of Medicine, Szentgyörgyi Albert University Medical School, Szeged, Hungary

Sixty patients underwent radiofrequency catheter ablation at our department since the introduction of that method. Most of the patients presented with left free wall accessory pathway, AV nodal reentry tachycardia or atrial fibrillation. Transseptal approach for left sided pathways proved to be safe and made the ablation of these accessory pathways the easiest task among these arrhythmias. A learning curve was evident by the success rate and mapping time for left free wall accessory pathways. In our series, localization of the target for slow pathway ablation was somewhat difficult and inadvertent complete AV block occurred in 2 cases (11%). In contrary to DC shock ablation of the AV junction, frequently more than 1 RF application was necessary to achieve complete AV block in patients with chronic atrial fibrillation.

1 Introduction

After 10 years of AV junctional ablation using DC shock[1] and transcoronary chemical ablation of accessory pathways and the AV junction[2], radiofrequency (RF) catheter ablation was started at our laboratory 18 months ago. RF application was proved to be safe and effective originally for ablation of accessory pathways[3] and slow pathway for AV nodal reentry tachycardia[4,5], later the technique was applied to other arrhythmias like atrial flattern, atrial tachycardia, and idiopathic ventricular tachycardia. For the introduction of this new method in our laboratory, arrhythmias with the best chance to be cured safely and effectively by RF ablation were treated: mostly left free wall accessory pathways, AV nodal reentry tachycardia and AV junction ablation to control chronic atrial fibrillation.

The aim of this study was to evaluate our experiences with the treatment of the first 60 patients (pts) by RF ablation.

2 Methods

Between October 24, 1995 - April 22, 1997, 60 patients (27 male, 33 female, age 17-77 years) underwent a total of 65 RF ablation sessions at our laboratory. Diagnosis was orthodromic AV reentry tachycardia in 27 pts, typical AV nodal reentry tachycardia in 19 pts, chronic atrial fibrillation in 11 pts, atrial tachycardia in 1 pt and idiopathic ventricular tachycardia in 2 pts.

Standard electrophysiologic study was performed in each patient prior to ablation in the same sitting. Quadripolar catheter electrodes (Bard) were introduced to the right ventricular apex, His-bundle position and high right atrium via the right femoral vein, and a decapolar electrode (Daig) to the coronary sinus via the left subclavic vein under fluoroscopic guidance (C-arm, GE). Programmed electrical stimulation was performed by an EP-2 digital stimulator. Signals were recorded by a 16-channel CardioLab System, version 3.1 (Prucka Engineering), and data were stored on optical disk.

After diagnosis was established, a thermistor ablation catheter was introduced (EPT). Accessory pathways were ablated from their atrial insertion site, for left sided pathways we applied the transseptal approach using standard Mullins introducers (Bard)[6]. In the cases of AV nodal reentry tachycardia, slow pathway ablation was performed using anatomical approach first, then mapping guided by the electrogram („m"-form atrial wave and A/V ratio 0.1-0.3). To control heart rate in patients with drug resistant tachycardia due to chronic atrial fibrillation, complete AV junction ablation (9 cases) or AV junction modification (2 cases) was performed. RF energy application was temperature controlled at 60 Celsius. For all the arrhythmias, a single pulse of RF energy was applied for 60 s if it was considered successful during the test period (max. 15-20 s). Insurance RF energy application was used only in selected cases of AV junction ablation to achieve complete AV block. Thirty min after successful RF energy application, a control electrophysiologic test was performed to confirm the success of the procedure.

3 Results

3.1 Patients with the Wolff-Parkinson-White syndrome

Twenty seven pts with the WPW syndrome underwent RF ablation. Twenty two of the pathways were overt, 5 were concealed. Most of the pathways (22) were located on the left free wall (due to specific pt selection), the other locations were right posteroseptal in 2 pts, left posteroseptal in 1 pt, anteroseptal in 1 pt and right anterior in 1 pt.

For left free wall accessory pathways, the first session was successful in 86% (19/22) of the pts, later the tachycardia recurred in 3 pts (15%). Two of the 3 unsuccessful cases were the first 2 pts who underwent RF ablation at our laboratory. The mapping time (time from the transseptal puncture to the successful RF application), X-ray time and number of RF applications for left free wall pathways were 36 (14-104) min, 25 (8-53) min, and 2.7 (1-7), respectively. The mapping time /21 (14-41) min vs 53 (15-104) min, $p<0.05$/ and X-ray time /14 (8-24) min vs 40 (13-53) min, $p<0.05$/ were favorable for the last 9 successful interventions than for the first 10 ablations, while the number of RF applications was not significantly different /2.9 (1-7) vs 2.5 (1-7)/, indicating, that there was difference in the time required to find the target, but once it was found, its prediction for success was similar in both groups.

In the cases of Kent pathways with location other than left free wall, only 2/5 (40%) were successfully ablated, 1 of them only at a 2nd session, and later it recurred, requiring a 3rd session, which was successful. The only serious complication occurred also in this series of pts: inadvertent AV block in the pt with anteroseptal accessory pathway. Other complications included uncomplicated atrial wall puncture with the Brockenbrough needle in 1 pt, transient sinus tachycardia in 1 pt following ablation of a right posteroseptal pathway, and a transient nonsustained ventricular tachycardia in 1 pt that was clinically well tolerated.

In overall, the immediate success rate for ablation of Kent pathways was 74%, the long-term success rate was 67%, and the recurrence rate was 19%.

3.2 *Slow pathway ablation in patients with AV nodal reentry tachycardia*

Slow pathway ablation was immediately successful in 84% of the pts (16/19). The tachycardia recurred in 2 pts (13%), thus the long-term success rate was 74%. In 2 pts (11%) out of the 3 unsuccessful cases inadvertent complete AV block developed, while we were unable to localize the electrocardiographic target of slow pathway in the third case, in a young athlete with tachycardia inducible only with very high dose of isoproterenol. The average X-ray time was 29 (4-90) min, and the number of RF applications was 3.7 (1-8) in these pts.

3.3 *Atrial fibrillation and miscellaneous tachycardias*

AV junction ablation to control heart rate in pts with chronic atrial fibrillation was successful in all 11 pts (100%), although complete AV block was achieved only at the 2nd session in 1 pt. Insurance RF application was frequently used to ensure permanent complete AV block. AV junction modification was performed in 2 pts, tachyarrhythmia recurred in 1 of them (recurrence rate 9%). Elevated CK level with normal MB fraction due to repeated external cardioversions were observed in 3 pts as the only complication in this series of pts. The average X-ray time was 14 (4-22) min, and the number of RF applications was 3.2 (1-7).

A case of atrial tachycardia originating from the low right atrium was successfully ablated in a young, otherwise healthy female pt.

We also tried to ablate two cases of idiopathic ventricular tachycardia (VT), one pt with VT originating from the right ventricular outflow tract, the other from the left posterior fascicle, but both attempts were unsuccessful.

4 Discussion

Provided the experience with transseptal catheterization, the atrial (transseptal) approach made ablation of left free wall accessory pathways a very effective and safe method, and probably the easiest ablation task in our first year. Due to the relatively high number of cases, we were able to demonstrate a learning curve for that procedure by the success rate and mapping time. A similar learning curve is expected for slow pathway ablation. At the beginning we had difficulties to find a good, reliable target, therefore the number of RF applications and X-ray time were both relatively high. Unfortunately, we had a high incidence of AV block (11%) in these pts. AV junction ablation might be difficult due to atrial fibrillation, hence lack of reliable His-potential recording.

In conclusion, the success rate, recurrence rate and number of complications are acceptable for our learning period of RF ablation for left free wall accessory pathways, slow pathway and AV junction. Septal accessory pathways, atrial tachycardia and idiopathic ventricular tachycardia constitute a more difficult task and require more experience with RF ablation.

Acknowledgments

This work was partly supported by grant No. F 021147 from the Hungarian National Research Found (OTKA).

References

1. K. Zámolyi et al., *Orvosi Hetilap* **32**, 1929 (1986).
2. L. Major et al., *LAM* **1**, 284 (1991).
3. H. Calkins et al., *N. Engl. J. Med.* **324**, 1612 (1991).
4. M.A. Lee et al., *Circulation* **83**, 827 (1991).
5. W.M. Jackman et al., *N. Engl. J. Med.* **327**, 313 (1992).
6. J.F. Swartz et al., *Circulation* **87**, 487 (1993).

SINUS NODE DYSFUNCTION IN CHILDREN

V.MILOVSKÝ

Postgraduate Medical School, Children's Cardiac Centre,Limbová 1, Bratislava, Slovak Republic

V.ŤAŽKÝ

Department of Medicine, Derer's Hospital, Limbová 5, Bratislava,Slovak Republic

We have studied a group of 35 children, 25 boys and 10 girls, at the age of 2 to 17, mean 12 years with various signs of sick sinus syndrome. 18 of them had operated congenital heart defects operated, in the rest the heart was structurally normal. Most of the patients had asymptomatic sinus bradycardia, 4 experienced syncope and three others effort dyspnea and presyncope. Five of them had sinus node function checked before pacemaker implantation because of congenital complete heart block. 16 patients receive no therapy, 3 are improved on atropine and/or sustained release isoprenaline, 2 with atrial flutter are treated by sotalol and 3 receive digoxin for diminished right ventricular function. 11 patients received pacemakers, 2 with VDD, 2 with AAIR and 7 with DDDR modes of stimulation.

1 Introduction

Sinus node dysfunction in children may be idiopathic, or caused by vagotonia, unoperated, or by operated congenital heart defects, postinflammatory, cardiomyopathies, or by other causes. It implies both depressed sinus nodal automaticity,sinoatrial conduction,or a combination of the two with a number of escape rhythms from lower pacemakers. This can lead to a variety of clinical symptoms from fatigue, diminished exercise tolerance, to cardiac failure, syncope and eventually to sudden death. Incidence and prevalence of patients with this syndrome has been increasing in the recent time, mainly because of survival of patients with some types of operations, that have inherent risk for this late complication. Most frequently this occurs after atrial switch for transposition of great arteries, older types of Fontan operations, but also suture of atrial and/or other septal defects(1,2).

2 Material nad Methods

25 boys and 10 girls at the age of 2 to 17 years, mean 12 years, were sent to our hospital because of suspected sinus node dysfunction. 18 had congenital heart defects operated: atrial switch for transposition of great arteries in 11, in three defects of ventricular, in one atrial septum. One had redirected total anomalous pulmonary veins connection, and one repaired complete atrioventricular septal defect. One patient with tuberous sclerosis underwent right ventricular tumour extraction in the newborn period.

17 patients without structural heart disease were referred to our hospital because of syncope and/or presyncope in four of them, and effort dyspnea in three. Seven

had complete and or advanced heart block , one had rate dependent bundle branch block and two others were sent for sinus bradycardia, inappropriate for their age. Half of the patients with operated congenital defects especially transpositions of the great arteries, had slightly diminished exercise tolerance.

On *Ecg* signs for sinus node dysfunction were looked for:

- sinus bradycardia:	< 7 years	50 bpm
	< 11 years	45 bpm
	older	40 bpm

- Intermittent junctional rhythm with AV dissociation
- sinus pauses/ sinoatrial block
- other arrhythmias

Atropine testing was done by administration of 0,02 mg/kg bw of atropine during one minute with continuous registration of Ecg. Ecg was then registered every minute for 10 seconds, to measure sinus/AV node acceleration. At least 25-50% rate increase was considered normal.

Exercise testing was performed on a bicycle ergometer according to James′ protocol. Ecg was monitored for heart/sinus rate acceleration, and occurrence of other arrhythmias.

For *24 hour ecg recording* three chanel tape recorder (Circadian) was used and the recordings were analyzed hourly for minimum, mean and maximum heart rates and for occurence of other arrhythmias as on Ecg.

Transoesophageal stimulation was performed by a stimulator (Medico), capable of incremental and extrastimulus pacing. Sinus nodal automaticity was assessed by overdrive suppression, AV nodal conduction by incremental pacing,atrial ERP and induction of atrial arrhythmias by atrial extrastimulus technique. Normal corrected sinus nodal recovery times were 275 msec(2,3,4,5,6).

3 Results

Ecg findings in our group of patients are in the table 1.

Table 1. Summarisation of Ecg findings

Sinus bradycardia/pronounced arrhythmia	18 pts
- Atrial flutter	2 pts
- AV nodal reentry tachycardia	1 pt
- Atrial extrasystoles	1 pt
- Atrial rhythm with bundle branch block	1 pt
Slow escape junctional rhythm	9 pts
Congenital complete heart block	5 pts
Borderline sinus arrhythmia	3 pts

Atropine testing

Atropine was given to seven patients,to check the ability of sinus node to accelerate. Five of them had slow escape junctional rhythm with AV dissociation. After atropine, at first sinus node slowly accelerated,but at the rate of 90 to 100 bpm accelerated junctional focus took over and junctional rhythm dominated untill dissipation of atropine effects. Two other patients with sinus bradycardia had less than 25% acceleration of sinus node.

Exercise test

Ten children were tested on a bicycle ergometer. Sinus node accelerated adequately in four, in another four sinus response during peak exercise was blunted and inadequate. In one patient during exercise junctional rhythm alternated with that of sinus, while in the last one, second degree AV block did not change.

24 hour Ecg monitoring

Holter monitoring was performed in 25 patients. Borderline findings had four of them. Marked sinus arrhythmia with longest PP interval more than twice of the shortest interval was found in six, profound sinus bradycardia with slow escape rhythm in another three. Four patients had multiple sinus pauses longer than 3 seconds during the night and one had frequent episodes of sinoatrial block. Two patients had persistent first and second degree AV block without pauses. All patients with congenital complete heart block had minimum heart rates below 40 bpm. Sinus nodal function was normal in two, in four was abnormal.

Transoesophageal stimulation

All 35 patients underwent transoesophageal electrophysiology.It consisted of incremental atrial pacing to assess sinus node recovery times and AV nodal conduction times, and of atrial extrastimulus techniques for assessment of atrial and AV nodal refractory periods,as well as for induction of intraatrial or other reentrant tachycardias.Sinus nodal recovery times were normal in 10 patients, while in 25 were abnormal, ranging from 300 to 1010 msec, mean 475msec. In three, first postpacing beat was always from the AV junction, with subsequent restoration of slow sinus rhythm.

Five children had binodal involvement with sinus and concomitant AV nodal dysfunction. Wenckebach conduction through AV node occured at the rates of 100 to 130 bpm and long AV nodal ERP were found in all of them.

From five patients with congenital complete heart block, sinus nodal function was normal in two, in three both sinus and AV nodal functions were abnormal.

4 Treatment

In 16 patients the signs of sinus nodal dysfunction were mild, so they receive no therapy, being only closely followed up regularly. In three sinus nodal function improved on medication with atropine alone in one, or in combination with sustained release isoprenaline in two other patients. Two patients with repetitive paroxysms of atrial flutter are treated by sotalol,while regularly checking sinus node function.Three patients receive digoxin to improve right ventricular function after operation for transposition of the great arteries. In eleven patients permanent pacemakers were implanted, all functioning in physiological mode of stimulation.From five patients with congenital complete heart block two with normal sinus function received single pass VDD systems (Phymos 3-Medico), and three dual chamber pacemakers with rate responsiveness (Thera DR-Medtronic). Dual chamber pacemakers were implanted also to the four children with AV dissociation and slow AV junctional rhythms, in whom dysfunction of both sinus and AV node was found. In two other children single chamber atrial pacemakers with rate responsive mode were implanted.

5 Discussion

Sinus node dysfunction is well known to occur after some type of cardiac operations. In our group there was almost half of the patients without congenital heart defects, a relatively high number, maybe due to the selection of the patients referred to our hospital. As in other reports, we have found relative high number (5 patients) of children with dysfunction of both sinus and AV nodal functions, requiring pacemaker implantation.

At present, ecg recording, Holter monitoring and transoesophageal stimulation are simple and reliable methods for recognition of sinus node dysfunction and decision for appropriate therapy.

References

1. SM Yabek, RE Swensson,JM Jarmakani, Circulation 56,235 (1977)
2.R Oberhofer et al., Kardiologie 83,812 (1994)
3. EP Walsh, JP Saul, in Nada s pediatric cardiology, p.377, ed.DC Fyler (Hanley and Belfus Inc, Philadelphia, 1993,)
4. EP Walsh, in Nadas pediatric cardiology, p.117, ed.DC Fyler (Hanley and Belfus Inc, Philadelphia, 1993)
5. HH Kramer et al., Internat.J.Cardiol. 32, 5 (1991)
6. DW Benson et all., Clin. Prog. Pacing Electrophysiol. 2,360 (1984)

AUTONOMIC NEUROPATHY AND HYPERTENSION INCREASE QT DISPERSION IN DIABETICS

B. KRAHULEC, L. ŠTRBOVÁ, I. BALAŽOVJECH
2nd Department of Internal Medicine, Faculty Hospital, Mickiewiczova 13, 813 69 Bratislava, Slovak Republic

We measured QT interval, corrected QT interval (QTc) and QTc dispersion on the standard 12 lead electrocardiograms in 72 Type-1 diabetics. The investigation with a battery of cardiovascular reflexes (deep breathing, active orthostasis, Valsalva maneuver) revealed 21 diabetics (29,2%) with autonomic neuropathy. These patients had higher systolic blood pressure, higher heart rate, prolonged QTc interval and higher QTc dispersion as diabetics without autonomic neuropathy. 85,7% diabetics with autonomic neuropathy had hypertension or borderline hypertension. QTc dispersion in hypertensive patients was significantly higher than in non-hypertensive patients. QTc dispersion correlated significantly with both systolic and diastolic blood pressures. Hypertension may be therefore important predictor of high risk of arrhytmogenicity and effective lowering of blood pressure should be the main goal of pharmacological intervention in diabetics.

1. Introduction

It is well known from the study of Ewing et al (1), which was performed in the year 1976, that diabetics with cardiac autonomic neuropathy have a poor prognosis. 50% of them were dead within the period of 2,5 years. More recently Rathmann et al (2) estimated mortality rate of 23% during the period of 8 years. Both studies found some patients, who died suddenly. Bellavere et al (3) found prolonged QT interval in diabetic autonomic neuropathy patients and it has been speculated that this could provide a possible explanation for the sudden deaths. Ewing et al (4) showed, those time changes in QT interval lenght vere in parallel with time changes in autonomic function and those diabetic subjects with autonomic neuropathy who died within 3 years had longer QT intervals than those who survive. Prolonged QT interval could lead to condition of increased myocardial electrical instability and this might predispose diabetic subjects with autonomic neuropathy to potentially fatal ventricular arrhythmias. QT dispersion represents variations in repolarisation in different regions of myocardium, and increased dispersion of ventricular recovery time may provide the substrate for ventricular arrhythmias. The study of Day et al (5) evaluated the usefulness of QT interval dispersion as a predictor of sudden death and risk of ventricular tachyarrhythmias. Hypertension is common in diabetic patients, seems to have a close relationship to diabetic autonomic neuropathy, sustained pressure overload lead to concentric left ventricular hypertrophy and patients with this condition are susceptible to sudden death (6).

Therefore, the purpose of this study was to test relationships between QT interval lenght, QT interval dispersion, blood pressure and autonomic neuropathy in our diabetic patients.

2. Patients and Methods

We studied 72 Type-1 diabetics (38 men, 34 women) with mean of age 36.5 years (95% confidence limits 34.1-38.9 years), diabetes duration 14.4 (11.9-16.9) years.
Standard 12 lead electrocardiograms were recorded at 25 mm/s with Hewlett-Packard (USA) Page writer II machine. The QT intervals were measured from the onset of the QRS to the end of the T wave, defined as a return to thc T-P baseline. When U waves were present the QT was measured to the nadir of the curve between the T and U waves. Whenever possible, three consecutive cycles were measured in each of the 12 electrocardiogram leads and from the three values a mean QT and corrected QT (QTc) was calculated using Bazett formula (7) $QTc=QT/\sqrt{RR}$. QTc dispersion was defined as the difference between the maximum and minimum QTc occuring in any of the 12 electrocardiorgam leads in which it could be reliably measured.
We performed three cardiovascular autonomic reflex tests according to Ewing et al (8):

1. Deep-Breathing Test. After 5 min at rest in the supine position, an ECG was recorded while the patient was breathing at a rate of 6 breaths/min (inspiration and exspiration lasting 5s each). The R-R intervals were converted in heart rate and the result of the test was expressed as the mean of the three best differences between the highest and the lowest heart rate during each respiratory cycle. Differences over 15 beats/min are considered normal, under 10 abnormal.
2. The 30:15 Ratio Test. After a further period of resting, the patient was invited to quickly assume the upright posture. Immediately after, the longest R-R interval (which is usually located around the 30th beat after standing) and the shortest one (around the 15th beat) were identified and the 30:15 ratio calculated. Normal values are greater than 1.03.
3. Valsalva Maneuver. After a 5-minute rest in the sitting position, the subject blew into a mouthpiece at a pressure of 40 mmHg for 15 s. The ratio of the longest R-R interval immediately after exspiratory effort and the shortest R-R interval during the effort was calculated. Normal values are greater than 1.21.

The diagnosis of diabetic cardiac autonomic neuropathy was made, when minimally one test was abnormal.
Statistical Analysis. The results are expressed as the mean and 95% confidence limits. The variables were tested with non-parametric Wicoxon test. The Chi-square test was used when appropriate. Spearman correlation coeficients were also tested.

3. Results

Autonomic neuropathy was diagnosed in 21 (29.2%) of 72 Type-1 diabetics. Patients with autonomic neuropathy had higher systolic blood pressure (149.6, 140.7-158.5 vs. 135, 131.2-138.8 mmHg, $p < 0.005$), higher heart rate (92.8, 85.7-99.8 vs. 78.4, 74.6-82.1 beats/min, $p< 0.001$), prolonged QTc interval (462, 451-473 vs. 435, 443-447 ms, $p< 0.005$) and slightly higher QTc dispersion (50.9, 41.6-60.4 vs. 39.6, 32.7-46.5 ms, $p < 0.05$).
18 of 21 (85.7%) diabetics with autonomic neuropathy had hypertension, or borderline hypertension in comparison to 20 of 51 (39.2%) diabetics without autonomic neuropathy ($p< 0.05$).
QTc dispersion in 38 hypertensive diabetics was significantly higher than in 34 non-hypertensive patients (63.3, 46.4-80.1 vs. 36.04, 29.6-42.5 ms, $p< 0.001$), but lenght of the QTc interval was not significantly different in both hypertensive and non-hypertensive diabetics (447, 439-455 vs 441, 425-457 ms, ns).
QTc dispersion correlated linearly with systolic blood pressure ($r=0.50$, $p < 0.001$) and diastolic blood pressure ($r=0.42$, $p < 0.005$).

4. Discussion

Cardiac autonomic neuropathy is a common complication of diabetes (17% Type-1 diabetics), althought yet it has mostly an asymptomatic course (9). Patients suffering from cardiac autonomic neuropathy are at risk of unstable blood pressure during anesthesia (10), higher occurrence of silent myocardial ischaemia (11), as well as at a high risk of sudden death (1). There is some link postulated by Bellavere et al (3) between cardiac autonomic neuropathy, prolonged QT interval and sudden death. We found in our study not only prolonged QTc interval in diabetics with cardiac autonomic neuropathy, but also higher QTc dispersion, which may be a marker of arrhythmogenic potential. Recently Wei et al (12) and Shimabukuro et al (13) also showed an increse in QTc dispersion in diabetics with autonomic neuropathy. It suggest, that such patients have a greather inhomogeneity of repolarisation that may be of prognostic significance, but still is not evidence, that QT dispersion in diabetics really increases the risk of arrhytmogenicity through autonomic dysfunction (12).
Airaksinen et al (14) referred about the strong association between high blood pressure and diabetic autonomic neuropathy and O´Brien et al (15) revealed, that supine systolic blood pressure was weak predictive factor of death in diabetics with autonomic neuropathy in 5-year follow-up study on 484 diabetics. We also found higher systolic blood pressure in diabetics with autonomic neuropathy and hypertension was very close to autonomic neuropathy. Recently, Liao et al (16) really suggested, that cardiac autonomic function is associated with prevalent hypertension, and that reduced vagal function and the imbalance of sympatho-vagal function are associated with the risk of developing hypertension. The classic cardiac adaptation to

a sustained pressure overload is concentric left ventricular hypertrophy and Mayet et al (17) referred, that QT dispersion is increased in association with an increased left ventricular mass index in hypertensive individuals and Belanescu et al (18) referred about elevated QT dispersion in association with more severe ventricular arrhythmias in hypertensive subjects with left ventricular hypertrophy. To our knowledge, the present report is the first to evaluate of QT dispersion in diabetic patients with hypertension and the good correlations between QTc dispersion and both systolic and diastolic blood pressure in our study shows very close relationship between QTc dispersion and hypertension in diabetic patients.

In conclusion, the poor prognosis of diabetics with autonomic neuropathy may be related to hypertension, and therefore treatment of hypertension seems to be the main target in these patients.

5. References

1. D.J. Ewing et al, Lancet 1, 7960 (1976)
2. W. Rathmann et al, Diabetic Med 10, 820 (1993)
3. F. Bellavere et al, Br Heart J 59, 379 (1988)
4. D.J. Ewing et al, Diabetologia 34, 182 (1991)
5. C. Day et al, Br Heart J 63, 342 (1990)
6. F.H. Messerli et al, Am J Med 77, 18 (1984)
7. S. Ahnve, Am Heart J 109, 568 (1985)
8. D.J. Ewing et al, Diabetes Care 8, 491 (1985)
9. D. Ziegler et al, J Diab Comp 6, 49 (1992)
10. L.G. Burgos et al, Anesthesiology 70, 591 (1989)
11. D.P. Murray et al, Diabetic Med 7, 580 (1990)
12. K. Wei et al, JACC 26, 859 (1995)
13. M. Shimabukuro et al, Am J Cardiol 78, 1057 (1996)
14. K.E.J. Airaksinen et al, Am J Noninvas Cardiol 6, 242 (1992)
15. I.A. O'Brien et al, Q J Med 79, 495 (1991)
16. D. Liao et al, Am J Hypertension 9, 1147 (1996)
17. J. Mayet et al, Hypertension 28, 791 (1996)
18. S. Balanescu et al, Arch Mal Coeur 89, 987 (1996)

PERIODICITY OF SEVERE ARRHYTHMIAS IN CHRONIC RESPIRATORY FAILURE AT ALTITUDE ABOVE 1,000 M

Š. KUJANÍK

Department of Physiology, Medical Faculty, Šafárik University,

Trieda SNP 1, 040 66 Košice, Slovakia

E-mail: kujanik@kosice.upjs.sk

M. MAYER

Institute of Tuberculosis and Respiratory Diseases,

059 84 Vyšné Hágy, Slovakia

M. SNINČÁK

Department of Internal Diseases, Military Airforce Hospital,

Murgašova ulica, 040 00 Košice, Slovakia

Z. RICHTÁRIKOVÁ

Department of Physiology, Medical Faculty, Šafárik University,

Trieda SNP 1, 040 66 Košice, Slovakia

I. VOKAĽ

Research Institute of Human Bioclimatology,

059 85 Štrbské Pleso, Slovakia

In our previous studies it was found that in the patients with chronic respiratory failure (CRF) at the moderate altitude over 1,000 m the single extrasystoles were not rare and had an expressed 24-hour periodicity. The occurence and periodicity of the following severe arrhythmias are compared in this study: ventricular tachycardia (VT), bigeminia (BG), pairs of ventricular extrasystoles (PES), and runs of ventricular extrasystoles (RES). The number and periodicity of these arrhythmias were evaluated during 24-hour Holter ECG monitoring (7 a.m. - 7 a.m.) in 43 men over 50 (53 - 73) years with CRF at the altitude 1180 m. The control group (CG) included 9 men of similar age at the altitude 1350 m, without cardiopulmonary diseases and any medication. In the CG no severe arrhythmia, only single supraventricular or ventricular extrasystoles occured. In CRF the highest occurence of VT was at 2 p.m., that of BG at 1 a.m., of PES at 9 a.m., of RES at 9 p.m. It is concluded that in CRF at the altitude above 1,000 m not only the single extrasystoles but also the severe arrhythmias (VT, BG, PES, RES) can occur and they show a periodical course. Except for BG the highest occurence of those arrhythmias is in daytime only, dispersed between 9 a.m. and 2 p.m.

In our previous studies at the moderate altitude 1,180 - 1,400 m (Kujaník and Mayer, 1994, Kujaník et al. 1995, 1996) we found that in the patients with chronic respiratory failure (CRF) the single supraventricular and ventricular extrasystoles were not rare and had an expressed 24-hour periodicity.

The supraventricular extrasystoles at the moderate altitude were evidently more frequent than at the lowland area (Košice, the Slovak republic - 200 m above the sea level) with the highest occurence around midnight and the lowest one at 2 a.m. The ventricular extrasystoles at the moderate altitude were evidently more frequent than at the lowland area (Košice, altitude 200 m) with the highest occurence between 9 a.m. till 1 p.m. and the lowest one at 3 a.m.

The occurence of single supraventricular and ventricular extrasystoles did not correlate (the coefficient of the simple correlation was always below 0.28) with the factors as follows - type of respiratory failure (partial or global), inhalation of oxygen (free accessable or no oxygen), values of the four acid-base balance parametres (Astrup - PaO_2, $PaCO_2$, pH, standard bicarbonates), and values of five spirometric parametres (FEV_1, FVC, MEF-50, TGV, Raw).

The occurence and periodicity of four severe arrhythmias - ventricular tachycardia (VT), bigeminia (BG), pairs of extrasystoles (PES), runs of extrasystoles (RES) are compared in this paper. The number and periodicity of these arrhythmias within each hour in 43 men over 50 years (the range 53 - 73) with chronic respiratory failure (partial and/or global) were evaluated during 24-hour Holter ECG monitoring (the apparatuses Memoport C Hellige and Hewlett-Packard Ambulatory ECG Monitoring System) since 7 a.m. till 7 a.m. next day in the Institute of Tuberculosis and Respiratory Diseases Vyšné Hágy (altitude 1180 m). The patients were hospitalized and acclimatized to that altitude at least two weeks. They were treated neither by beta-blockers, amiodarone or sotalol known to depress the periodicity of cardiac arrhythmias, nor by beta-2 stimulatory drugs known to produce hypokalemia and hypomagnesiemia. The treatment included some of drugs as follows: the bronchodilatory agents, calcium blockers, corticosteroids, cardiotonics, nitrates, and other indicated drugs, oxygen was free accessable. The results were processed separately for subgroups of partial and global respiratory failure at first. Because no significant differences in the occurence of arrhythmias between both subgroups were obtained, they were taken together as one group of respiratory failure.

The control group included 9 at least two weeks acclimatized healthy men over 50 years, of similar age, hospitalized in the Research Institute of Human

Bioclimatology at Šrbské Pleso (altitude 1350 m). Their history was without any cardiopulmonary diseases, they showed the normal findings of the physical cardio-pulmonary examination, acid-base balance (Astrup), ECG curve, blood pressure valid for that altitude and their age, no drugs were taken by these persons during Holter monitoring.

In the control group no severe arrhythmia, only single supraventricular or ventricular extrasystoles (classes 0 and I according to the Lown classification) occured. Both types of extrasystoles were rare, usually in the range 1 - 2 per hour.

In chronic respiratory failure not only single supraventricular and ventricular extrasystoles but also higher classes (II, III, IV, V) of cardiac arrhythmias according to Lown occured. The ventricular fibrillation was not recorded. The highest occurence of ventricular tachycardia (VT) was at 2 p.m. (7 times in all patients of that group), the summary occurence per 24 hours was 37 times, VT was substantially more frequent during daytime (6 a.m. - 8 p.m.) than during nighttime. The R on T extrasystoles were not very rare, too.

The highest occurence of bigeminia (BG) was at 1 a.m. (10 times in all patients), the summary occurence per 24 hours was 64 times, but BG was substantially more frequent during night period (8 p.m. - 6 a.m.).

The highest occurence of pairs of extrasystoles (PES) was at 9 a.m. (45 times in all patients of that group), the lowest one at 12 p.m. (2 times), the summary occurence per 24 hours was 396 times, PES were substantially more frequent in daytime.

The highest occurence of runs of extrasystoles (RES) was at 9 a.m. (16 times in all patients), the summary occurence per 24 hours was 104 times, RES were substantially more frequent in daytime.

Mechanisms of detected arrhythmias can be summarized as follows:

(a) Influence of hypoxia, (b) Influence of hypercapnia and hypoventilation, (c) Influence of hyperventilation and hypocapnia, (d) Influence of ventricular hypertrophy and heart failure, (e) Increased activity of the autonomic nervous system, (f) Ionic changes of various origin, (g) Dependence on sleep and sleep apnea syndrome, (h) Influence of applicated drugs, (i) Presence of ischemic heart disease, (j) Influence of altitude and acclimatization, (k) Dependence on biological rhythms, (l) Other factors.

The changes produced by chronic pulmonary diseases may frequently be contradictory, they can either stimulate or inhibit the origin of cardiac arrhythmias. Due to high cleanliness of air the moderate altitude is used for the treatment of respiratory diseases, especially asthma. This altitude is not harmful for healthy persons but the number of cardiac arrhythmias is progressively increasing in them with increasing altitude and age.

Our results indicate that even severe arrhythmias (classes II to V according to Lown) can occur in chronic respiratory failure at the moderate altitude. All of those arrythmias show an expressed 24 hour periodicity usually with several peaks. Except for bigeminia their highest occurence is in daytime, but it is dispersed between 9 a.m. and 2 p.m. In healthy persons and in patients with CRF at the lowland area only the single supraventricular or ventricular extrasystoles occur. It is assumed that the cause of higher occurence of cardiac arrhythmias at the moderate altitude is increased adrenergic activation of the heart. It can be elicited by hypoxia (decrease in the partial pressure of oxygen in the air is more than 20 mm Hg at the altitude of 1,400 meters compared to a lowland area).

Conclusions

- Cardiac arrhythmias in chronic respiratory failure can arise as a result of diverse mechanisms. The changes produced by chronic pulmonary diseases may frequently be contradictory.
- The moderate altitude is used for the treatment of respiratory diseases, especially asthma but the number of cardiac arrhythmias is progressively increasing with increasing altitude and age
- For patients with the cardiovascular or respiratory diseases over 50 years already the altitude 1,000 - 3,000 m can be a risk factor for occurence of cardiac arrhythmias, especially after the sudden ascent and accompanied physical activity
- recommendation for a stay at the moderate altitude and for flying in plains should be made strictly individually

References

1. Š.Kujaník and M.Mayer, *Folia Fac. Med. Univ. Safarik. Cassov.* V **51** (1), 227 (1994).
2. Š.Kujaník *et al, J. Moll. Cell. Cardiol.* V **27** (6), A 195 (1995).
3. Š.Kujaník *et al, Eur. J. Physiol.* V **430** (4), R 143 (1995).
4. Š.Kujaník, *Stud. Pneumol. Phtiseol.* V **57** (1), 27 (1997).

COMPARED STUDY TO HOLTER-SA-ECG WITH LEFT VENTRICULAR FUNCTION USING MULTIPLE GATED ACQUISITION CARDIAC BLOOD POOL IMAGING IN PATIENTS WITH MYOCARDIAL INFARCTION

L.X.ZHAO, K.HORIUCHI, Y.OZAWA, S.SAITO, N.TANIGAWA, I.WATANABE, K.NAKAYAMA, Y.KASAMAKI, Y.TAKAHASHI, M.MORIUCHI, K.KANMATSUSE.

The 2nd Department of Medicine, School of Medicine, Nihon University.
30-1, Oyaguchi-Kamimachi, Itabashi-ku, Tokyo, Japan.

Summary: The purpose of this study is to evaluate the relationship between left ventricular function and Holter-signal averaged ECG (H-SA-ECG) in patients with myocardial infarction(MI). We have determined the prognostic significance of Left ventricular function from multiple gated acquisition (MUGA) cardiac blood pool imaging in patients with MI. 30 patients were followed with intravenous administration of 99m-Technetium labeled human serum albumin-DTPA for study MUGA cardiac blood pool imaging; And every patient carried a 24h Holter monitor. The data were recorded by Del Mar Avionics Model 459 3-channel Cardio Corder and Model 563 strata scan-Holter ECG analysis system. We used peak filling rate (PFR) to evaluate early diastolic filling function, and an ejection fraction (EF) to evaluate the systolic function of left ventricular in these 30 patients. Rusults: 1). PFR in Group of positive H-SA-ECG was lower than that group which had negative H-SA-ECG. 2).Otherwise, there was no significant difference of EF between two groups.

Backgrouds and purpose

The Holter-signal averaged electrocardiogram (H-SA-ECG) has emerged as an accurate, reliable and noninvasive method to identify the patients at risk of a malignant arrhythmic event, particulary, sustained ventricular fibrillation or ventricular fibrillation which as the harbingers of sudden cardiac death after a myocardial infarction.[1,2,3] On the other hand, the management of patients with MI often depends upon clinical assesment of left ventricular (LV) function. Both of these are important for determination of medical treatment plan of MI. It is interesting to evaluate the relationship between LV function and late potential with H-SA-ECG in two groups, which had positive and negative H-SA-ECG in patients with MI.

Patients and Methods

30 patients (mean age of positive H-SA-E 52.1y/negative H-SA-E 64.9y,period

from on set 3.1ys/3.5ys,each group 13male and 2 female) with old myocardial infarction were studied , all patients were in normal sinus rhythm at the time of study.Every patient carried a 24h Holter monitor. The data were recorded by Del Mar Avionics Model 459 3-channel Cardio-Corder and analysis by Model 563 strata scan-Holter ECG analysis system. The criteria of H-SA-ECG: QRSd>114ms, RMS40<12 uV, LAS40>38ms. An abnormal H-SA-ECG (Late potential positive) is defined as the presence of at least 2 of 3 parameters. QRSd: Filtered QRS duration. RMS40: Root mean square voltage of the signals in the last 40 ms of QRS. LAS40: The duration of low amplitude signals (<40uV) in the latter part of the QRS.All patients were followed with intravenous administration of 740 MBq of 99m-Technetium labeled human serum albumin (99mTc-HSA) for study muitiple gated acquisition (MUGA) cardiac blood pool imaging.[4] 15minutes after injection, started imaging which anterior oblique (ANT), left anterior oblique (LAO) and left posterior oblique (LPO). For the analysis of quantitative left ventricular function, we chose the LAO view and calculated left ventricular ejection fraction (LVEF) as an index of systolic function and peak filling rate (PFR) to evaluate diastolic function.

Results

The correlation coefficient between values of PFR in group of H-SA-ECG negative and group of positive H-SA-ECG were showed difference significantely (P<0.05). The value of PFR in group had negative H-SA-ECG was higher than that group which had positive H-SA-ECG. However, LVEF was showed no significant difference (Fig.1 and Fig.2)

Conclusion

1:LVEF showed no significant difference both in patients with positive and negative H-SA-ECG.2:PFR in group with positive H-SA-ECG was lower than that group which had negative H-SA-ECG. It had stronger evidence for that LV early diastolic dysfunction was due to myocardial injury in patients with positive H-SA-ECG. These results suggested that PFR was the manifestation of cardiac diastolic dysfunction and had the possibility after that to frequently develop systolic dysfunction.3:MUGA cardiac blood pool imaging as a noninvasive, an reliable, safety and had reproducible means to quantify LV function in patients with MI.

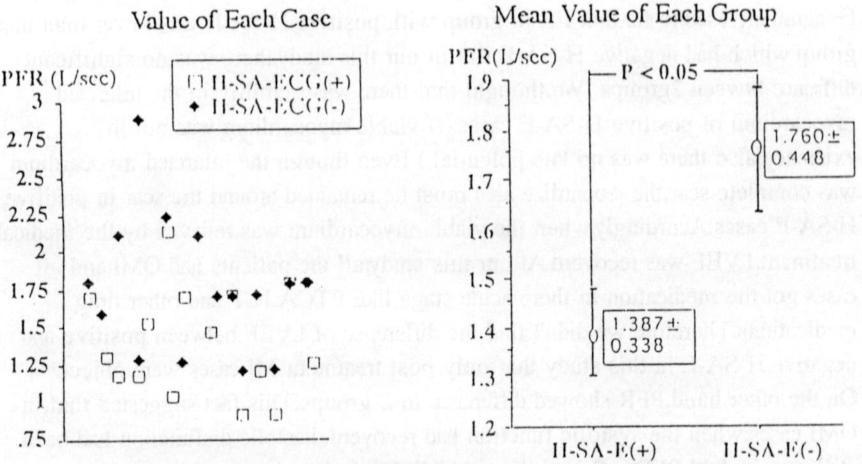

Fig 1 The correlation coefficient between values of PFR in group of H-SA-ECG negative and positive were showed differenee significante (p<0.05)

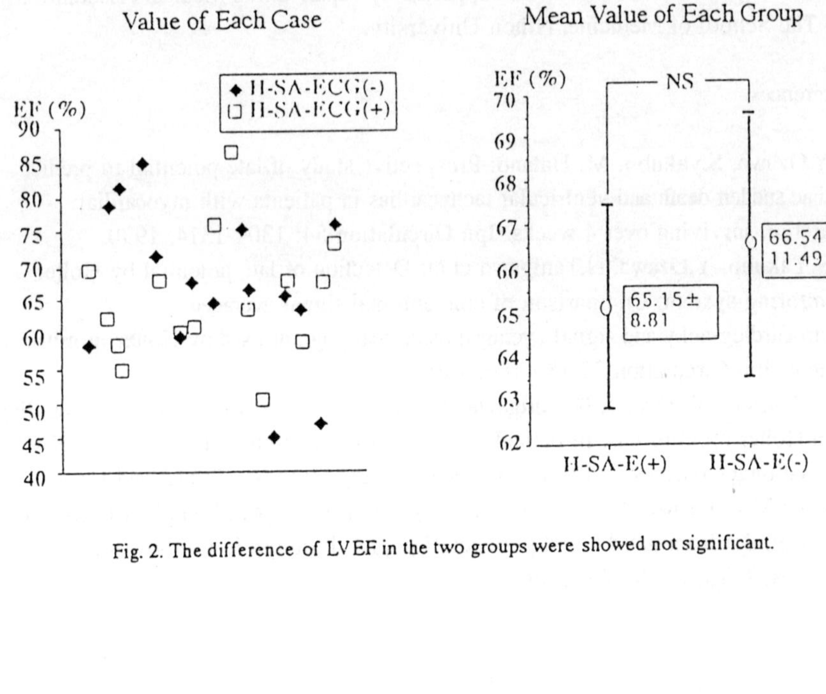

Fig. 2. The difference of LVEF in the two groups were showed not significant.

Discussion

Generally,it used to be that EF in group with positive H-SA-E was lower than that group which had negative H-SA-E.But in our this study,there was no significant diffrence btween 2groups .We thought that there was viability in the infarcted myocardium of positive H-SA-E cases.(If viable myocardium was not in existence,also there was no late potential.) Even though the infarcted myocardium was complete scar,the jeopardize area must be remained around the scar in positive H-SA-E cases.Acordingly,when the viable myocardium was relieved by the medical treatment,LVEF was recoverd.At our this study,all the patients had OMI,and all cases got the medication in there acute stage like PTCA,ICT and other drug medications.Therefore we didn't find the difference of LVEF between positive and negative H-SA-E in this study that only post treatment MI cases were object.
On the other hand,PFR showed difference in 2 groups.This fact suggested that,in OMI cases,when the systolic function had recoverd,diastolic disfunction had been still remain.And PFR reflected the post MI LV disfunction much more sensitively, and correlated with H-SA-E more strongly.

Acknowledgment: This study was supported by Japan-China Medical Association and The School of Medicine, Nihon University.

References

1. Y.Ozawa, S.yakubo, M. Hatano: Prospective study of late potential to predict cardiac sudden death and ventricular tachycardias in patients with myocardial infarction surviving over 4 weeks. Jpn Circulation 54: 1304-1314, 1990.
2. S.Yakubo, Y.Ozawa, N.Tanigawa et al: Detection of late potential by Holter monitoring system. Comparison of conventional signal averaged electrocardiography and signal averaged electrocardiogram used by Holter monitoring system. Jpn Circulation 32:180-186, 1992.
3. L.X. Zhao, Y. Ozawa, N.Tanigawa et al: Signal-averaged ECG directly recording from Holter monitor tape in patients with ventricular arrhthmia. Abstract of XXIII International Confress on Electrocardiology. Aug, 1996 in Cleaverland USA.
4.Green MV, Bacharach SL: Function imaging of the heart: Methods, Limitation, and examples from gated blood pool scintigraphy. Progress in Cardiovascular Diseases, 28 (5) : 319-348, 1986.

INFLUENCE OF THE INFARCT SITE ON THE IDENTIFICATION OF PATIENTS WITH VENTRICULAR TACHYCARDIA AFTER MYOCARDIAL INFARCTION BASED ON THE TIME -DOMAIN AND SPECTRAL TURBULENCE ANALYSIS OF THE SIGNAL- AVERAGED ELECTROCARDIOGRAM

Tobias, N.; Moffa, P.; Moraes, A.; Pastore, C.; Sanches, P.C.; Bellotti, G.; Pileggi, F.
Heart Institute- University of São Paulo, Brazil.

ABSTRACT

In a significant proportion of patients with sustained ventricular tachycardia (SVT) following anterior myocardial infarction, the areas of slow conduction are activated early during cardiac depolarization.Therefore, they may not be detected by the presence of late potentials (LPs) in the signal-averaged electrocardiogram (SAECG). Spectral turbulence analysis of the SAECG is a new technique which examines the whole QRS complex and may improve identification of patients with SVT following anterior infarction. We compared the results of the time- domain and spectral turbulence analysis of the the SAECG in 40 postinfarction patients with SVT, 23 with anterior myocardial infarction (AMI), 17 with inferior infarction (IMI) and 40 age and infarct site- matched patients without SVT. The presence of LPs was admitted, with 40 Hz filter, in patients without bundle branch block (BBB) when the filtered QRS duration ≥ 114 ms, the duration of the terminal QRS ≥ 38 ms and the root -mean -square amplitude of the last 40 ms (RMS) ≤ 20 μV. In the patients with BBB, RMS ≤ 14 μV was considered as a pointer of LPs. Using fast Fourier transformation, spectral turbulence across the entire QRS region was analysed using the technique of Kelen. Results: AMI : sensitivity (Sn) was 47.8% and 69.5%, specificity (Sp) was 97.3% and 30.4% and accuracy (Ac) was 50% and 50% for Lps and spectral turbulence, respectively. IMI: Sn was 88.2% and 58.8%, Sp was 82.3% and 35.2% and Ac was 85.2% and 47% for Lps and spectral turbulence, respectively. Conclusions : The time domain analysis resulted in better identification of patients with SVT following inferior than following anterior infarction, whereas the spectral turbulence analysis performed better in the anterior site of infarction.

INTRODUCTION

The signal-averaged electrocardiogram (SAECG) is a well-established technique for identification of patients at risk for sustained ventricular tachycardia (SVT) following myocardial infarction (MI).[1] Late potentials (LPs) detected by the time-domain analysis of SAECG are believed to reflect myocardial areas of slow conduction that might have arrhythmogenic properties[2-3] However, the limitations of this analysis of the SAECG have been recognized. Indeed, the conventional time-domain analysis of the SAECG is confined to the terminal region of the QRS and ST segment; thus, abnormality buried in other QRS regions cannot be detected. It has been shown that the prevalence of LPs is higher in patients after inferior infarction compared with patients after anterior infarction.[4]

Spectral turbulence analysis of the SAECG is a new technique for the detection of late potentials which examines inhomogeneity of conduction throughout the whole QRS complex and may therefore be capable of detecting "late" potentials within the QRS complex and improve identification of patients with SVT following anterior infarction.[5]

The purpose of this study was to compare the results of both time-domain and spectral turbulence analyses of the SAECG in postinfarction patients with and without SVT with respect to the infarct site.

METHODS

PATIENTS

The study group consisted of 80 postinfarction patients of two pair -matched groups. The SVT group (Group I) consisted of 40 patients (23 with anterior infarction, 17 with inferior infarction) with a spontaneous SVT, documented on the 12-lead electrocardiogram .

The control group (Group II) consisted of 40 postinfarction patients without any arrhythmic event. These patients were age-, gender- and site pair-matched with the patients from the SVT group.

SIGNAL -AVERAGED ELECTROCARDIOGRAM

The SAECG was recorded with the Arrhythmia Research Technology model 1200 EPX using standard bipolar orthogonal X, Y and Z leads. Signal average of 200 to 300 beats was performed to achieve a noise level of 0.3 μV or less.

All recordings were subsequently analysed using the CEWS software package (Del Mar Avionics, model 183).

The time-domain analysis of the SAECG was performed at high-pass filter settings of 40 Hz. The presence of late potential in the groups without bundle branch block (BBB), when at least two of three variables were out of range: the duration of the total QRS complex (QRSd) ≥ 114 ms, the duration of the low amplitude (< 40 μV) signals at the terminal portion of the QRS complex (LAS) ≥ 38 ms and the root mean square voltage of the last 40 ms of the QRS complex (RMS40) ≤ 20 μV.[6] Late potentials were defined as signals with RMS40 ≤ 14 μV in the patients with BBB.[7]

Spectral turbulence analysis was performed using the method of Kelen et al.[5] The spectral turbulence was abnormal, when at least three of four indices were abnormal: 1-low-slice correlation ratio (LSCR) ≥73,5, 2- interslice correlation mean (ISCM) ≤ 92,3, 3- interslice correlation standard deviation (ISCSD) ≥104,8, and 4- spectral entropy (SE) -≥14,4. The recordings were scored between 0 and 4,and an abnormal spectral turbulence analysis was defined as a score of 3 or 4 .

STATISTICS

Continuous variables are presented as the mean and ± SD. The statistical analysis was performed using the Fisher's exact test. Values less than 0.05 were considered to be significant. The following definitions were used for calculating the Sensitivity (Sn), Specificity (Sp) and Accuracy (Ac) of SAECG for spontaneous SVT : 1- true positive, patients with abnormal SAECG. and with SVT; 2- false positive, patients with abnormal SAECG and no SVT; 3- true negative, patients with normal SAECG and no SVT; 4- false negative, patients with normal SAECG and with SVT.

RESULTS

The time domain analysis of SAECG was abnormal in 26 (65%) patients with SVT versus 5 (12.5%) controls ($p < 0.05$). The spectral turbulence analysis was abnormal in 26 (65%) patients with SVT compared with 22 (55%) patients without SVT (p=NS).

Table I expresses the comparative performaces of time domain anlysis and spectral turbulence anlysis in patients with anterior infarction and in patients with inferior infarction.

Table I - Sensitivity (Sn), Specificity (Sp) and Accuracy (Ac) of Late Potentials and Spectral Turbulence for spontaneous Sustained Ventricular Tachycardia in patients with anterior infarction and patients with inferior infarction.

	AMI		IMI	
	LP	ST	LP	ST
Sn	47.8	69.5	88.2	58.8
Sp	97.3	30.4	82.3	35.2
Ac	50.0	50.0	85.2	47.0

LP= late potentials ST= spectral turbulence AMI= anterior myocardial infarction IMI= inferior myocardial infarction

Figure 1 is a bar graph illustrating the data showed in Table I

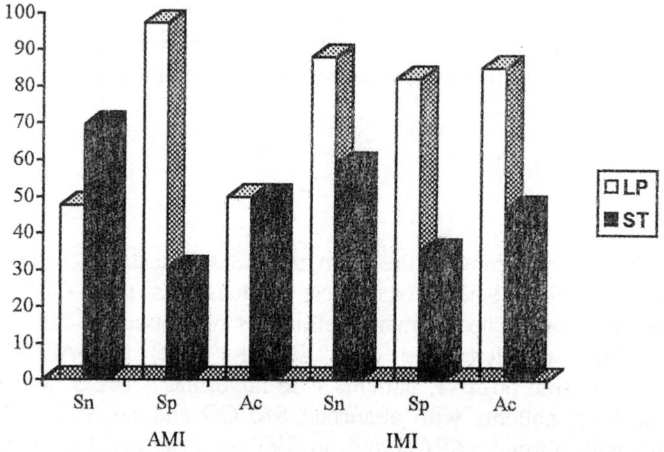

Figure 1. The bar graphs illustrate the comparative effectiveness of time-domain analysis (TDA) and spectral turbulence analysis (STA) as expressed by Senstivity (Sn), Specificity (Sp) and Accuracy (Ac) in distinguishing the SVT from the no SVT patient.

DISCUSSION

One of the concerns about the utilization of time domain analysis of the SAECG for risk stratification has been that its most effective performance has been limited to patients whose MI are dominantly expressed in the late part of the ventricular excitation. When the MI is confined to the beginning of the ventricular excitation, the electrical expression of arrhythmogenic substrate is overwhelmed by the QRS complex. Indeed, it has been shown that the site of infarction influences the results of the time domain analysis of the SAECG.[4] On the other hand spectral turbulence anlysis of the SAECG which examines the entire QRS complex is capable of detecting the inhomogeneity of conduction and may improve identification of patients with SVT following anterior infarction.[8-10]
This study shows that in inferior infarction, time domain analysis is a very sensitive and specific technique for identification of patients with SVT, and spectral turbulence anlysis does not offer any significant improvement. This probably is because the inferopostero-basal region of the left ventricle, which is usually involved in inferior infarct, is activated later, and late potentials even of short duration extend beyond the QRS complex are detected by the conventional time domain analysis.
Although spectral turbulence analysis slightly improved the identification of

patients with SVT following anterior infarction, the change was very small. This may be due to the high number of false positive recordings in the patients with anterior MI and left ventricular aneurysm. More extensive fibrosis and scarrings may explain these results [8]. The combination of the two methods may nevertheless improve identification of patients with SVT following anterior infarction.

CONCLUSION

The time domain analysis resulted in better identification of patients with SVT following inferior than following anterior infarction, whereas the spectral turbulence analysis performed better in the anterior site of infarction.

REFERENCES

1. Simson, M.B. Use of signals in the terminal QRS complex to identify patients with ventricular tachycardia after myocardial infarction. Circulation 64: 235-242, 1981.
2. Breithardt, G.; Becker, R.; Seipel, L.; Abendroth, R.R.; Ostermeyer, J. Noninvasive detection of late potentials in man. A new marker for ventricular tachycardia. Eur. Heart J. 2 : 1-11, 1981.
3. Breithardt, G.; Borggrefe, M.; Fetsch, T.; Böcker, D.; Mäkijärvi, M.; Reinhardt, L. Prognosis and risk stratification after myocardial infarction. Eur. Heart J. 16: 10-19, 1995. Supplement G.
4. Gomes, J.A.; Winters S.L.; Martinson, M.; Machac, J.; Stewart, D.; Targonski, A. The prognostic significance of quantitative signal-averaged variables relative to clinical variables, site of myocardial infarction, ejection fraction and ventricular premature beats: a prospective study. J. Am. Coll. Cardiol., v. 13: 377-84, 1989.
5. Kelen, G.J.; Henkin, R.; Starr, A.M.; Caref, E.B.; Bloomfield, D.; El-Sherif, N. Spectral turbulence analysis of the signal-averaged electrocardiogram and its predictive accuracy for inducible sustained monomorphic ventricular tachycardia. Am. J. Cardiol. 67: 965-975, 1991.
6. Breithardt, G.; Cain, M.E.; El-Sherif, N.; Flowers, N.C.; Hombach,V.; Janse, M.; Simson, M.B.; Steinbeck, G. Standards for analysis of ventricular late potentials using High-Resolution or Signal-Averaged Electrocardiography: A statement by a Task Force Commitee of the European Society of Cardiology, the American Heart Association, and the American College of Cardiology. J. Am. Coll. Cardiol. 17: 999-1006, 1991.
7. Moraes, A.P.; Moffa, P.J.; Sosa, E.A.; Belloti, G.M.V.; Pastore, C.A.; Lima, E.V.; Chalela, W.H.; Grupi, C.J.; Pileggi, F.J.C. Signal-averaged

electrocardiogram in chronic Chagas' heart disease. São Paulo Medical Journal (Rev. Paul. Med.) 113: 851-855, 1995.

8. Malik, M.; Kulakowski, P.; Hnatkova, K.; Staunton, A.; Camm, J. Spectral turbulence analysis versus time-domain analysis of the signal-averaged ECG in survivors of acute myocardial infarction. J. Electrocardiol. 27: 227-32, 1995. Supplement.
9. Kulakowski, P.; Hnatkova, K.; Bashir, Y.; Heald, S.C.; Staunton, A.; Malik, M.; Camm, J. Influence of the infarct site on the identification of patients with ventricular tachycardia after myocardial infarction based on the time-domain and spectral turbulence analysis of the signal-averaged electrocardiogram. Clin. Cardiol. 18: 39-44, 1995.
10. Turitto, G.; Rao, S.; Ahuja, R.K.; Caref, E.B.; El-Sherif, N. Time-domain and frequency-domain analyses of the signal-averaged ECG in patients with ventricular tachycardia and ischemic versus nonischemic dilated cardiomyopathy. J. Electrocardiol. 27: 213-8, 1995. Supplement.

SIGNAL AVERAGED ELECTROCARDIOGRAM IN CHRONIC CHAGAS' HEART DISEASE

Moraes, Ap; Moffa, Pj; Sosa, Ea; Bellotti, G; Pastore, Ca; Lima, Ev; Chalela, Wa; Tobias, N; Pileggi, F. *Heart Institution Of Hc Fmusp,São Paulo, Brazil.*

ABSTRACT

The aim of the study was to register the prevalence of late potentials (LP) in patients with chronic Chagas' heart disease (CCD) and the relationship with sustained ventricular tachycardia (SVT). 192 patients (96 males), mean age 42.9 years, with CCD were studied through a Signal Averaged ECG using the time domain analysis. According to presence of bundle branch block (BBB) and SVT, four groups of patients were created: **Group I** (n=72): without SVT (SVT-) and without BBB (BBB-): **Group II** (n=27); with SVT (SVT+) and BBB; **Group III** (n=63): SVT- and BBB (BBB+); and **Group IV** (n=30): SVT and BBB+. The LP was admitted, with 40 HZ filter, in the groups without BBB using standart criteria of the method. In the group with BBB, the root-mean-square amplitude of the last 40 ms (RMS) $\leq 14\ \mu V$ was considered as an indicadtor of LP. Results: In groups I and II, LP was present in 21 (78%) of the patients with SVT and in 22 (31%) of the patients without SVT ($p < 0.001$), with Sensitivity (S) 78%; Specificity (SP) 70% and Accuracy (Ac) 72%. LP was present in 30 (48%) of the patients without and 20 (67%) of the patients with SVT, in groups III and IV. p= 0.066, with S= 66%; SP= 52%; and Ac= 57%. In the follow-up, there were 4 deaths unrelated to arrhythmic events, all of them did not have LP. Eight (29.6%) of the patients from group II and 4 (13%) from group IV presented recurrence of SVT and 91.6% of these patients had LP. Conclusions: LP occurred in 77.7% of the patients with SVT and without BBB. In the groups with BBB, there was association of LP with SVT in 66.6% of the cases. The recurrence of SVT was present in 21% of the cases from which 91.6% had LP.

INTRODUCTION

The signal-averaged electrocardiogram constitutes a noninvasive method whose purpose is to detect low voltage and high frequency potentials that occur at the end of a QRS complex and/or in the ST segment. These are called late potentials and they have presented presumed as noinvasive markers of the arrhythmogenic setting [1,3,5,6,10]. In chronic chagasic cardiopathy (CCC), the congestive cardiac failure is the final stage of its clinical progression. The occurrence of ventricular arrhythmias of the sustained ventricular tachycardia type and ventricular fibrilation or thromboembolic phenomena may interrupt this progression leading the patient to death [13,16]. The tachycardiac syndromes may occur as a consequence of changes in the formation (automatism) and/or in the conducting of electrial stimuli (reentry) [18,23]. The mechanism of reentry, habitually found in ventricles depends, from the electrial point of view, on the slow conduction component, unidirectional block and on the recovery of the excitability distal to the block zone, thus favoring the genisis of ventricular ectopic rhythms [24,26]. The prevalence of SVT or ventricular fibrilation in the chronic chagasic cardiopathy is unknown: as it is episodic, the recording of these findings during noininvasive examinations is rare [7,9,17]. The relationship between late potentials and CCC has not been previously investigated. This study aimed at recording the prevalence of late potentials, by means of signal-averaged electricardiogram in patients with chronic chagasic cardiopathy and their relationship to sustained ventricular tachycardia.

PATIENTS

One hundred and ninety two subjects with positive serological tests for chagasic cardiopathy were studied. Ninety six subjects were male patients, age range from 17 to 75 with an age average of 42.93 years. The patients were subjected to the following exams: electrocardiogram, stress testing, long term electrocardiogram and signal-averaged electrocardiogram. The follow-up period ranged from 9 to 57 months, with an average of 39.83 months. The reccurence rate of SVT was recorded and the causes of death were rigorously investigated. According to the electrocardiographic findings showing the presence or abscence of bundle branch block (BBB + and BBB-) and the presence or absence of sustained ventricular tachycardia (SVT+ and SVT-), all patients were divided into four groups:

Group I (SVT-, BBB-): was made up of 72 patients, 41 (75%) were female. Age ranged from 17 to 75 (with and age average of 41.06 years).

Group II (SVT+, BBB-): was made up of 27 patients, 13 (49%) were female. Age ranged from 28 to 64 (with an age average of 46.74 years).

Group III (SVT-, BBB+): was made up of 63 patients, 31 (49%) were female. Ages raged from 21 to 63 (with an age average of 40.84 years).

Group IV (SVT+, BBB+): was made up of 30 patients, 11 (37%) were female. Ages ranged from 23 to 70 (with an age average of 48.36 years).

All four groups were subdivided into late potential negative and late potential positive when the presence or the absecence of late potentials was respectiveky considered.

METHODS

The System Art (Arrhythmia Research Technology Inc.), with a unit of 1200 EPX, a computadorized analysis system. Standard 10 Mhz, PC-AT with 40 MB, hard disk and EGA graphics and a Hewlett-Packard Laser Jet printer with memory expansion were used for the recording of the signal-averaged electrocardiogram in the 192 patients sample. It also contained the operation program of filters by computers including patients data management.

The electrocardiographic signals were captured by bipolar derivations x, y and z wich are represented by a vector whose magnitude is computer-calculated by making use the root-mean-square method. This vector is known as QRS filters.

Subsequently, there variables were evaluated in the filtered QRS complex[8]:

a) the duration of QRS (DQRS);

b) the root-mean-square voltage of the last 40 ms (VM 40); and

c) the duration of the signal below 40 μV (SBA).

In this research, the presence of late potentials was admitted in the group of patients without bundled branch block when at least two of the following criteria were present: DQRS ≥ 110 ms; SBA ≥ 35 mm and VM40 ≤ 20 μV.

In this study, the criterion VM40 ≤ 14 μV was used to define the presence of late potentials in the patients with BBB. This value was obtained from the analysis of data concentration, related to different levels of cut point values (from 12 to 18 μV) with calculation of sensitivity and specificity for all levels.

The records were obtained during the clinical follow-up carried at InCor. The cut of frequency (CF) - lower value used was 40 Hz. The final noise value was accepted when ≤ 0.3 μV with a gain of 2.000/4.000.

The statistical analysis was carried out through proportion tests, Fisher's exact test and chi-square test, always perceptive of the conditions of applicability.

The probability of occurence of an error of the first kind (Type I Berquo), the only relevant error to the present study was fixed at 5% for all the tests.

All the calculations were made using the statistical software "Statgraphics"(Statistical Graphics System).

The statistical analysis also inclued the calculations of the operacional variables, sensitivity, specificity and accuracy, according to the elaborate formulas.

RESULTS AND DISCUSSION:

The analysis of the findings of the signal-averaged electrocardiogram and its relationship with SVT are::

Group I: Patients without BBB and without SVT. This group corresponded to 72 (37.5%) patients of the sample. Fifty (69.4%) patients presented no late potentials and 22 (30.6%) had late potentials. At is was observed, the prevalence of late potentials without SVT, in this series of patients with CCC, is higher than the rate of 15% of patients with coronary artery disease. It is also higher than the rate of 14% of patients with dilated cardiopathy of other origins, both without SVT[20].

The eletrophysiologic changes found in the chronic chagasic cardiopaty due to the functional disorganization, may contribute to the emergence of late potentials, but without the background to sustain a reentry.

Group II: Patients without BBB and with SVT. This group corresponded to 14% of the sample. Late potentials were found in 21 (77.7%) of patients, while it was absent in 6 (22.3%). The prevalence of late potentials in patients with SVT in CCC in this study is similar to the findings described by Poll and cols.[20] in patients with dilated cardiopathy of other etiologies. It was also found to be within the average rate observed in patients with coronary artery disease, that is, 70% to 93% [19].

There were false-negative results - absence of late potentials and SVT. This observation may be related to: a) presence of a small extension of the arrhythmogenic setting and/or its intermitent manifestation; b) arrhythmogenic mechanism of an anormal automatism kind [21].

Thc influence of the Autonomic Nervous System imbalance may be associated to these two possibilities wich may be verified in such condition [11].

The value of late potentials a marker of SVT in patients with CCC in the groups I and II showed a sensitivity degree of 78%, a specificity degree of 70% and an accuracy rate of 77%. The relationship betwwen patients without BBB with and without SVT and the presence or absence of late potentials was statistically significant ($p<0.0001$).

Group III: Patients with BBB and without SVT corresponded to 32.8% of the sample, 33 (52.4%) patients did not have late potentials in the signal-averaged electricardiogram while its presence was reported in 30 patients (47.6%).

This findings concerning the present of late potentials in a high number of patients without SVT may be attributed to the following facts:

a) Out of the 30 patients with late potentials, 96.7% had ventricular arrhythmias with a predominance of non-SVT. They are prone to have the anatomic settings for the occurence of SVT, but they may not have had conditions to develop it.

b) In the case of dilated cardiopathies of other etiologies, as well as the chagasic one, the presence of BBB generates an asynchronous ventricular activation. This generates a signal that may be recorded as a late potential in the absence of actual background to the reentrant tachyarrhytmia [25].

Group IV: Patients with BBB and SVT. This group comprises 30 patients who represent 15.6% of the sample. Twenty (66.6%) had the late potentials and 10 (33.4%) did not. The percentage of individuals with late potentials as well as CCC was close to the average found in patients with coronary artery disease without BBB [4,19,22].

The false negatives (33.4%) could possibly be accounted for:

a) the involved mechanism in the tachyarrhythmia event may be that of an abnormal automatism and not that of reentry. Although the latter may be present, but with an arrythmogenic setting of low magnitude, preventing its manifestion in the signal-averaged electrocardiogram;

b) the imblance of a central or of a reflex origin, amid the sympathetic and parasympathetic autonomic activies, becomes an important hypothesis as an attempt to explain the arrhythmogenic disordes in CCC.

The cardiac autonomic dysfunction in chagasic cardiopathy may play an important role in the changes of the eletrophysiologic properties of the heart, wich may or may not be associated with lesions in the myocardium or in the conduction system [12].

For these 2 groups of patients with CCC and BBB, the late potentials as a marker of risks for SVT showed the following values: sensitivity 66%; specificity 52%; accuracy 57%. The relationship between the number of patients of these two groups who had or did not have SVT and late potentials was not statistically significant with a p value of 0.0666. This is probably due to the results obtained in the group III (patients without SVT, 33 without late potential and 30 with late potential), contrasting to the group IV which shwoed an agreement of findings in 66.6% of the cases and disagreement in 33.4%.

The clinical follow-up of the 192 patients was carried out in a period of time wich varied from 9 to 57 months. During that period, four deaths occured. All belonged to group III (SVT-, BBB+) and according to the information from the medical reports and relatives, such deaths did not relate to arrhythmic events. They did not show late potentials.

Recurrence of SVT was observed in 8 (29.6%) of the patients in group II and in 4 (13%) of the patients in group IV. There was, however, reccurence in 21% of the cases. It is important to stress that out of 12 patients belonging to group II and IV who had SVT, even in the period they were on antiarrhythmic drugs, late potentials were recorded in 11 (91.6%) of them.

CONCLUSIONS

The analysis of the signal-averaged electrocardiogram carried out in patients with CCC showed that the occurrence of late potentials in patients with SVT and without BBB was 77%. In the groups with BBB, there was an association of late potentials with SVT in 66.6% of the cases and the recurrence of SVT was present in 21% of the cases; out of which 91.6% had late potentials.

REFERENCES

1. Berbari, E.J.; Scherlag, B.J.; Hope, R.R. & Lazzara, R. - Recording from the Body Surface of arrhytmogenic ventricular activity during the ST segment. **Am J Cardiol** 1978, 41:697-702.
2. Berquo, E.S.; Souza, J.M.P. & Goltlieb, S.I.D.- Bioeatatística. São Paulo: EPU, 1980.
3. Boineau, J.P. & Cox, J.L.- Slow ventricualr activation in acute myocardial

infarction: a source of reentrant premature ventricular contraction. **Circulation** 1973, 48: 702-6.

4. Breidhardt, G.; Becker, R.; Seipel, L.; Abendroth, R.R. Ostemeyer, J.- Noinvasive detection of late potentials in man. A marker for ventricular tachycardia. Eur Heart J 1981, 2:1-11.
5. El-Sherif, N.; Ursell, S.N.; Bekneit, et al.- Prognostic significance of the signal-averaged electrocardiogram depends on the time of recording in the post infarction period. **Am Heart J** 1989, 118: 256-64.
6. Fontaine, G; Frank, L.; Gallais, H.F.; Allali, I. & Phan Thuc, H.G. - Electrocardiografie des potentiels tardifs du syndrome de post-excitation. **Arch Mal coeur** 1978; 71: 854-64.
7. Grupi, C.- Variabilidade espontânea da arritmia ventricular da cardiopatia chagásica crônica. São Paulo, 1984, 88p. [Tese de doutorado - Faculdade de Medicina da Universidade de São Paulo].
8. Haal Pax, A.J.E.; Myers, J. & Froelicher, V.F.- The signal-averaged surface electrocardiogram and the identification of late potentials. **Prog Cardiovasc Dis** 1989, 31: 295-317.
9. Hernandez, M.I.R.- Contribution de la electrocardiografia dinánica en el estudo de la miocardiopatia chagásica crónica. In: Acquatella, H.; Pulido, P.A. 1982, eds. **Miocardiopatias**. Barcelona, Salvat 1982, p.71-6.
10. Josephson, M.E.; Horowitz, L.N. & Farshidi, A.- Continuos local eletrical activity: a mechanism of recurrent ventricular tachycardia. **Circulation** 1978, 57: 659-65.
11. Junqueira J.R., L.F- Sobre o possível papel da disfunção autonômica cardíaca na morte súbita inesperada do chagásico. In: Reunião Anual Sobre Pesquisa Aplicada em Doencá de Chagas. **Resumos**. Araxá, 1988. 100p.
12. Junqueira, J.R.; L.F.; Soares, J.D.; Beraldo, P.S.S.; Jesus, P.C- Equivalentes efeitos arritmogênicos e disfunção autonômica cardíaca em pacientes chagásicos e em ratos com infecção chagásica experimental. In: reunião Anual sobre Pesquisa Aplicada em Doença de Chagas. **Resumos**, Araxá, 1988, 100p.
13. Köberle, F.- Cardiopatia chagásica. **Hospital**, 1958; 53: 311-46.
14. Kuchar, D.L.; Thorun, C.W. & Sammel, N.L.- Prediction of serious arrhythmic events after myocardial infarction: signal-averaged electrocardiogram, holter monitoring and radionuclide ventriculography. **J. Am Coll Cardiol** 1987; 9: 531-8.
15. Mendonza, I.; Camardo, J.; Moleiro, F. et al- Sustained ventricular tachycardia in chronic chagasic myocardits: eletrophysiologic and pharmacologic characteristics. **am J Cardiol** 1986, 57: 423-7.
16. Mendonza, I.; Moleiro, F. & Marques, J.- Morte súbita na doença de Chagas. **Arq Bras de Cardiol**, 1992, 50: 3-4.
17. Molina, A.; Carrasco, H.; Milanés, J.; Molina, C.; Pacheco, A. & Fuenmayos, A. La prueba esfurezo en la miocardiopatia chagásica crónica su valor en el diagnóstico precoz. El comportamiento de las arritmias

ventriculares y los transtornos de conductión al ejercício en las fases más avanzadas de la enfermedad. **Arq Bras de Cardioln** 1981, 36: 95-100.

18. Motte, G; Laine, J.; Slam, M.S.C. & Davis, J.M.- Pathophysiology of ventricular tachyarrhytmias. **Pace** 1984, 7: 1129-36.

19. Paylos, J.M.- Promediado de senales del eletrocardiograma de alta resolution. Potenciales tardios ventriculares. **Rev. Esp Cardiol** 1990, 43:591-603.

20. Poll, D.S.; Marchlisnski, F.E.; Falcone, R.A.; Josephson, M.E. & Simson, M.B.- Abnormal signal-averaged electrocardiograms in patients with nonischemic congestive cardiomyopathy: relationship to sustained ventricular tachyarrhythmias. **Circulation** 1985, 72: 1308-13.

21. Rubio, A.M.; Borggrefe, M.; Soldevilla, J.G.; Bayes de Luna, A. & Breithardt, G.- Potenciales tardios ventriculares que son, como se detectan y que representan. **Rev Lat Cardiol** 1989, 10: 218-32.

22. Simson, M.B.- Use of signals in the terminal QRS complex to identify patients with ventricular tachycardia after myocardial infarction. **Circulation** 1981, 64: 234-42.

23. Wellens, H.J.J. - Pathophysiology of malignant ventricular tachycardia in man. **Arch. Int. Med** 1975, 135: 475-81.

24. William, D.O.; Sherlag, B.J.; Hope, R.R.; El-Sherif, N. & Lazzara, R. - The pathophysiology of malignant ventricular arrhythmias during acute myocardial ischemia. **Circulation** 1974, 50:1163-72.

25. Winters, S.L.; Stewart, D. & Gomes, J.A.- Signal averaging of the surface QRS complex predicts inducibility of ventricular tachycardia in patients with syncope of unknown origin. A prospective study. **J Am Coll Cardiol** 1987; 10: 775-81.

26. Zipes, D.P.- Electrophysiological mechanism in ventricular fibrilation. **Circulation** 1975, 52(3): 120-30.

SIGNAL-AVERAGED ECG IN THE EVALUATION OF ANTHRACYCLINE CARDIOTOXICITY IN SURVIVORS OF CHILDHOOD CANCER

B. MLADOSIEVICOVA, M. BERNADIC, P. HUBKA, H. PETRASOVA, I. HULIN
Institute of Pathological Physiology, School of Medicine, Comenius University, Sasinkova 4, 811 08 Bratislava, Slovak Republic

A.FOLTINOVA, J.PUSKACOVA
Children's University Hospital, Limbova 1, 833 40 Bratislava, Slovak Republic

Anthracycline cytostatics play an important role in achieving progressive improvement in the prognosis of children with cancer. However, the incidence of anthracycline cardiotoxicity represents a new clinical problem in these patients (pts). Continued loss of myocytes, progressive fibrosis and poor myocardial growth may lead to dilated cardiomyopathy, heart failure and fatal arrhythmias. Late clinical manifestations and potentially progressive subclinical cardiac damage have been demonstrated in high percentage of these pts. This study analyzes the correlates of anthracycline-induced myocardial alterations in the frequency content of signal-averaged ECG (SAECG). SAECG was performed in 45 pts (mean age 15,6+/-3,5 years) 3 months-12 years following completion of anthracycline therapy. The total cumulative doses of anthracyclines were 90-555 (median 230) mg/m^2. The control group consisted of 30 healthy age-matched volunteers.

Using frequency-domain analysis in the terminal portion and within the QRS complex, area ratio 1 (area of 20 to 50 Hz/ area of 0 to 20 Hz) and area ratio 2 (area of 40 to 100 Hz/area of 0 to 40 Hz) were calculated. Area ratios 1 and 2 of pts after anthracycline therapy were significantly higher than those in control group in the terminal portion and within the QRS complex.

In our group of 45 pts, 16% had abnormal area of 40 to 100 Hz/area of 0 to 40 Hz within QRS complex when tested less than 4 years after therapy, 25% when tested from 5-8 years after therapy and 56% when tested from 9-12 years after therapy.

Our results suggest that chemotherapy with anthracyclines, even in low dosage, is associated with increased incidence of SAECG abnormalities. Serial SAECG monitoring could be helpful in risk stratification and the long-term management of these patients.

1 INTRODUCTION

Long-term effects of anticancer therapy on the heart have been the source of growing concern in the past decade. The incidence of late cardiac complications-induced by cytostatics and radiotherapy becomes alarming with the increased number of cancer survivors and with length of survival of oncologic patients. Risk of serious cardiac disease is particularly related to therapy with anthracycline cytostatics - doxorubicin and daunorubicin. Since the 1970s anthracyclines have been used in more than half pediatric oncologic patients. These agents are highly effective in leukemias, lymphomas and solid tumors in children. Anthracycline-induced cardiac damage may be clinically manifested as dilated cardiomyopathy, progressive heart failure and fatal arrhythmias several years after completion of anthracycline therapy. Late clinical manifestations of anthracycline cardiotoxicity have been recently reported in about 5-20% of long-term cancer survivors (1-4). These patients have required hospitalization, intensive care, pacemakers, internal defibrillators and cardiac transplantation. In most instances, clinical manifestation of cardiotoxicity appears to be only the " top " of subclinical myocardial alterations, starting during the time of active therapy. Several leading clinical researchers have found potentially progressive subclinical myocardial abnormalities in about 30 to 60 % of children and young adults who received anthracyclines. (1) Development of late cardiac disease from these minimal abnormalities is potentiated by substantial somatic growth, pregnancy, childbirth, heavy weight lifting, strenous exercise and other factors (5). Untill now, the optimal simple approach for monitoring of anthracycline cardiotoxicity has not been found.

The aim of this study was to 1) to establish incidence of frequency-domain abnormalities of the SAECG in patients after anthracycline therapy and 2) to investigate the vulnerability of patients treated with anthracyclines according to the length of elapsed time after therapy using frequency-domain FFT analysis.

2 PATIENTS AND METHODS

SAECG was performed in 45 patients (mean age 15,6+/-3,5 years), 3 months-12 years following completion of chemotherapy containing 90-555 mg/m^2 doxorubicin or daunorubicin. 43 patients were off succesful therapy. 53% of patients had 2-5 serial SAECG examinations. The control group consisted of 30 age- and gender-matched healthy subjects.

Fast Fourier transform analysis (FFT) was performed in a 120 ms interval, starting 20 ms before the QRS offset and in a 140 ms interval starting at the QRS onset. Results were expressed as area ratio 1(AR1) 20-50Hz/0-20 Hz and area ratio 2 (AR 2) 40-100 Hz/ 0-40 Hz.

3 RESULTS

Significantly higher AR 1 and AR 2 were observed in patients after completing anthracycline therapy than in control subjects (p=0,045 and p=0,035, respectively) in the terminal QRS complex.

Significantly higher AR 1 and AR 2 were also observed in patients than in controls (p=0,0187 and p=0,0043, respectively) within the QRS complex.

During follow up two patients unsuccesfully treated died. Left ventricle dilation in 8-year-old boy and dispersed myocardial fibrosis in 14-year-old girl was found in autopsy. Echocardiographic examinations were not able reveal abnormalities before death in those patients. Both patients had abnormal area ratios.

The incidence of AR abnormalities in our study increased with the time elapsed from the last anthracycline dose. 16% patients had abnormal area of 40 to 100 Hz/area of 0 to 40 Hz within QRS complex when tested less than 4 years after therapy, 25% when tested from 5-8 years after therapy and 56% when tested from 9-12 years after therapy.

4 DISCUSSION

Untill now, optimal strategy for posttherapy cardiac monitoring of patients treated with potentially cardiotoxic anticancer agents has not been accepted. Many studies have demonstrated that detection of abnormal time and frequency-domain parameters in the terminal part and within the whole QRS complex is helpful in differentiation of patients with normal and abnormal myocardial architecture and also in identification of arrhythmia-prone patients in various clinical settings (6,7). Because anthracycline-induced heart failure and fatal arrhythmias are associated with microstructural alterations in ventricular architecture, signal-averaged ECG (SAECG) revealing such discrete myocardial abnormalities in various clinical settings, might be also helpful in cardiac risk stratification of cancer survivors. To our knowledge only two previously published studies have analyzed the usefulness of time-domain SAECG in detection of cardiac effects of anthracycline cytostatics. We are not aware of the existence of any study using frequency-domain SAECG analysis in monitoring of anthracyline therapy.

5 CONCLUSION

We can conclude that chemotherapy with anthracyclines, even in recommended dosage, is associated with increased incidence of frequency-domain SAECG abnormalities. These abnormalities may perhaps represents the initial stage of anthracycline-induced cardiac damage. The potential of this noninvasive method to detect progressive subclinical cardiac alterations and facilitate prognostic stratification of cancer survivors is promising, however, must be established in a larger and longer study with concurrent Holter monitoring, echocardiography, resp. radionuclide angiography.

REFERENCES

1. Lipshultz, S.E., Colan, S.D., Gelber, R.D., Perez-Atayde, A.K., Sallan, S.E., Sanders, S.P. Late cardiac effects of doxorubicin therapy for acute lymphoblastic leukemia in childhood. New Engl J Med, 324, 1991,808-815.
2. Steinherz, L.J., Steinherz, P.G., Tan, Ch.T.C., Heller, G., Murphy, L. Cardiac toxicity 4 to 20 years after completing anthracycline therapy. JAMA, 266, 1991,1672-77.
3. Steinherz, L.J., Steinherz, P.G., Tan, Ch. Cardiac failure and dysrrhythmias 6 -19 years after anthracycline therapy: A series of 15 patients. Med Ped Oncol., 24, 1995,352-361.
4. Steinherz, L.J. Anthracycline cardiomyopathy - a growing clinical concern. Proceedings from Satellite Symposium during the 28th International Society of Paediatric Oncology Meeting in Vienna, Austria, 1996, 8-9.
5. Davis, L.E., Brown, C.E. Peripartum heart failure in a patient treated previously with doxorubicin. Obstet. Gynecol., 71, 3 pt 2, 1988, 506-508.
6. Kinoshita, O., Fontaine, G., Rosas, F., Elias, J., Iwa, T., Tonet, J., Lascaut, G., Frank, R. Time- and frequency-domain analyses of the signal-averaged ECG in patients with arrhythmogenic right ventricular dysplasia. Circulation., 91, 1995, 715-721.
7. Keeling, P.J., Kulakowski, P. Yi. G., Slade, A.K.B., Bent, S.E., McKenna, W.J. Usefulness of signal-averaged electrocardiogram in dilated cardiomyopathy for identifying patients with ventricular arrhythmias. Am J Cardiol, 72, 1993, 78-84.

IV. Body Surface Potential Mapping

SPHERICAL-QUASIEPICARDIUM POTENTIAL MAPPING IN ESTIMATION OF SURGICAL TREATMENT FOR WOLFF-PARKINSON-WHITE SYNDROME

L.I.TITOMIR., V.G.TRUNOV, E.A.I.AIDU, N.E.BARINOVA
Institute for Problems of Information Transmission,
Russian Acad. Sci., B. Karetny 19,
Moscow 101447, Russia

I.P.POLJAKOVA, A.Sh.REVISHVILI
Bakulev Institute of Cardiovascular Surgery,
Russian Acad. Med. Sci., Leninsky prosp. 8,
Moscow 117049, Russia

This study demonstrates possibilities of a straightforward estimation of changes in the ventricular depolarization process after surgical treatment in patients with WPW syndrome, using noninvasive mapping of the potential on a spherical quasiepicardium. The method is illustrated with several cases of WPW syndrome observed before and after the radiofrequency ablation procedure.

1. Introduction

The body surface potential mapping has proved itself in topical diagnosis of preexcitation sites in patients with WPW syndrome (e.g., see [1]). However, a straightforward estimation of the depolarization events in the heart from the body surface potential distribution itself is complicated, because the measurement region is situated asymmetrically with respect to the electric generator region (excitable myocardium), thereby a simple correspondence between the body surface potential maps and the spatial configuration of the generator is distorted. An approach to overcome this difficulty is based on transformation of the measured body surface potential into the potential produced by the same generator on a sphere concentric with and completely enclosing the heart, i.e., on the so-called spherical quasiepicardium.

An analysis of the quasiepicardium potential distributions in patients undergoing a surgical treatment for ventricular preexcitation can be used to assess the results of operation.

2. Subjects and Methods

We observed 10 men and women, aged 10 to 43 years, with WPW syndrome identified by invasive electrophysiological mapping. All patients were treated by radiofrequency catheter ablation. The initial data of body surface potential were acquired by means of the 80-lead device CARDIAG 128.1 (VELTECH Ltd., Czechia) prior to the treatment procedure and several days after the procedure. Then the potential distributions on the spherical quasiepicardium were calculated using the multipole expansion. In addition, a projection of a hypothetical major depolarization front onto the quasiepicardium was determined (the required mathematical relations are given in [2]).

Several lower-order multipole components of the cardioelectric generator are calculated from synchronous multiple-lead measurements of the potential on the body surface and coordinates of this surface approximated by a standard torso model. Then the potential on the spherical quasiepicardium with an optimal radius is calculated from the multipole components. The quasiepicardium center is placed at the ventricle geometrical center determined from the X-ray picture or from empirical relationships for given external parameters of the chest. The medium is assumed to be a homogeneous conductor inside of the quasiepicardium with mean conductivity of the body, and to be nonconducting outside of it (the exposed heart condition). Our previous investigations on simplified mathematical models of the cardioelectric generator (combinations of double-layers during depolarization and distributed sources during repolarization) showed that under the aforementioned conditions the multipole expansion terms of three lower orders, namely, the dipole, quadrupole, and octupole, suffice to obtain a reasonable accuracy of potential approximation (comparable with the actual errors of the measurement procedure).

The region on the quasiepicardium where the hypothetical depolarization front is projected is defined by the absolute values of potential exceeding a level Δ_t which for the time instant t is calculated by the formula

$$\Delta_t = \delta + 0.5(U_{Mt} - \delta)\left[1 + \frac{(U_M - U_{Mt})^2}{U_M^2}\right],$$

where δ is the peak-to-peak noise threshold, U_M is the global peak-to-peak potential maximum over the quasiepicardium surface and ventricle depolarization time interval, and U_{Mt} is the instantaneous peak-to-peak potential maximum over the quasiepicardium at t. The potential is measured from the global minimum if the absolute value of the global maximum exceeds that of the global minimum, and measured from the global maximum otherwise.

The instantaneous quasiepicardium potential distributions with the depolarization front projections indicated (instantaneous depolarization topograms, abbreviated as IDT) are depicted in the form of plane maps preserving the elementary areas of the quasiepicardium, with the heart anatomical landmarks projected onto the same surface.

A conventional approach to qualitative, as well as quantitative, interpretation of the potential distribution is based on an evaluation of the potential extrema. Therefore the mathematical description of the potential distribution should retain the total number and absolute values of the potential maxima and minima with an allowed accuracy.

Our studies on a mathematical model have shown that the proper choice of the quasiepicardium radius, which renders the structure of the true potential extrema, corresponds to the maximal eccentricity of the elementary cardioelectric generators no more than 0.42 of this radius.

The approximation can be further improved by optimally choosing the origin of the multipole expansion.

3. Results and Conclusion

The instantaneous quasiepicardium potential distributions with the depolarization front projections indicated (IDT) were depicted and comparatively estimated for the states prior to and after the treatment in each particular case. The visual estimation is based on the presumption that the negative potential or positive potential dominates in a quasiepicardium region, if the region is faced by the negative side or positive side of the depolarization front, e.g., for solitary subepicardial or subendocardial excitation focuses, respectively.

It is found that the configuration of the depolarization fronts upon the treatment has changed to that more normal, since the accessory pathway has vanished. The instantaneous body surface maps and IDT for the initial part of the QRS complex of the WPW patients are presented in Figure.

Thus, it is shown by particular clinical examples that the proposed technique of spherical quasiepicardium potential mapping with depicting the IDTs facilitates explicit visual estimation of the results of surgical treatment.

Acknowledgements

This work was in part supported by the Russian Foundation of Fundamental Research, Project No. 96–01–01080.

References

1. D.W.Benson *et al*, *Circulation*, 65, 1259 (1982).
2. L.I.Titomir, P.Kneppo, *Bioelectric and Biomagnetic Fields. Theory and Applications in Electrocardiology* (CRC Press, Boca Raton etc., 1994).

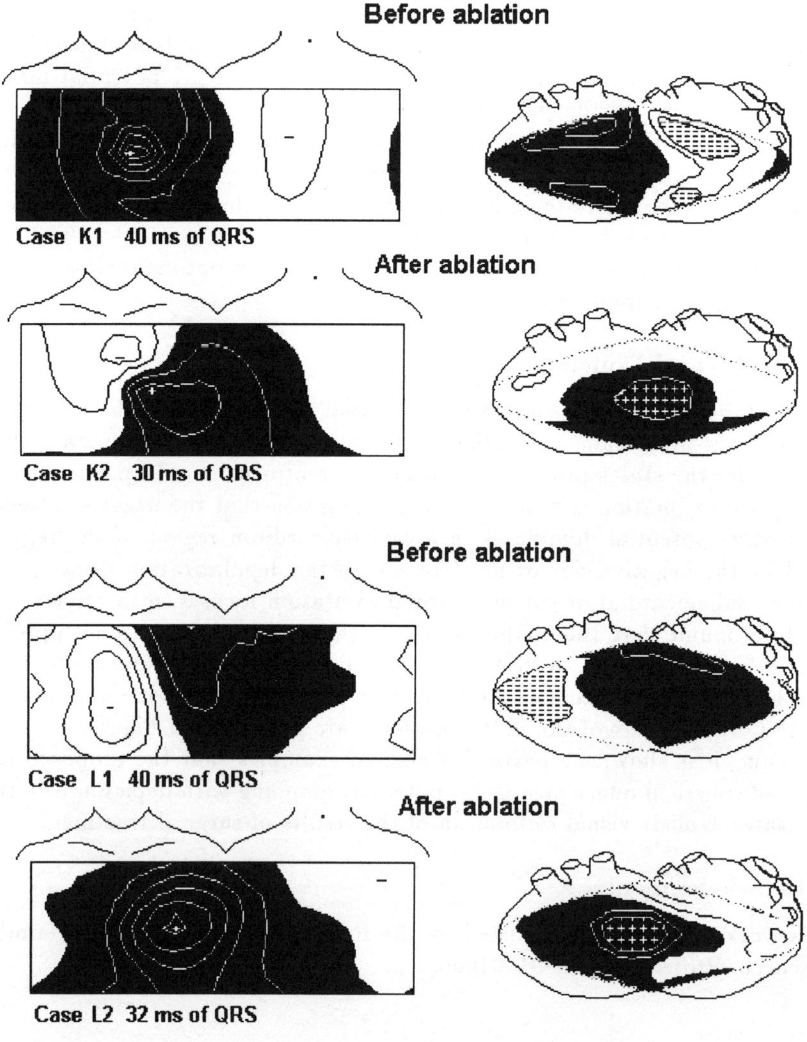

Figure: Body surface and spherical quasiepicardium potential distributions in two patients treated for WPW syndrome.

Case K, left-lateral localization of the preexcitation pathway; normalized ventricular depolarization after the operation. Case L, right-posterior-lateral localization of the preexcitation pathway; partly normalized ventricular depolarization after the operation (revealed signs of intraventricular conduction disturbances).

NONINVASIVE LOCALIZATION OF PREEXCITATION SITES USING EXPERIMENTAL BSPM DATA

M. TYŠLER, M. TURZOVÁ, J. ŠVEHLÍKOVÁ, M. TIŇOVÁ
Institute of Measurement Science SAS, Dúbravská cesta 9, 842 19 Bratislava, Slovakia
E-mail: umertysl@ savba.sk

K. KOZLÍKOVÁ
Institute of Pathophysiology, Medical Faculty, Comenius University, Sasinkova 2, 811 08 Bratislava, Slovakia
E-mail: kozlikova@med.uniba.sk

In the paper, results of preoperative noninvasive localization of single accessory pathway (AP) on the atrio-ventricular (AV) ring obtained by a model based approach are presented. Body surface potential maps (BSPM) from 9 patients were measured before rf catheter ablation (RFCA) using the 24-lead system according to Barr and submitted to the localization procedure. Two types of equivalent cardiac electric generator were used in the inverse calculations: a multiple dipole (MD) and a single "jumping" dipole (JD). In both cases analytical heart model with 39 dipole locations and realistic heart model with 29 dipole locations were used. For MD model, the maximal integral of segmental dipole moment computed over the initial 25 ms of activation was chosen as the criterion for AP localization. For JD model, the AP was localized in position where the RMS difference between measured and by JD model generated surface potentials summed over the first 25 ms was minimal. One realistically shaped inhomogeneous torso with estimated heart position and orientation were used as the patient geometry approximation.
With the analytical heart model, the MD generator approach located the AP in 4 cases correctly, in 3 cases into the first, in 2 cases into the second neighboring segment and there was no localization failure. With the JD approach, respective results were obtained in 4, 2 and 1 case, there were 2 failures. With the realistic heart model, the MD generator approach located the AP in 2 cases correctly, in 5 cases into neighboring segment and in 2 cases the localization failed. With the JD approach the respective numbers of cases were 3, 3 and 3 failures. The results indicate that the MD approach was in most cases able to determine the approximate position of the AP within predefined 11 or 12 regions on the AV ring. The success rate is in correspondence with previously reported results achieved on simulated ecg. The JD approach had difficulties to identify preexcitations in right ventricle and mid septum.

1 Background

On simulated data we have previously demonstrated[1] the ability of multiple dipole based inverse localization method to identify single accessory pathway (AP) under realistic conditions (noise in ecg 5 mV, inaccuracy of heart position less than 1 cm). Satisfactory localization with mean localization error of 1.7 cm and 86% of AP located into correct or first neighboring segment was achieved when ecg from 63 leads were used. For simulated ecg from 24 leads (electrode positions according to

Barr), the mean localization error was 2.8 cm and 65% of AP were localized near the exact position. The aim of this study was to test the performance of the method on available real ecg data.

2 Method and Material

Two cardiac electric generator models: multiple dipole (MD) and "jumping dipole" (JD) were examined for noninvasive localization of single AP. For both generators, two different heart shapes were used: analytically defined heart divided into 39 segments (22 of them in the basal level) and realistic heart divided into 29 segments.

For the MD model, real cardiac generator was approximated by a set of dipoles located in the centers of predefined heart segments. Components of segmental dipole moments $\boldsymbol{M}$ were estimated from surface potentials $\boldsymbol{\Phi}$ using the formula $\boldsymbol{M}=\boldsymbol{T}^{+}\boldsymbol{\Phi}$. The pseudo-inverse matrix $\boldsymbol{T}^{+}$ was obtained using the truncated singular value decomposition of the transfer matrix $\boldsymbol{T}$, which represents the relationship between torso geometry used in the computations and segmental dipoles[2]. The maximal integral of segmental dipole moment computed over the initial 25 ms of activation was considered to indicate the segment with earliest activation containing the initial activation point.

For the JD model, single best fitting dipole was calculated at each possible source location for initial 25 ms of activation. For all dipole locations, the RMS errors between the measured ecg and ecg corresponding to the obtained dipole was computed. The dipole with minimal sum of RMS errors over the 25 ms interval was selected as the best "jumping dipole" approximation of the real generator.

In the inverse computations, one realistically shaped torso model with main electrical inhomogeneities (lungs, heart cavities) and with heart position defined for each heart geometry was used as the approximation of chest geometry of all patients.

Body surface potential maps (BSPM) from 9 patients (3 male, 6 female, age 18 to 51) who later underwent successful RFCA were measured using the 24-lead system according to Barr and submitted to the noninvasive localization. In 5 patients, basic torso dimensions were measured and individual chest circularity C_i defined as the ratio between antero-lateral and left-right torso diameter was computed. Similarity between individual geometry and the model torso was estimated by the ratio C_i/C_m, where C_m is the circularity of the model torso. No geometry data was available for the other 4 patients.

Successful RFCA indicated left lateral (LL) AP in 4 patients, left antero-lateral (LAL) AP in 2 patients, left postero-lateral (LPL), right lateral (RL) and mid-septal (MS) AP in 1 patient.

3 Results and Discussion

Results of the noninvasive localization using the analytical heart model (Fig. 1) are summarized in Table 1. The MD generator approach located the AP in 45% cases correctly, in 33% cases into the first, in 22% cases into the second neighboring segment and no localization failed. With the JD approach, respective results were 45%, 22%, 11% and 22% of failures.

Results with the realistic heart model (Fig. 2) are summarized in Table 2. The MD generator approach located the AP in 22% cases correctly, in 56% cases into the neighboring segment and in 22% cases the localization failed. With the JD approach, respective results were 33%, 33% and 33% of failures.

The localization results were less satisfactory in patients with torso shapes more different from the used torso model (C_i/C_m ratio differing from 1).

In one patient, localization at individual time instant before the end of delta wave gave correct result, while the standard 25 ms interval failed. In some patients, individual selection of evaluated time interval would probably improve the localization results.

Similar results were obtained when homogeneous torso model was used in inverse calculations, the number of localization failures did not increase.

Reconstruction of full grid maps (in 15 x 10 points) and inverse computations from 150 approximated leads did not improve the localization results.

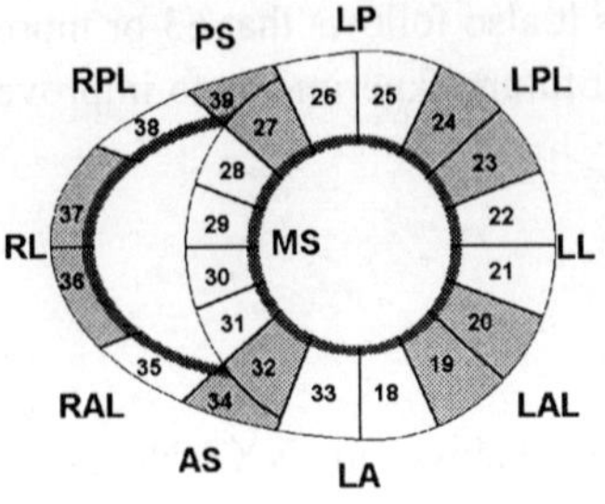

Figure 1: Segmentation of the analytically defined heart in the A V plane.

*Table 1: Results of localization in the analytically defined heart using MD and JD model. In cases marked with *, the second or third maximal dipole (first located in the A V plane) was taken. Failures of localization are shaded.*

patient	Ci/Cm ratio	AP site	segment	localized MD	localized JD
FA45	0.88	LPL	23-24	21 *	23
F460	1.02	LL	21-22	21	22
F530	1.03	LL	21-22	19 *	20
F780	1.06	LL	21-22	21	20
AF49	0.82	LAL	19-20	20 *	22
BISC	-	LL	21-22	21	21
SCHN	-	LAL	19-20	21 *	20
FICH	-	RL	36-37	35	33
BICH	-	MS	28-31	35 *	18

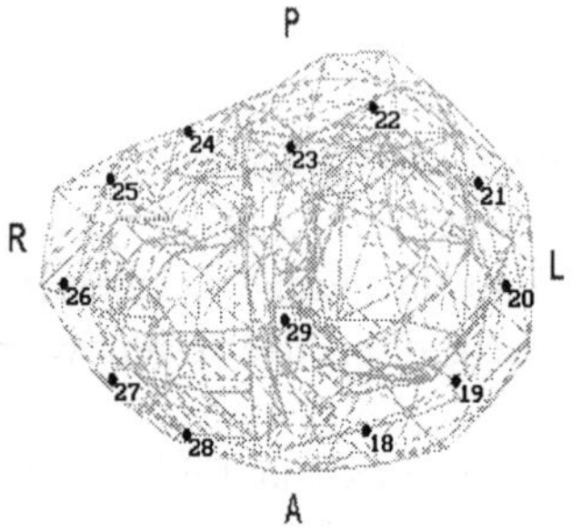

Figure 2: Segmentation of the realistic heart model in the AV plane.

*Table 2: Results of localization in the realistic heart using MD and JD model. In case marked by * second maximal dipole (first in AV plane) was taken, in case + individual time interval was used, failures of localization are shaded.*

patient	Ci/Cm ratio	AP site	segment	localized MD	localized JD
FA45	0.88	LPL	21	21+	21
F460	1.02	LL	20	21	21
F530	1.03	LL	20	19 *	20
F780	1.06	LL	20	21	20
AF49	0.82	LAL	19	28	21*
BISC	-	LL	20	26	21
SCHN	-	LAL	19	19 *	20
FICH	-	RL	26	25	18
BICH	-	MS	29	28	19

4 Conclusions

The presented results indicate that the MD approach was in most cases able to determine the position of the AP within 11 or 12 regions on the AV ring. The JD approach had difficulties to identify preexcitations in right ventricle and mid septum.

The success rate was in correspondence with previously reported results achieved on simulated ecg data. From the simulations it also follows that 63 or more leads and individual torso geometry should be tried in future experiments to improve the localization accuracy.

References

1. M. Tyšler, M. Turzová, J. Švehlíková, M. Tiňová in XX. Neumann Kollokvium, ed. Gy.Kozmann (NJSZT, Budapest 1996).
2. R.M. Gulrajani, F.A. Roberge, P.Y. Savard eds., Comprehensive Electrocardiology (Pergamon Press, New York 1989).

Acknowledgments

Presented work was supported by grant 1216/97 from the Scientific Grant agency of the Slovak Republic.

THE INCIDENCE OF MULTIPOLAR DISTRIBUTION IN THE BODY SURFACE QRST ISOINTEGRAL MAPS IN PATIENTS WITH POSTINFARCTION LEFT VENTRICULAR ANEURYSM

D. JAGIELSKI[1], D. KAŁKA[2], W. BANASIAK[2], T. HIRNLE[3],
M. SOBIESZCZAŃSKA[1], K. NAMIĘTA[3], A. FUGLEWICZ[2],
A. TELICHOWSKI[2], K. WIĘCH[2]

[1] *Department of Patophysiology, Wroclaw University of Medicine, Marcinkowskiego 1, 50-368 Wroclaw, Poland*
[2] *Department of Cardiology, Military Hospital, Weigla 4, 53-114 Wroclaw, Poland*
[3] *Department of Cardiosurgery, Wroclaw University of Medicine, Sklodowskiej-Curie 58, 50-368 Wroclaw, Poland*

The multipolar distribution of QRST isointegral maps (I-maps) has been proposed to be an indicator of regional disparity of recovery properties playing important role in the genesis of ventricular arrhythmias. The purpose of this study was to evaluate the usefulness of the body surface I-maps in detecting regional disparity of recovery properties in patients with left ventricular aneurysm and to compare them with the I-maps acquired from the same patients after surgical intervention.

15 subjects (12 men, 3 women) in II-IV NYHA class (mean age 57±8 years; 1 with one vessel disease; 12 with two vessels disease and 1 with three vessels disease) were examined. The diagnosis of left ventricular aneurysm was confirmed by echocardiography and ventriculography testing. Body surface potential mapping system HPM-7100 Fukuda Denshi was used in this study. The surface potentials were measured simultaneously from 87 electrodes arranged over the torso (59 on anterior and 28 on posterior chest wall) with Wilson's central terminal as a reference. The QRST I-maps with 3 or more extrema were considered abnormal and described as multipolar. Each subject underwent left ventricular reconstruction surgery using Jatene`s or Dor`s technique with coronary artery bypass grafting. Body surface I-maps were recorded again within 4-8 weeks after surgical intervention.

Results: As compared to the control group (35 age-matched subjects) demonstrating in the whole a dipolarity of QRST I-maps, multipolar distribution in the QRST I-maps was observed in 7 of 15 (46.7%) patients with ventricular aneurysm before surgery. The mean number of extrema found per QRST I-map was 4.1±1.13. After cardiac surgery procedures the incidence of the multipolar distribution in the QRST I-map was as follows: 0 of 15 patients (0%) with $p<0.001$ as compared to results before surgery.

Conclusions: Patients with left ventricle aneurysm tend to have multipolar distribution in QRST I-maps. Cardiac surgery seems to alleviate the multipolar content in the QRST I-map. Body surface potential mapping may provide a new and noninvasive tool to detect a substrate for cardiac arrhythmias and to improve the evaluation of the results of surgical treatment in the patients with postinfarction left ventricular aneurysm.

Introduction

A body surface potential mapping (BSPM) has been proved to be a very interesting noninvasive approach to study cardiac electric field which offers many advantages over a conventional 12-lead electrocardiography. BSPM is more sensitive to regional cardiac events, puts emphasis on spatial features of cardiac field and allows evaluation of cardiac equivalent generator models.

Many attempts have been made to search for the correlation between the multipolar distribution of QRST isointegral maps (I-maps) and regional disparity of recovery properties which play important role in the genesis of ventricular arrhythmias (1-5). It is well known that the patients with postinfarction left ventricular aneurysm are at higher risk for lifethreatening arrhythymias than other survivals of myocardial infarction.

There is very limited data available concerning the value of BSPM in evaluation of patients with ventricular aneurysm (6). The aim of the present study was to assess the usefulness of body surface potential mapping in detecting regional disparity of recovery properties in patients with left ventricular aneurysm and to compare the I-maps before and after surgical intervention in order to confirm a good result of the surgery.

Material

A group of 15 subjects (12 male and 3 females) in II-IV NYHA class (mean age 57±8 years; 1 with one vessel disease; 12 with two vessels disease and 1 with three vessels disease) were examined. All of them had a ventricular aneurysm clearly documented by echocardiography and ventriculography testing as well as confirmed by visualization at surgery. Each subject underwent left ventricular reconstruction surgery using Jatene`s or Dor`s technique with coronary artery bypass grafting.

Patients with bundle branch block, long QT syndrome or abnormalities of serum electrolyte (K, Na, Ca, Cl) were excluded from the study. A group of 35 age-matched subjects (25 males and 10 females) with no history of documented cardiovascular system disorders were also studied as a control.

Informed consent was given by all subject before their participation in the study.

Methods

Body surface potential mapping system HPM-7100 Fukuda Denshi was used in this study. The surface potentials were measured simultaneously from 87 electrodes placed over the torso (59 on anterior and 28 on posterior chest wall) with Wilson's central terminal as a reference, at a rate of 1000 samples/sec/channel. Frank leads X, Y, Z and space magnitude lead were recorded simultaneously with body surface maps and served as reference for identification of onset and offset of the QRST interval. Standard 12-lead ECGs were also sampled when recording from 87 electrodes.

The time integrals of QRST waves were calculated at each lead as the sum of all potentials from the onset of QRS wave to the offset of the T wave and displayed by indicating as units of microvolt•seconds.

A QRST I-map with 3 or more extrema or a map with one or more pseudopods were considered abnormal and described as multipolar. Body surface I-maps were recorded again within 4-8 weeks after surgical intervention.

Each patient underwent left ventricular reconstruction surgery using Jatene`s or Dor`s technique with concomitant coronary artery bypass grafting.

Statistical analysis was performed using the Fisher's test. P value < 0.05 was considered as statistically significant.

Results

Both males and females in the control group demonstrated in the whole a smooth dipolar distribution of the QRST I-maps with positive values located over the precordium and negative values over the right chest and back. Example of the dipolar distribution is shown in Fig. 1. In contrast, the multipolar distribution in the QRST I-maps was observed in 7 of 15 (46.7%) patients with ventricular aneurysm before cardiac surgery (see Fig. 2A). The mean number of extrema found per QRST I-map was 4.1 ± 1.13.

After cardiac surgery procedure the incidence of the multipolar distribution in the QRST I-map was reduced and was presented as follows: 0 of 15 patients (0%) with $p<0.001$ as compared to results in the same patient before surgery (see Fig. 2B).

The example of the influence of cardiac surgery on distribution in the QRST I-maps is presented in Fig. 2 and 3.

Discussion

The presented results shows that the patients with left ventricle aneurysm tend to have multipolar distribution in the QRST I-maps. The QRST I-maps has been proposed to be an indicator of regional disparity of recovery properties which play important role in the genesis of ventricular arrhythmias.

Intraoperative mapping studies demonstrated that the earliest activation occurs in the endocardial border of the aneurysm indicating the origin of the arrhythmia (7). During the cardiac surgery procedure this areas are often removed which seems to alleviate the multipolar content in the QRST I-maps.

In conclusion, body surface potential mapping may provide a new and noninvasive tool in detecting a substrate for cardiac arrhythmias and to improve the evaluation of the results of surgical treatment in the patients with postinfarction left ventricular aneurysm. However, more research is needed to establish the best approach to the interpretation of nondipolar contest of the isointegral maps and to confirm our findings.

References

1. L.S. Green, *Circulation*, 66, II-337 (1982).
2. G.M. Vincent, *Circulation*, 68, III-352 (1983).
3. M.J. Gardner, *Circulation*, 73, 684 (1986).
4. H. Tsunakawa, JACC, 14, 1530 (1989).
5. L. De Ambroggi, Am J Cardiol, 68, 614, (1991).
6. C.A. Pastore, Proceedings from XXIII Congres on Electrocardiology, 44, (1996).
7. L.N. Horowitz, *Circulation*, 61, 1227 (1980).

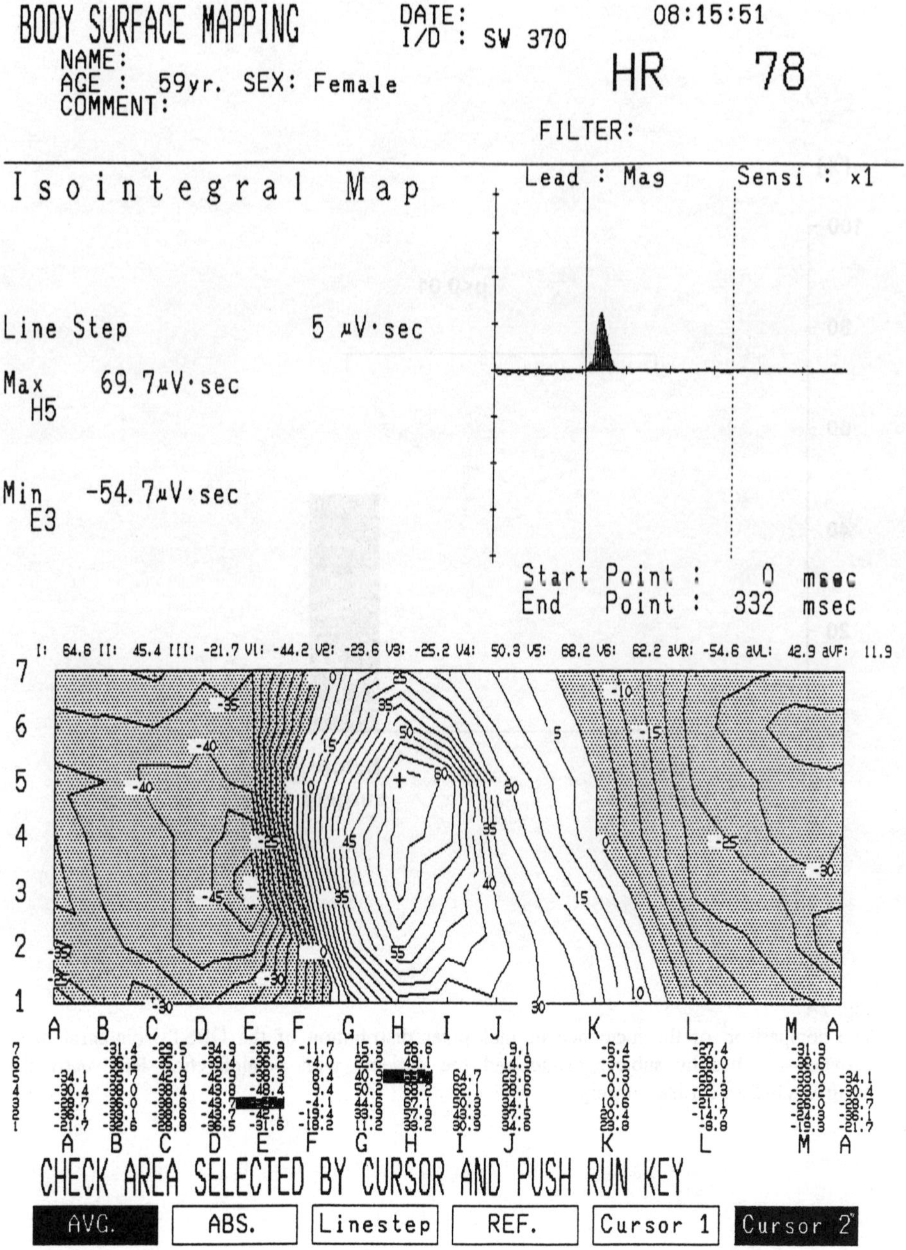

Fig. 1. Typical pattern of dipolar distribution of the QRST isointegral map in healthy subject.

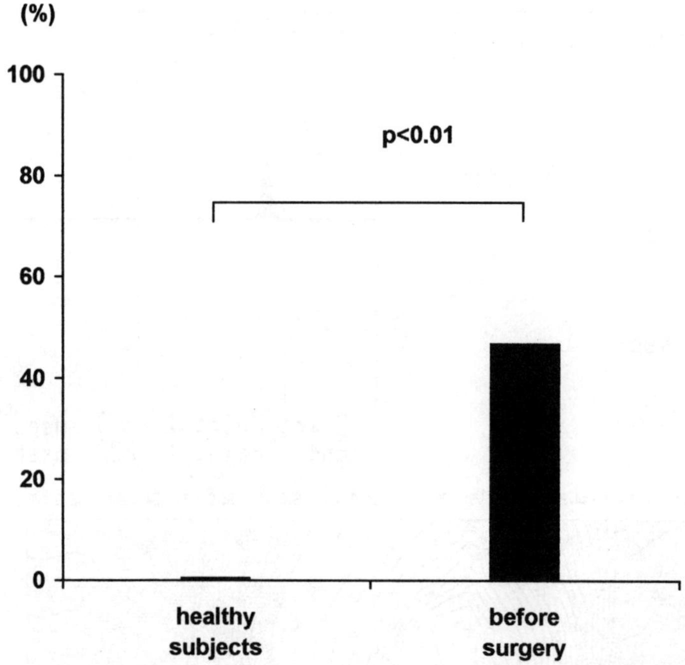

Fig. 2A
The comparison of the incidence of multipolar distribution of the QRST isointegral maps between the healthy subject group and the patients with postinfarction left ventricular aneurysm before cardiac surgery.

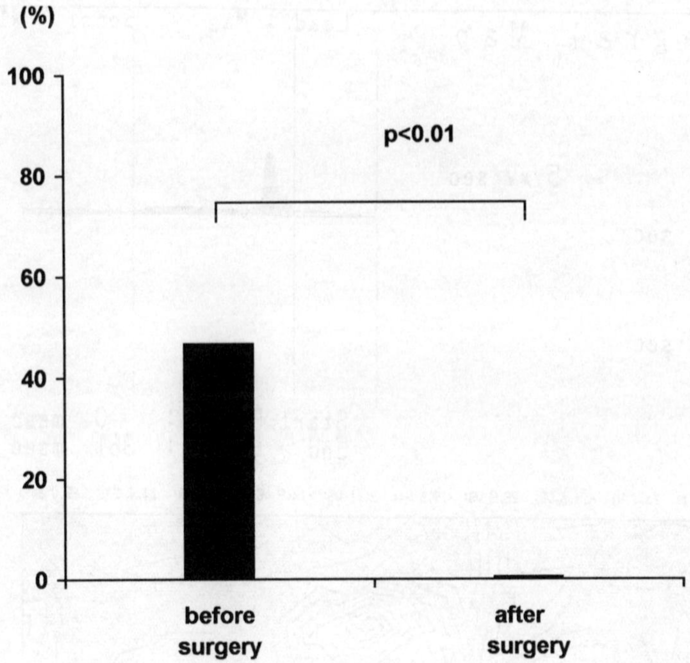

Fig. 2B
The comparison of the incidence of multipolar distribution of the QRST isointegral maps between the patients with postinfarction left ventricular aneurysm before and after cardiac surgery.

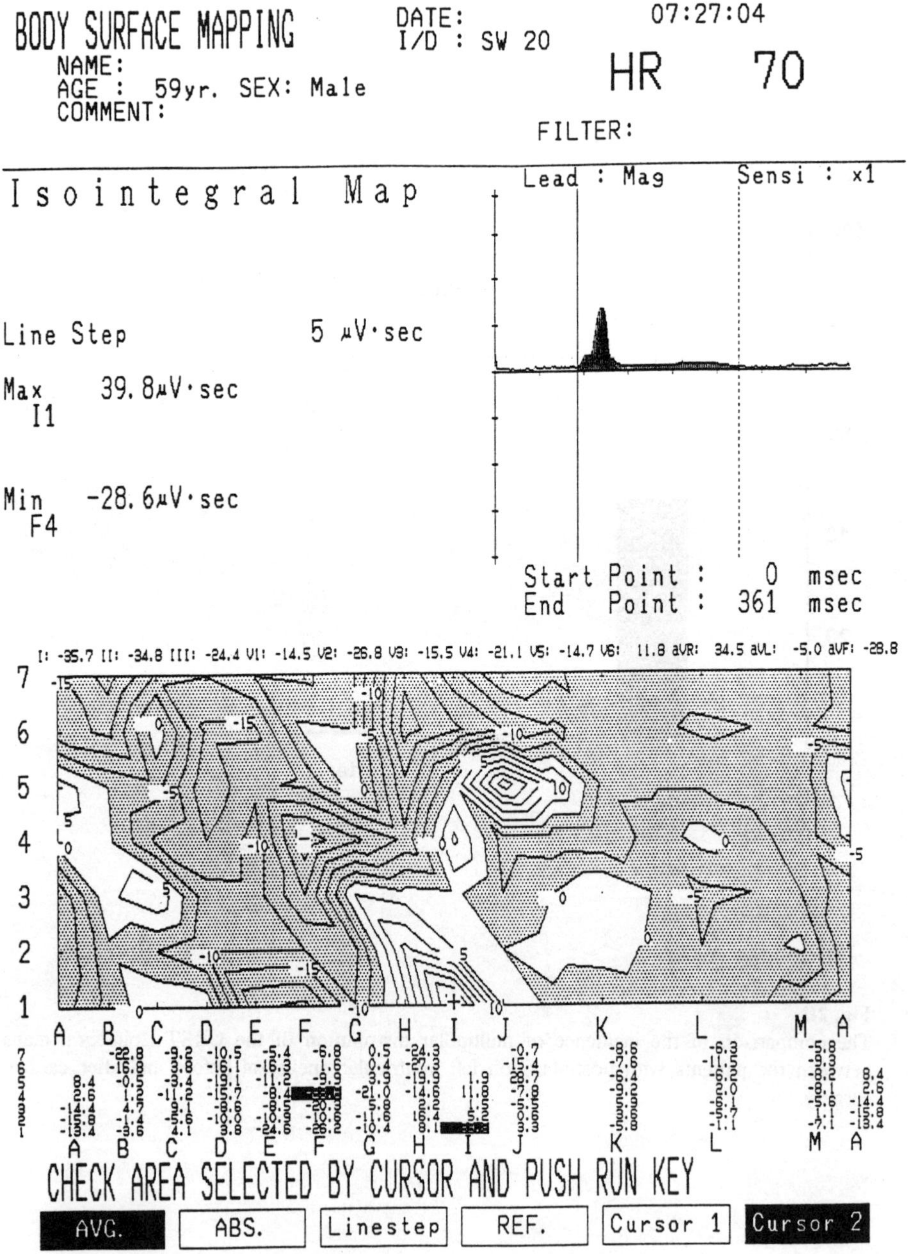

Fig. 3. Pattern of multipolar distribution of the QRST isointegral map in 59 year old patient before cardiac surgery.

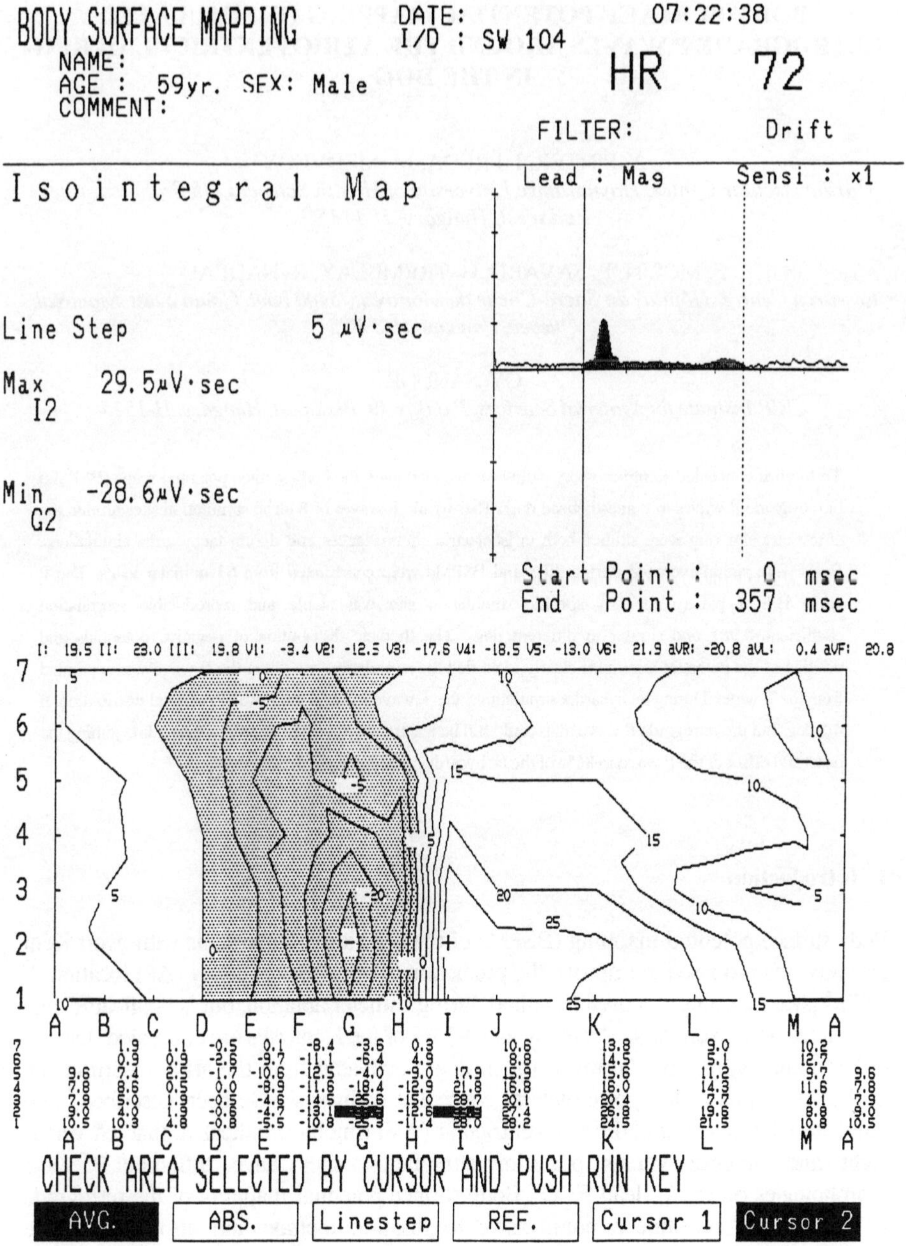

Fig. 4. Pattern of dipolar distribution of the QRST isointegral map in the same patient as in Fig. 3 but after cardiac surgery.

BODY SURFACE POTENTIAL MAPPING OF SIMULATED RETROGRADE P WAVES AROUND THE ATRIOVENTRICULAR RING IN THE DOG

A. PINTÉR, I. PRÉDA, M. MEDVEGY
Cardiovascular Center, Haynal Imre University of Health Sciences, 35 Szabolcs street, Budapest, Hungary, H-1135

F. MOLIN, P. SAVARD, G. TREMBLAY, R. NADEAU
Research Centre, Hôpital du Sacré-Coeur de Montréal, 5400 boul. Gouin ouest, Montréal, Québec, Canada H4J 1C5

GY. SÁNDOR
CRIP Institute for Material Sciences, P.o.Box 49, Budapest, Hungary, H-1525

To localize concealed Kent accessory pathways, we evaluated the body surface potential maps (BSPMs) of retrograde P waves in 8 anesthetized dogs. Retrograde P waves of 8 atrial stimulation sites around the atrioventricular ring were studied both in isoelectric circumstances and during tachycardia simulations. Beats were signal-averaged during 30 s and BSPMs were constructed from 63 unipolar leads. The P wave BSPM pattern for any specific stimulation site was stable and reproducible (correlation coefficient>0.98), and similar in different dogs. The thoracic distribution of negative potentials and position of the potential minimum clearly identified the stimulation site when the P wave was separated from the T wave. During tachycardia simulations, the T wave masked the P wave potential distribution in 4/8 dogs but the retrograde P wave map could still be accurately extracted by subtracting a line joining the onset and offset of the P wave in 86% of the tachycardia simulations in these 4 dogs.

1 Introduction

Body surface potential mapping (BSPM) of the delta wave in patients with overt Kent pathway was proposed to improve the prediction of accessory pathway (AP) location.[1-5] BSPM pace mapping is a useful method during catheter ablation, but is applicable only to patients with overt APs.[6] As many as 20-30% of the Kent APs are concealed. During orthodromic tachycardia however, the atria are activated from the atrial insertion site of the AP. Signs of left posterolateral concealed pathways have been described,[7] and atrial stimulations around the atrioventricular (AV) ring have indicated, that left versus right and anterior versus posterior stimulation sites have different P wave morphologies on the 12-lead ECG.[8] Body surface potential mapping of the retrograde P wave could constitute a noninvasive localisation method and also could guide ablation at the atrial insertion site in patients with concealed APs.

A major difficulty of the P wave BSPM is its small potential in comparison to the ventricular potentials. Therefore, first we investigated the BSPMs of simulated retrograde P waves separated from the T wave in a dog model. The aims of this study were to determine: 1) the reliability of retrograde P wave detection with BSPM, 2) the BSPM patterns corresponding to different AP sites and 3) the effects of T wave potentials on the detection of the retrograde P wave during tachycardia.

2 Methods

2.1 *Canine preparations and experimental protocol*

Eight mongrel dogs of both sexes weighing 22 to 30 kg were anesthetized and median sternotomy was performed. Eight pairs of silver wire electrodes were sutured to the atrial epicardium along the AV ring in anterior, anterolateral, posterolateral and posterior positions on both atria with a distance of 15 to 40 mm. Then the chest was closed and the body surface mapping electrodes were mounted on the shaved torso. Surface ECG (standard lead II), heart rate, right ventricular electrogram and systemic arterial pressure were recorded.

Orthodromic reentry was simulated by atrial stimulation coupled to the detected ventricular activation. Long coupling time stimulations (250-300 ms) resulted in retrograde P wave occurring after the preceding T wave. Short coupling time stimulations (100-130 ms) simulated tachycardias (P wave occurring during the preceding T wave). The protocol was approved by the local Animal Care Committee.

2.2 *Body surface potential mapping*

The body surface potentials were measured with 63 unipolar leads referenced to the Wilson central terminal using the Montréal configuration.[9] The signals were amplified by programmable-gain amplifiers with 0.05-450 Hz bandwidth, sampled at 1000 sample/sec and converted to a 12 bit format. Signal averaging of a 30 sec period (40-80 beats) was used to improve the signal-to-noise ratio and to eliminate beat-to-beat variability in P wave morphology. After baseline correction, isopotential maps were generated at every 1 ms starting from the beginning of the P wave. On these maps, the torso surface is represented by a rolled-out cylinder cut along the right midaxillary line.

3 Results

3.1 *P wave potential mapping when P wave is separated from T wave*

Retrograde P wave duration was 60-85 ms. During the middle of the P wave the BSPM pattern was stable for at least 15 ms. This map was selected as the typical pattern for that specific stimulation site. The correlation coefficient for repeated stimulation with slightly shorter coupling time was always higher than 0.98.

3.2 Comparison of BSPM patterns for different stimulation sites

The map for each stimulation site from a representative preparation is shown in Figure 1. The distribution of negative potentials and location of the minimum reflects the location of the stimulation site: negativity over the inferior part of the map reflecting posterior sites; over the superior part for anterior sites; over the left part for right sites and over the right part for left sites. The maps of neighbouring stimulation sites could always be discriminated visually. Quantitatively, the correlation coefficient of neighbouring maps was always below 0.90. The corresponding maps from different dogs were qualitatively similar to these maps.

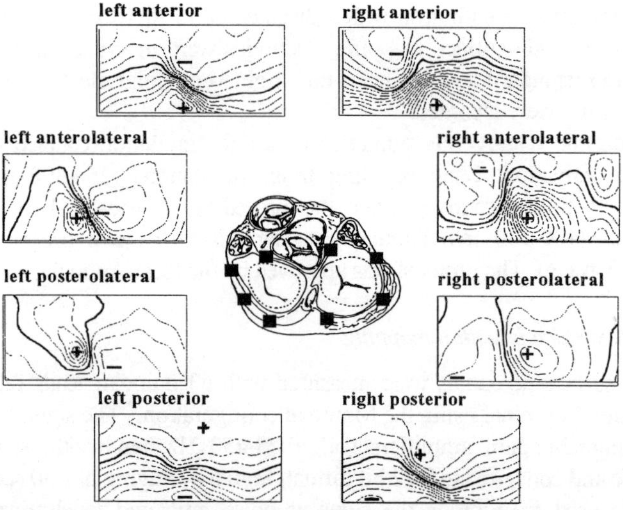

Figure 1: BSPM patterns for free wall retrograde P waves separated from the T wave. Isoline: 30 mV, heavy line: zero isopotential line, +/-: location of the maximum/minimum

3.3 Influence of the T wave during tachycardia

When the retrograde P wave occurred during the preceding T wave, in 4/8 of the preparations the T wave potential values (<200 mV) were in the range of the P wave potentials, and the retrograde P waves were discernable with BSPMs similar to those of presented in Figure 1. In the other 50% of the preparations the T wave potential values were significantly higher (400-500 mV) and the T wave masked the P wave. In these cases the baseline was corrected by subtracting a line joining the onset and offset of the P wave. With this subtraction technique, in 24 of the 28 stimulation sites (86%) in these 4 dogs, the map pattern indicated the correct stimulation site.

4 Discussion

Map reproducibility (corr. coeff.>0.98) and the existence of a stable map pattern throughout the middle of the P wave are important features for reliable retrograde P wave mapping. The reproducibility at different cycle lengths suggests that maps recorded during orthodromic tachycardia would be comparable to those recorded after atrial stimulation during pace mapping regardless of the cycle length of the stimulation. The stability of the typical pattern throughout at least a 15 ms period during the middle of the P wave is helpful as it makes it unnecessary to determine the exact onset of the P wave, which would be difficult during orthodromic tachycardia.

The retrograde P wave BSPM patterns for different stimulation sites are similar to those for ventricular preexcitation at corresponding sites.[10] With this method, the location (right or left, anterior, anterolateral, posterolateral or posterior) of free wall AP can be determined. However, the T wave can mask the BSPM pattern of the retrograde P wave during tachycardia. In our experiments, a simple subtraction method helped to extract the correct BSPM pattern of the retrograde P wave in 86% of these cases.

Acknowledgements

This study was supported by grant from the Medical Research Council of Canada and partly by grant No. F 021147 from the National Research Found (OTKA).

References

1. K. Yamada et al., *Am. Heart J.* **90**, 721 (1975).
2. L. de Ambroggi et al., *Circulation* **54**, 251 (1976).
3. R.A. Nadeau et al. in *Electrocardiographic Body Surface Potential Mapping*, eds. R.T. van Dam and A. van Oosterom (Martinus Nijhoff, Boston, 1986).
4. M. Lorange and R. Gulrajani, *Trans. Biomed. Eng.* **33**, 862 (1986).
5. C. Giorgi et al., *Am. Heart J.* **121**, 1445 (1991).
6. M. Dubuc et al., *Circulation* **87**, 135 (1993).
7. P. Puech and R. Grolleau, *Arch. Mal. Coeur* **70**, 49 (1977).
8. D.M. Fitzgerald et al., *J. Electrocardiol.* **29**, 1 (1996).
9. P. Savard et al., *J. Electrocardiol.* **18**, 211 (1985).
10. D.W. Benson et al., *Circulation* **65**, 1259 (1982).

CARDIAC ELECTRIC FIELD ON VENTRICULAR EPICARDIUM AND BODY SURFACE IN THE DOG UNDER VENTRICULAR ENDOCARDIAL STIMULATION

K.K. MOSTIVENKO, M.P. ROSHCHEVSKY, D.N. SHMAKOV,
I.M.ROSHCHEVSKAYA, T.V. KIRUSHEVA
Institute of Physiology of the Komi Science Centre, Ural Division, Russian Academy of Sciences, Syktyvkar, Komi, Russia
E-mail: compcard@online.ru

V.P. NUZHNY
The Komi Republic Cardiological Centre, Syktyvkar, Komi, Russia

The reflection of ectopic activation sequence on the cardiac electric field on the torso we studied by comparison between epicardial potential map (EPM) and body surface potential map (BSPM) under identical pacing foci at corresponding time instants of ventricular depolarization. Ectopic foci were produced by the use of electrical stimulation.

1 Introduction

Investigation of the ventricular excitation wave spread with a known source of ectopic activation is necessary for addressing the forward problem of electrocardiology both in mathematical simulations and in clinical practice.

2 Methods

Experiments were performed on 15 adult mongrel dogs anaesthetized with sodium pentobarbital. The trachea was intubated and the lungs were ventilated by a pump respirator. The chest was open through the left thoracotomy. The heart was exposed and suspended in pericardial cradle. Electric cardiac field under various right endocardial pacing sites was investigated with epicardial and body surface potential mapping. Isopotential and isochronal maps were constructed on the basis of 64 simultaneously recorded electrocardiosignals. Duration of ectopic ventricular activation was determined with respect to artifact of stimulus. The electrodes were distributed regularly over the heart ventricles' and torso surfaces. Epicardial electrode array was performed in the form of grid. Electrical stimuli were delivered by the use of the catheter inserted through the right jugular vein in the right ventricular cavity and by means of intramural needle electrodes. Extrasystoles were produced by single restangular impulses (amplitude 0,4 - 2 V, duration 2 ms).

3 Results

3.1 Sequence of the epicardial ventricular depolarization under ectopic excitation

The epicardial potential distributions and the sequence of epicardial activation under various ectopic foci were analyzed. The excitation breakthrough on the epicardium appeared approximately in the site of epicardial projection of the endocardial stimulation area in 16±2,2 ms after delivering of the ventricular stimulus (fig. 1). Under the epicardial stimulation the earliest activation was observed in the area of pacing site with latent period 11±1,1 ms. The significant slowing-down of depolarization wave spread occured in the area of the interventricular septum projection onto the epicardium. The higher density of isochronal and isopotential lines in this area in comparison with that on the epicardium of free ventricular walls confirms it. This phenomenon was more expressed under stimulation of the right ventricle as compared with that of the left one and wasn't expressed under the stimulation of the interventricular septum. The contralateral ventricle was excited first in the apical area, then ventricular depolarization on epicardium had been completed in the base of this ventricle.

The stimulation of free ventricular walls was characterized by successive spread of excitation wave from the zone of pacing, while at the pacing of interventricular septum there was a complicated spread of depolarization wave with several epicardial breakthroughs and a significant shift of areas of breakthroughs in respect to the pacing site.

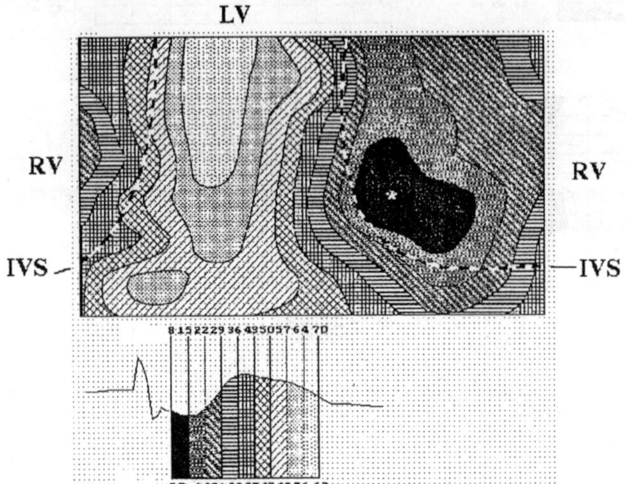

Figure 1: Chronotopographic map of activation sequence of right ventricle under endocardial stimulation. Dotted line - the projection of interventricular septum onto the epicardium, reference time point is artifact of stimulus (ms), RV - right ventricle, LV - left ventricle, IVS - interventricular septum, * - pacing site.

3.2 Relationship between potential distributions over torso and ventricular surfaces under ectopic foci in the right ventricle

The excitation spread from endocardium towards epicardium forms a maximum on the epicardium as well as on the body surface. The location of this maximum corresponds to the projection of the pacing site onto the body and heart surfaces. The right ventricular breakthrough of the excitation resulted in a clearcut potential minimum development on EPMs in 12-16 ms after the stimulation onset (fig.2). At that moment a simple potential pattern with a minimum, corresponding to the stimulation site, over projection of the right ventricle and with a maximum over that of the left ventricle is forming on body surface.

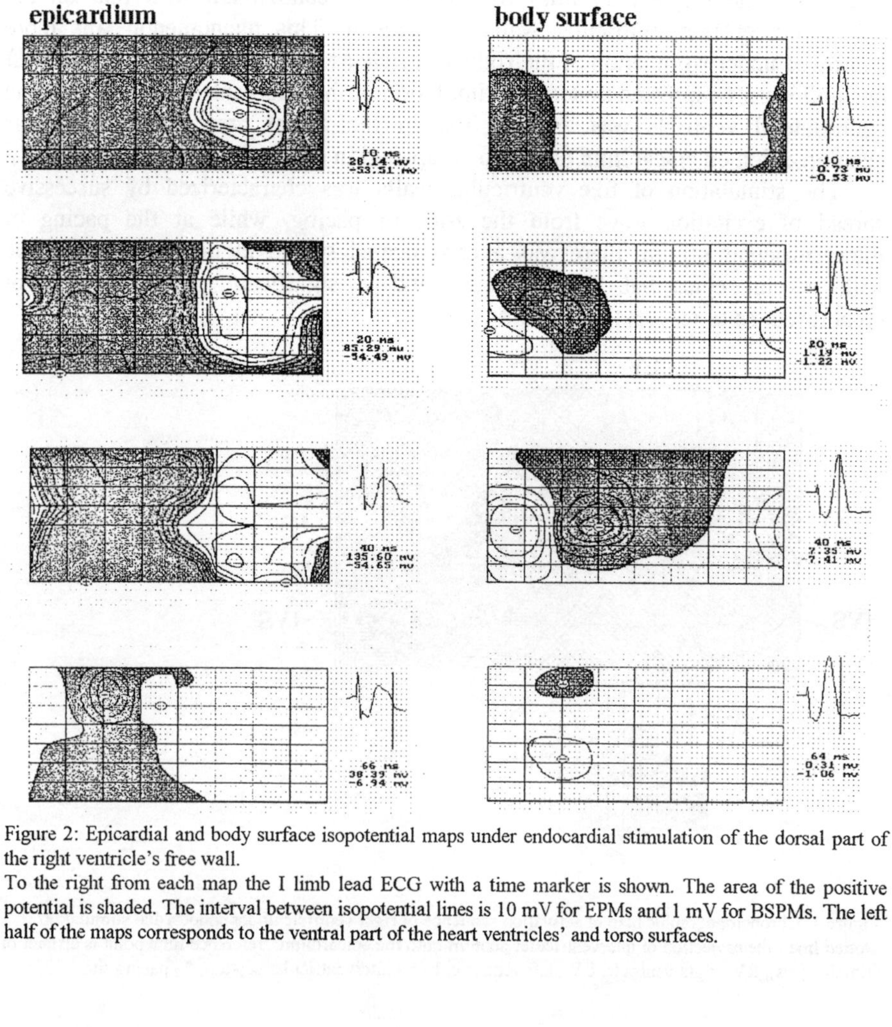

Figure 2: Epicardial and body surface isopotential maps under endocardial stimulation of the dorsal part of the right ventricle's free wall.

To the right from each map the I limb lead ECG with a time marker is shown. The area of the positive potential is shaded. The interval between isopotential lines is 10 mV for EPMs and 1 mV for BSPMs. The left half of the maps corresponds to the ventral part of the heart ventricles' and torso surfaces.

Under the endocardial stimulation of the dorsal part of the right ventricular free wall the positive and negative potential extrema on body surface shifts laterally and to the left. While stimulating the ventral part of the right ventricular free wall the potential extrema shifts in the same direction but to a less degree.

When the apical area of the heart is excited, an inversion of positive and negative potential zones is observed on BSPMs: the positive zone moves cranially and the negative one - caudally. Thus, the period of inversion depends on the distance between the location of the ectopic focus and the apical zone. At the moment of termination of ventricular depolarization that occurs in the base of the left ventricle the maximum on body surface is located more cranially as compared to the minimum. Duration of the process of ectopic depolarization was 66,8 ± 2,2 ms, that is approximately 160% of normal activation duration.

Variations of stimulation sites effect the spatio-temporal features of ventricular depolarization during the initial stages of excitation.

4 Conclusion

Thus, the localization of the ectopic stimulus determines the sequence of heart activation, the location of positive and negative potential zones on body surface and the period of the inversion of these zones, the place of potential extrema appearence and their shift trajectory. The determination of this parameters of cardio-electric fields permits noninvasive localization of ectopic foci in the myocardium.

CARDIAC ELECTRIC FIELD ON BODY SURFACE IN PATIENTS WITH IMPLANTED ARTIFICIAL CARDIAC PACEMAKERS

M. P. ROSHCHEVSKY, D. N. SHMAKOV, I. M. ROSHCHEVSKAYA,
T. V. KIRUSHEVA, K.K. MOSTIVENKO
Institute of Physiology of the Komi Science Centre, Ural Division, Russian Academy of Sciences, Syktyvkar, Kommunisticheskaya, 24, Komi, 167610, Russia
E-mail: compcard@online.ru

V.P. NUZHNY
The Komi Republic Cardiological Centre, Syktyvkar, Komi, Russia

The investigation of body surface potential distribution in patients with known position of the ectopic focus allows an estimation of the informativity of cardioelectric field and development of the noninvasive method of cardiac diagnostics. The body surface cardiac electric field was investigated in patients before and after an implantation of pacemaker systems functioning in regimen of the ventricular R-prohibiting stimulation (VVI) with standard parameters. Pacing was applied to the endocardium of the right ventricular apex. A current source was located subcutaneously in the right or left subclavicular areas. An analysis of the equipotential momentous maps provides a suggestion that the trajectory of the extrema shift is dependent on the pacing electrode position. On the basis of the cardiac electric field studies we may also speculate that the heart ventricular excitation waves spread from the ectopic activation focus in a myogenic way.

1 Introduction

The ECG investigation is considered to be a basic method of the implanted cardiostimulating system observation in patients. At the artificial rhythm the clinical interpretation of ECG in 12 leads is made difficult due to influence of the stimulus artifact on morphology of the QRS complex. Stability of the artificial complex form is used as a criterian of normal cardiostimulation system functioning. However, it is the sustaind deformed morphology QRS complex, that makes difficult diagnostics of pathological myocardial alterations, that can appear in patients with implanted cardiostimulators.

2 Materials and methods

Cardioelectric field was investigated on body surface in 11 patients in seven days and during a year after the artificial pacemaker had been implanted. The analysis of standard lead ECGs carried out according to NYNA classification in all the patients before pacemaker implantation did not reveal any symptoms of heart ventricles' pathology. The cardiostimulating system functioning in regimen of the ventricular R-prohibiting stimulation (VVI) with standard parameters. Pacing was applied to the endocardium of the right ventricular apex. A current source was located subcutaneously in the right or left subclavicular areas. The electrode was implanted under the visual X-ray control. Body surface potential mapping in the patients was carried out in reclining position with the aid of the original array of 64 electrodes. The leading electrodes were located regularly on human torso surface from the level of clavicles and the scapula upper third to the chest lower border.

3 Results

The complicated complex formed by the artifact of the electrical stimulas and artifitial ventricular complex with changed morphology of the initial part was registered on ECG in conventional leads at ventricular pacing cardiostimulation. Cardioelectric field on chest surface in patients with implanted cardiostimulating system is characterized by development of the negative extremum on ventral body surface in the region of medioscapular line near the chest lower border after the cardiostimulating impulse on ECG in the I limb lead. At ventricular depolarization the negative extremum is shifted from the lower border of endocardial right ventricular area of stimulation to the left shoulder or to the left-lateral surface. The negative extremum is shifted mainly to the heart apex projection on ventral body surface. At ventricular depolarization the positive extremum is developed on ventral surface in the left-lateral area of the lower and upper parts of chest, shifting further to the chest upper border. At the final period of ventricular depolarization the positive extremum is located in the left axillary or left scapular areas, the negative one is in the area of sternal or apex projections on chest ventral surface. At the initial artificial ventricular complex during the ventricular depolarization extrema shift trajectories on BSPM are significantly shorter than those at normal spread of the excitation wave, and in some patients the shift of extrema was not observed.

Cardioelectric field in dogs with the implanted artificial pacemaker was investigated to reveal mechanisms of myocardial functioning at endocardial stimulation in humans. On the basis of investigations of cardioelectric field on human torso and on body surface and ventricular epicardium in dogs with implanted cardiostimulating system there were determined four periods of ventricular activation at endocardial stimulation of the right ventricular apex (fig.1):

The first period corresponds to time from stimulus to the initial artificial ventricular complex formation on ECG in limb leads. The positive extremum is formed on canine and human body surfaces in the area of the right ventricular projection on ventral body surface. Probably, in this period in the human as well as in the canine heart the wave of excitation spreads from the zone of stimulation, located on the right ventricular endocardium to epicardium.

The second period corresponds to the upstroke phase of the artificial initial ventricular complex on ECG in limb leads. It lasts from the instant of the excitation wave breakthrough on epicardium of the right ventricle to its complete depolarization. In this period on body surface of both dogs and men with the implanted cardiostrimulating system the negative extremum is formed on the right-lateral chest surface. The positive zone is located on the left-lateral chest surface with extremum in the region of the heart apex projection.

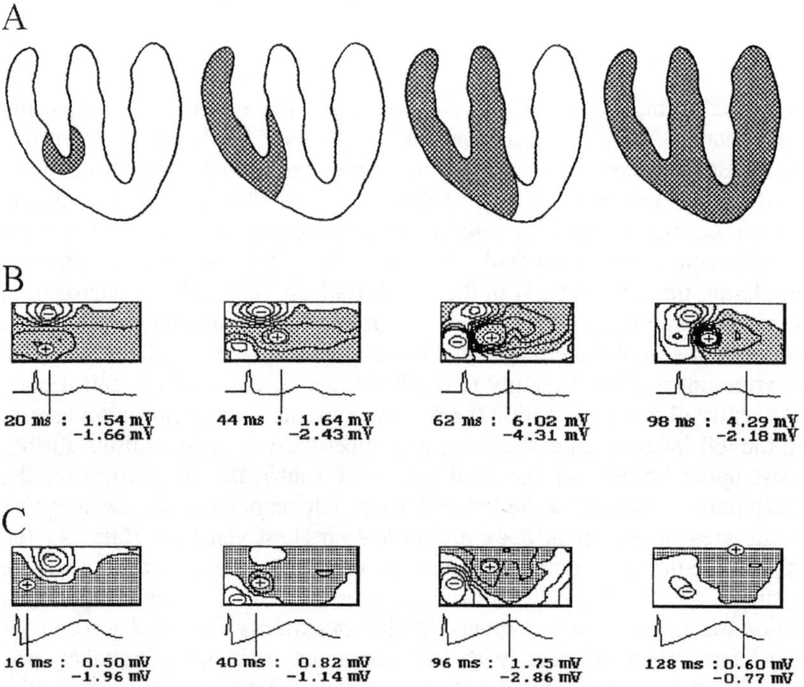

Figure 1. The relationship between the heart ventricles' depolarization sequence and body surface potential patterns under endocardial stimulation of the right ventricle.
A - the scheme of intramural activation at the time instants corresponding to the time markers on ECGs; B - equipotential momentous maps on canine body surface at time periods, corresponding to the final depolarization periods, shown by markers on ECG; C- equipotential momentous maps on chest surface in the patient with implanted cardiostimulating system at time moments, corresponding to the final depolarization periods, shown by markers on ECG.

The third period is in keeping with the apex part of the initial artificial ventricular complex on ECG in the I limb lead. Probably, it describes the slow excitation wave spread through the interventricular sternum with the excitation of His-Purkinje system. In this period general direction of the excitation wave spread on ventricular epicardium changes, that leads to reversion of positive and negative extrema zones on body surface in men and dogs with the implanted pacemarkers system.

The fourth period corresponds to the downstroke phase of the initial artificial ventricular complex on ECG in the I limb lead and, probably, reflects the excitation wave spread by the conductive system of the left ventricle. No changes in mutual location of positive and negative extrema on body surface in men and dogs with the implanted cardiostimulating system were observed.

Thus, it was shown, that we can localize the stimulation zone on endocardium of the right ventricle on the basis of position and trajectory of the positive extremum on body surface and mutual location of positive and negative potentials.

4 Discussion

It was found, that in patients with the implanted cardiostimulator there is only one reversion of potentials on BSPM in comparison with cardioelectric potentials in normal subject with two potential reversions at the initial ventricular activity. Probably, the presence of only one reversion of potentials reflects the myogenous way of the excitation spread from the stimulating electrode to the excitation wave breakthrough on epicardium of the right ventricle and alterations of depolarized myocardium correlation from the left to the right in interventricular sternum. After that the excitation spreads by a combined way, both myogenically and through the conductive system from the heart apex to its base, and the excitation wave spread direction does not, probably, change.

5 Conclusion

The precise determination of the pacing zone location on endocardium of the right ventricle by the initial artificial ventricular complexes of ECG in 12 conventional leads in men with the implanted cardiostimulating system in regimen VVI is impossible. The analysis of cardioelectric field on body surface in patients with implanted cardiostimulating system can be used as an additional method of control under the dynamic observation of the cardiostimulating system functioning and myocardial state.

PROPERTIES OF CARDIOPOTENTIAL DISTRIBUTION ON CHEST SURFACE IN HEALTHY PEOPLE AT THE PERIOD OF THE HEART VENTRICULAR DEPOLARIZATION

I.M. ROSHCHEVSKAYA, T.V. KIRUSHEVA, M.P. ROSHCHEVSKY, D.N.SHMAKOV
Institute of Physiology of the Komi Science Centre, Ural Division, Russian Academy of Sciences, Syktyvkar, Kommunisticheskaya, 24, Komi, 167610, Russia
E-mail: compcard@online.ru

V.P. NUZHNY
The Komi Republic Cardiological Centre, Syktyvkar, Komi, Russia

In subjects, having no cardiac deseases according to data of ECG in 12 conventional leads the cardioelectric activity during the heart ventricular depolarization was investigated by body surface potential mapping. It was found, that at the initial phase of the ventricular depolarization the properties of the positive extremum shift are correlated with various positions of the heart within the thorax. Similar changes of the positive extremum shift trajectory in the QRS complex onset are observed during the deep inspiration and expiration, when the heart position is changed.

1 Introduction

At present in the laboratory of physiological informativity of biophysical fields of the Institute of Physiology of the Russian Academy of Sciences the data base of cardioelectric field on body and heart ventricular surfaces, in intramural layers of heart ventricles in various classes of animals with different structures of heart and type of myocardial excitation is being worked out. The comparison of data on reflection of electrical activity of heart ventricles onto body surface in animals with that in humans is of great importance for the development of a theory of the electric field formation on body surface.

2 Methods

Cardioelectric field on chest surface was investigated in 53 healhy humans (male and female). Cardioelectric potentials were recorded on body surface of subjects in reclining position at various phases of respiration (quiet respiration, deep inspiration and expiration). Unipolar ECGs were simultaneously recorded from the original array of 64 electrodes, located regularly on human torso surface from clavicles and the upper scapular third to the lower chest border.

3 Results

The analysis of body surface potential maps in healthy subjects with the normal (fig.1, A), right (fig.1, B), and left (fig.1, C) direction of the electrical heart axis at

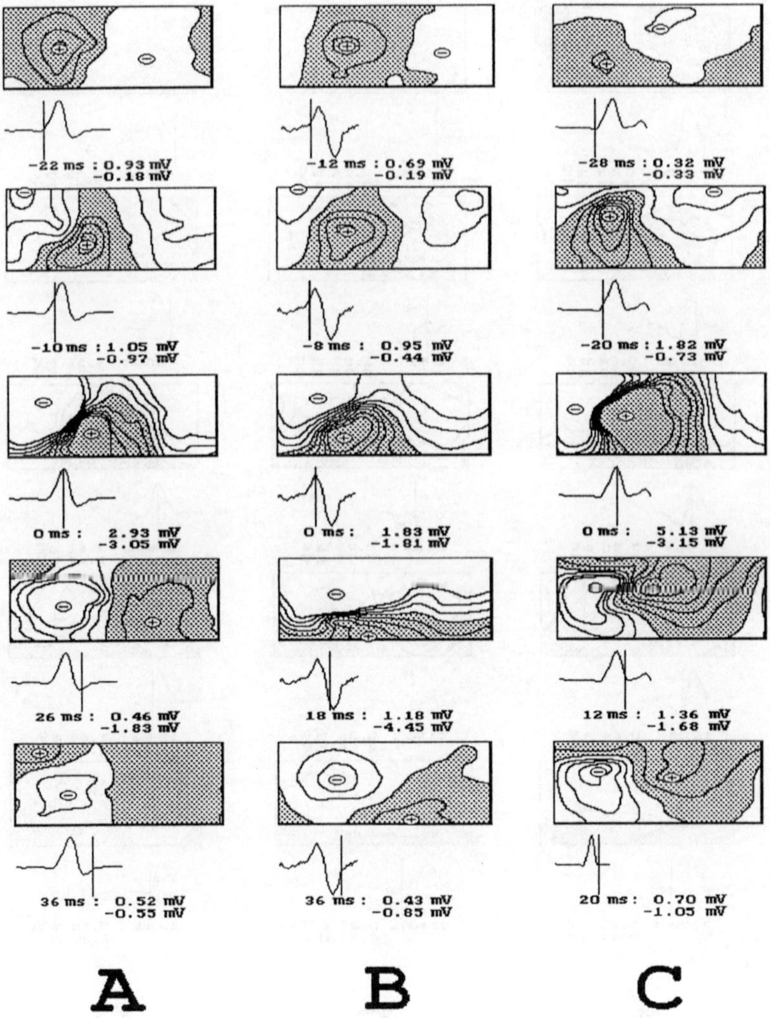

Figure 1. Equipotential momentous maps in healthy subjects at normal electrical heart axis direction (A), the right (B) and the left (C) deviations of the electrical heart axis direction (quiet respiration).
The electropositive zone is shaded, under the maps the I limb lead ECG with a time marker is qiven.

quiet respiration showed the pecularities of the position of positive and negative potentials zones and their extrema during the ventricular depolarization. At the initial moments of the ventricular depolarization the properties of the positive extremum shift are correlated with various anatomic positions of the heart within the thorax.

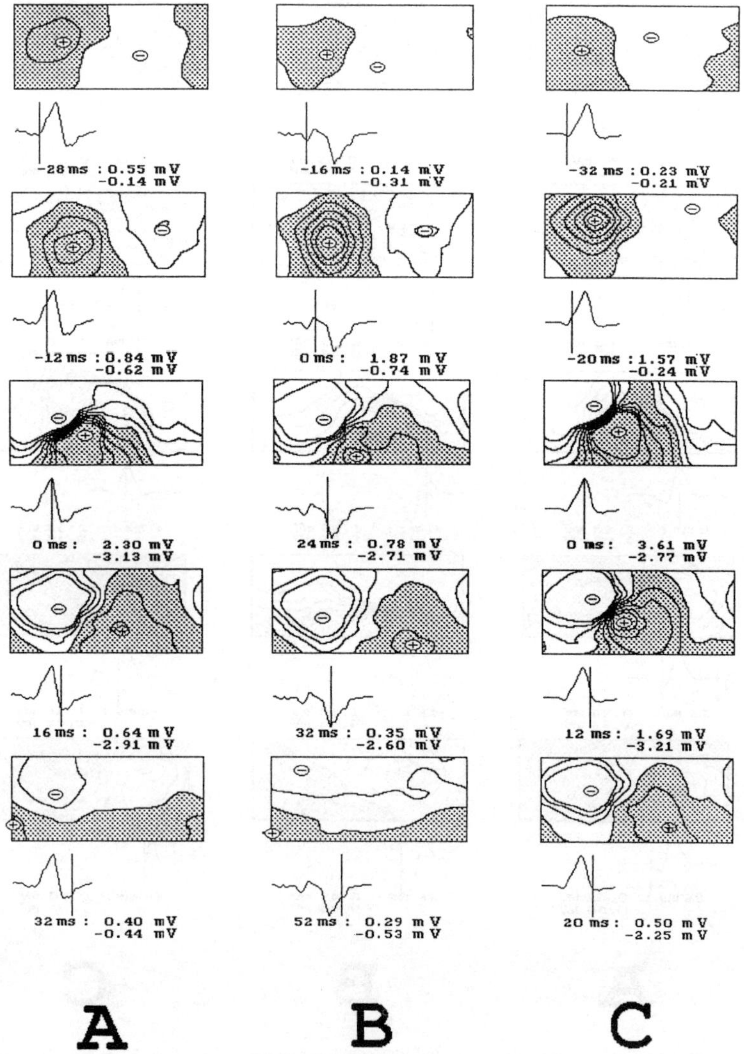

Figure 2. Equipotential momentous maps during the initial ventricular activity in the same patient at quiet respiration (A), deep inspiration (B) and deep expiration (C).
Conventional signes are the same as on figure 1.

At prominant deviations of the electrical heart axis at the period of inspiration and expiration the trajectories of the positive extrema on ventral surface of chest are changed (fig.2). At deep inspiration general direction of the movement of zones and extrema is not changed (fig.3,B). However, the positive and negative extrema at the initial depolarization are registered lower, than at quiet respiration. Moreover, the positive extremum is shifted almost vertically to its lower border. At deep inspiration the negative extremum at the initial depolarization is located in the left subscapular area (fig 3, C). At the next instance of the ventricular depolarization the direction of the negative extremum shift is similar to that at quiet respiration. At the initial depolarization the positive extremum is registered in the area of sternum. But at the period of the upstroke phase of the R wave it is shifted to the upper chest border , but at the moment of the R peak - in the apex area. At the final ventricular depolarization the positive extremum is registered on dorsal surface. At less pronounced deviations of the electrical heart axis at deep inspiration and expiration changes in cardiopotential distribution at the initial ventricular activity were slight or not observed at all.

4 Discussion

In some cases at deep inspiration the cardiopotential distribution at the period of the ventricular depolarization was similar to that in people, having at quiet respiration the deviation of the electrical heart axis to the right, while at deep expiration it was similar to the potential distribution in people, having at quiet respiration the deviation of the electrical heart axis to the left. The general direction of the negative extremum shift at the ventricular depolarization is similar in people with various positions of the electrical heart axis. There is a number of factors, that influence the changes of the shift of positive and negative extrema and the location of zones at various phases of respiration. They are: the change of heart position in chest, the heart shape, the area of the heart contact with extracardiac tissues, hemodynamics, electrical conductivity of extracardiac tissues.

5. Conclusion

In healthy people with various electrical heart axis directions at different phases of respiration trajectories of the positive extremum movement differ from each other at the initial ventricular depolarization, while the negative extrermum trajectories have no significant changes.

COMPARATIVE STUDY OF THE INFLUENCE OF SOMATOMETRIC VARIABLES ON VECTORCARDIOGRAPHIC AND BODY SURFACE MAPPING CHARACTERISTICS.

V. REGECOVÁ
Institute of Normal and Pathological Physiology,
Sienkiewiczova 1, 813 71 Bratislava, Slovakia,
E-mail: regecova@unpf.savba.sk

Direct chest measurements in addition to recording of conventional anthropometric variables, such as age, height, weight, can improve the efficiency of the prediction of normal individual data. In sum, endomorphic (pycnic) subjects with rounded chest tend to have more horizontal orientation of atrial and ventricular depolarization as well as repolarization vectors. They also have smaller amplitudes of atrial and ventricular maximum depolarization vectors. Rounded chest in males goes also hand in hand with increased spatial angle between integral QRS-STT vectors. Similarly to the behavior of vectors, the values of the maximum on isopotential QRS maps are influenced by body constitution. On the other hand, the localization of maxima are under the influence of chest parameter.

1. Introduction

Correlation between somatometric measures of the chest and electrocardiologic variables are not sufficiently reflected in studies dealing with current anthropometric characteristics, since the latter are usually confounded by such nongeometric factors as gender, age, weight, or height (1,2,3).

The aim of the present study was to give a complete quantitative evaluation of the influence of somatometrically characterized chest configuration as well as body constitution on the vectorcardiographic variables and body surface potential distributions obtained from one single heartbeat.

2. Subjects and Methods

The study group consisted of 95 healthy subjects (63 males, 32 females), aged from 10 to 68 years, median of age was 25 years.

The following constitutional measurements were taken into consideration: height, weight, mesosternal (MTC), and xiphosternal thoracic circumference (XTC), transversal (TTD) and sagittal thoracic diameter (STD), both taken in the mesosternal plane, thoracic index (TI): TI= STD/TTD.100 , Pignet index (PI): PI= height - (weight + MTC), (4), body mass index (BMI): BMI= weight.10^3/height^2.

Electrocardiologic parametres were obtained by means of the Cardiag 128. PC based electrocardiologic system (METE, Prague).Frank lead system vectors were recorded in seated persons in mid respiratory position of the chest from the same single heartbeat. Maximum magnitudes of spacial instantaneous vectors, as well as values of azimuth and declination of integral vectors were evaluated for atrial depolarization, ventricular depolarization and ventricular repolarization respectively. The spacial angle between the integral QRS and T vectors was also assessed.

Maximum positivity and negativity as well as their localization were computed on isopotential and isointegral maps.

3. Results and Discussion

3.1 Atrial Activation

As shown in Table 1 the magnitude of maximal P vector was independent of age and sex, but significantly related to chest measurements (STD). Even more pronounced was the association with BMI and PI in males. That means, that the amplitude of P vector is higher in taller, slim subjects with flat chest. Similarly to P max, maximum on the isopotential maps was influenced mainly by body constitution represented by height, BMI and PI ($p<0.001$), this relation is more pronounced in females.

Table 1. Correlation coefficients between anthropometric and electrocardiologic data during atrial activation.

	P max	BSPM max	BSPM min	P dec
	M / F	M / F	M / F	M / F
Age	- / -	- / -.36*	- / .40*	-.33** / -
Chest	-.29* / -	- / -.49*	- / .42*	-.49*** /-44**
Body	.39** / -	- / .49**	- / .38*	-.22 /-.55***

M - males, F - Females, * - p<0.05, ** - p<0.01, *** - p<0.001

The localization of maximum on BSPM as well as azimuth of integral P vector was not dependend of body constitution. Horizontal orientation of P vector is characteristic for endomorphic subjects with rounded chest. The strongest relationship with BMI and with weight means that in females the declination of the P vector is very strongly associated with the shape and ponderosity of the whole body, while as shown by thight correlation with thoracic measures (TI and with STD) in males, the chest configuration seems to be more important. This finding could not be ascribed to the effect of age.

3.2. Ventricular activation

Significant associations between the magnitude of maximal QRS vectors and somatic characteristics were observed only in males (Table 2). The decrease of magnitude of the QRS vector goes hand in hand with greater antero-posterior dimension of the chest, endomorphy and age.

Table 2. Correlation coefficients between anthropometric and electrocardiologic data during ventricular activation.

	QRS max	BSPM max	BSPM min
	M / F	M / F	M / F
Age	-.35* / -	-.33** / .19	.47*** / .28
Chest	-.33** / -	-.44** / -	.43*** / .33
Body	-.33** / -	-.48*** / -	.45*** / -

	QRS dec	BSPM max right - left	BSPM max up - down
Age	-.45** /-.35*	- / -	- / -.39*
Chest	-.37** /-.36*	- / .25	- / -.45**
Body	-.31** /-.20	.27* / .32	- / -.53**

M - males, F - Females, * - p<0.05, ** - p<0.01, *** - p<0.001

Also maximum positivity and negativity on the isopotential maps were greater in tall, slim subjects with flat chest and at the same time they decreased with age. Azimuth of the integral QRS vector was independent on age, or body characteristics, which had greater impact on declination of QRS as well as on the localization of maximum pozitivity on BSPM. With advancing age, the integral QRS vector shifted more horizontally. Among single body characteristics, only STD manifesteted significant influence on the declination of QRS in both sexes. This documents the role of the chest configuration in the variability of integral QRS vector orientation, which is more vertical in slim, asthenic subjects with flat chest. Also the maximum on isopotential maps was placed lower in these same somatotypes.

3.3 Ventricular Repolarization

The amplitude of the maximal T vector was related to sex, it was lower in females, and was not significantly influenced by body characteristics. Maximum on BSPMs was higher in males and generally in taller subjects ($p<0.001$) with narrow chest. As regards the body constitution parameters, only height and derived measures showed to be relevant to spatial orientation of T vector. T vector was oriented more forward in males, or taller subjects with wide chest. Localization of maximum positivity was related to height and STD ($p<0.01$) in the same way like the orientation of T vector. The integral T vector was shifted more horizontally with increasing age, STD and endomorphy (PI, BMI). On BSPM the orientation of maximum was not affected by age, sex or body constitution.

Less dependence upon anthropometric parameters was observed for the spacial QRS - T angle. The only significant correlation was found with STD ($p<0.05$). In males it also increased with age. Magnitude as well as localization of maxima on isointegral maps was related neither to age, nor to sex or somatotype.

Conclusion

This study has shown the relative independence of relations between some electrocardiologic variables and direct chest measurements from the relationships of this parameters to overal anthropometric measures. It follows that this fact should be taken into acount in constructing mathemathical expressions which will be useful for prediction of electrocardiologic variables from individually measured constitutional parameters.

References

1. E. Simonson and A. Keys, Circulation 9, 105 (1954)
2. H. V. Pipberger at al, Circulation 35, (1967)
3. Z. Drška et al, Ann. Med. Section of Polish Acad. Sci. 16 (1973)
4. R. Martin , K. Saller, Lehrbuch der Antropologie, Stuttgart, G. Fischer Verlag (1957)

LONG-TERM STUDY OF HEART ACTIVATION CHANGES DISPLAYED IN BODY SURFACE ISOCHRONE MAPS WITH THRESHOLD POTENTIAL

K. KOZLÍKOVÁ, I. HULÍN
Institute of Pathophysiology, Medical Faculty, Comenius University, Sasinkova 2, 811 08 Bratislava, Slovak Republic
E-mail: kozlikova@fmed.uniba.sk

J. MURÍN, J. BULAS
1st Medical Department, Faculty Hospital, Mickiewiczova 13, 813 69 Bratislava, Slovak Republic

M. TYŠLER
Institute of Measurement Science, Slovak Academy of Sciences, Dúbravská cesta 9, 842 19 Bratislava, Slovak Republic

We have introduced body surface isochrone maps (ICHM) with threshold potential (TP) several years ago as a method for reducing the measured data before analysis. They have been used for necrotic lesion detection in patients with myocardial infarction (MI). We are now giving the evidence that these maps really project the heart activation onto the body surface. From a group of 16 male patients with MI who were repeatedly examined 2 patients who died on heart failure have been chosen: 1 with anterior and 1 with inferior MI. For each examination ICHM with TP = 50 μV, 100 μV, 150 μV and 200 μV were constructed during the QRS complex. They were compared with corresponding mean ICHM of a control group consisting of 20 healthy men. Infarcted areas were established from the maps using the division of the left ventricle (LV) proposed by Selvester and confirmed by necropsy findings. The ICHM of the control group showed the beginning of activation in the chest areas corresponding to septal segments. It spread almost uniformly through the anterior chest. After reaching the back it turned upwards and rightwards. The ICHM of the patient with anterior MI revealed always blank map areas corresponding to the anterior segments. The activation began either in the apex of the LV or in the middle part of the posterior wall. He had a 2nd MI 21 months later that markedly changed the activation sequence. But the infarcted segments on maps remained the same and corresponded well with injured segments found by necropsy. The ICHM of the patient with inferior MI revelaed blank map areas corresponding to inferior segments 1 month after MI. Later, they became partially filled up and changed to crowds of isochrone lines. The activation began always in the midseptum as in controls but spread slowlier. Infarcted segments found in necropsy corresponded to map segments that were either blank, or displayed delayed activation or crowds of isochrones. According to our findings we conclude that the ICHM with TP really project the heart activation sequence onto the body surface.

1 Introduction

The body surface isochrone maps (ICHM) with threshold potential (TP) were presented as a method for reducing the data[1,2] before analysis and for the localization of the necrotic site[3]. It was assumed that they project the heart activation sequence onto the body surface. An experimental proof of this statement is given.

2 Theoretical background

We assume that the activation wavefront is represented by a uniform double layer of strength V_D. It can be shown[3] that the potential U on the body surface of an infinite homogeneous conductor is proportional to the squared radius r of the wavefront and inversely proportional to the squared distance R to body surface

$$U = -(V_D/4) \cdot (r/R)^2 . \qquad (1)$$

Waves of the electrocardiogram reach different amplitudes. For the construction of ICHM we choose one value of potential as a threshold. Then we look for all higher potential values. We can either find a time instant of the first higher potential value or there is no potential higher than the TP during the whole wave. Then in ICHM with TP the distribution of time values corresponding to the first higher potential value will be displayed. Areas of maps with potential always lower than the TP remain blank.

Correspondence between heart segments and the areas on the chest surface can be obtained using the model proposed by Startt/Selvester[4]. He divided the left ventricle (LV) into 12 segments of equal volume. Each segment was represented by a dipole the positive potential of which was displayed to a certain area on the chest surface.

We have combined this model with our ICHM to establish the necrotic sites in patients (pts) with myocardial infarction (MI). The location was based on the assumption that the electrically inactive necrotic site causes the split of activation wavefront. This leads to the decrease of its radius as well as of the potential according to Eq. 1.

3 Methods

We have repeatedly examined 16 male pts with MI (5 anterior, 2 anterior with right bundle branch block, 2 apical, 6 inferior and 1 posterior) during a body surface mapping (BSM) study. At the date of acute MI they were aged 40 to 70 years. During the study, 4 pts died and 2 of them who died on heart failure had detailed necropsy analysis - 1 with anterior MI (13 measurements, died 27 months after MI) and 1 with inferior MI (15 measurements, died 37 months after MI). Detailed clinical examination including BSM was performed before pts' discharge from hospital and were repeated at least once a year.

BSM were registered with the microcomputer-based mapping system ProCardio[5] which includes a limited 24-electrode system by Barr. Two to 4 successive records of 4 to 4.4 s duration were made at each session. The 2nd heart beat of the 2nd record was taken to compute ICHM. The onset and offset of the QRS complex was established from the root mean square signal. ICHM with TP = 50 μV, 100 μV, 150 μV and 200 μV were constructed during the QRS complex from each measurement.

A control group was taken to compare to patient's data. It was formed by 20 healthy young men aged 18 to 19 years. None of them had documented heart disease and all had normal standard 12-lead electrocardiograms.

4 Results

Mean ICHM of the control group showed the beginning of activation on the chest corresponding to septal segments. The activation spread almost uniformly through the anterior chest. After reaching the back it turned upwards and rightwards (Fig. 1 and 2). For the lowest TP = 50 μV almost the whole map was covered by time values in more than 90% of cases, for the highest TP = 200 μV only a part of the anterior chest was covered by values.

The above mentioned decrease of the potential caused by MI is of interest only in those parts of maps where there is high occurence of potential in controls. Therefore, we have focused our attention to the 100 μV threshold that covers all the chest areas belonging to the heart segments with at least 50% probability and the value of potential is over the noise.

The ICHM of the pt with anterior MI revealed blank map areas corresponding to the anterior segments during the whole study (Fig. 1). The activation began either in the apex of the LV or in the middle of the LV posterior wall but never in the septum as it did in controls. He had a 2nd MI 21 months later that markedly changed the activation. But the infarcted (blank) segments on maps remained the same and corresponded well with injured (necrotic) segments found by necropsy.

The ICHM of the pt with inferior MI revelaed blank map areas corresponding to inferior segments 1 month after MI (Fig. 2). Later, they became partially filled up with time values and changed to crowds of isochrone lines. The activation began always in the midseptum as in controls but spread slowlier. Infarcted segments found in necropsy corresponded to map segments that were either blank, or displayed delayed activation or crowds of isochrones.

5 Conclusion

According to our findings we conclude that we have given the evidence that the isochrone maps with threshold potential in fact project the heart activation sequence onto the body surface.

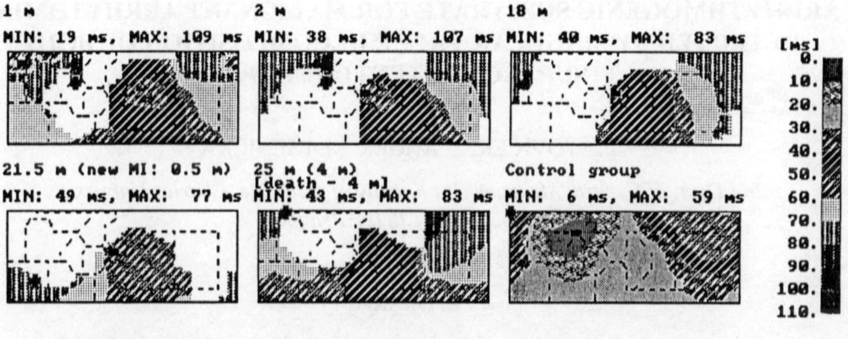

Figure 1: ICHM with TP = 100 μV in pt with anterior MI and in controls

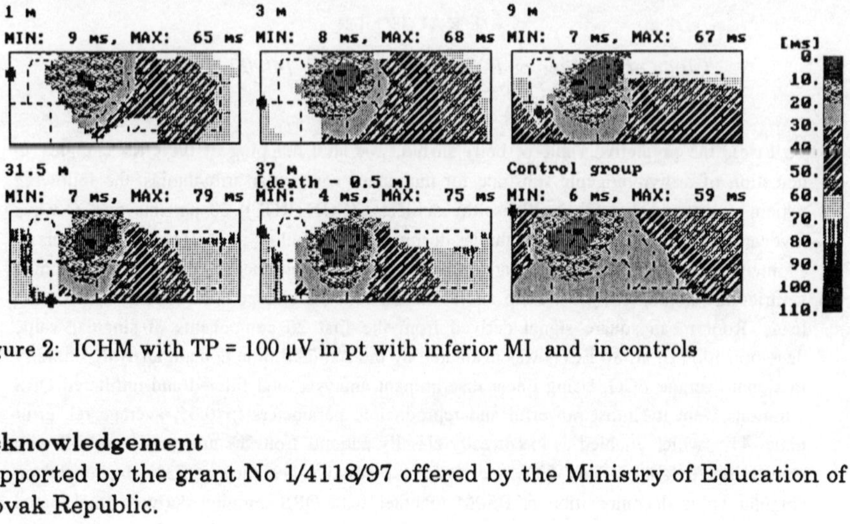

Figure 2: ICHM with TP = 100 μV in pt with inferior MI and in controls

Acknowledgement

Supported by the grant No 1/4118/97 offered by the Ministry of Education of Slovak Republic.

References

1. K Kozlíková and I Hulín, *Bratisl lek Listy 87, 194 (1987)*
2. K Kozlíková et al, in *BIOSIGNAL'94* (Brno, 1994)
3. K Kozlíková et al, *Lék Tech 25, 51 (1994)*
4. R H Startt/Selvester et al, in *Comprehensive Electrocardiology*, ed. R Th van Dam and A van Oosterom (Pergamon Press, New York, 1989).
5. V Rosík et al, in *Measurement'97*, ed. I Frollo and A Plačková (IMS SAS, Bratislava, 1997)

ARRHYTHMOGENIC SUBSTRATE FOR MALIGNANT ARRHYTHMIAS DETECTED BY SINGULAR VALUE DECOMPOSITION OF BODY SURFACE POTENTIAL MAPS

P. ŠŤOVÍČEK, Z. ANGER, M. PŠENIČKA

2nd Dept. of General Medicine, 1st Faculty of Medicine, Charles University, U nemocnice 2, 128 08, Prague, CR

Z. DRŠKA

Expert Laboratory of the Inspector of Air Forces and Air Defense of the Army of the Czech Republic, Mladoboleslavská 197 06, Prague, CR

J. KAUTZNER

Clinic of Cardiology, IKEM, Vídeňská 800, 140 00, Prague, CR

To assess the predictive value of body surface potential mapping of the QRS complex in detection of arrhythmogenic substrate for malignant ventricular arrhythmias, the following patient groups were studied: 20 healthy subjects, (CONTROL), 20 patients post Q-wave myocardial infarction and no arrhythmias during one-year follow-up (MI) and 18 survivors of spontaneous sustained ventricular tachyarrhythmia reproducible during programmed ventricular stimulation (VT). Each subject underwent simultaneous recording of 80 torso leads. Root mean square signal derived from the first 20 components of singular value decomposition of all 80 ECGs was evaluated by the standard time domain analysis similarly to signal-average ECG. Using linear discriminant analysis total filtered and unfiltered QRS durations were the most powerful and reproducible parameters ($p<0.05$, average rel. error under 4%), which enabled us to correctly classify patients from the groups VT and MI with sensitivity 70%, specificity 72% and positive predictive accuracy of 73%. In conclusion singular value decomposition of BSPM together with QRS duration derived from spatial amplitude curve appears to be a promising technique in detection of arrhythmogenic substrate.

1 Introduction

Late potentials detected noninvasively by the time domain analysis of the signal-averaged electrocardiogram (ECG) have been demonstrated to be a clinically useful predictor of susceptibility to ventricular tachyarrhythmias [1]. However, current techniques for detection of cardiac micropotentials are still imperfect, and this may contribute to relative low positive predictive accuracy of conventional signal-averaged ECG [2]. To overcome these shortcomings and improve clinical value of the method, novel techniques are being developed. One of these approaches employs body-surface potential maps (BSPM) [3]. The objectives of this study was to evaluate the performance of an approach using a singular value decomposition of BSPM to better describe all frequency, temporal, and spatial characteristics of cardiac micropotentials, and assess its predictive value in patients with inducible ventricular tachycardia.

2 Material and methods

2.1 *Study subjects*

20 asymptomatic subjects (2 women, 18 men, mean age 48±8 yrs) with normal 12 lead electrocardiogram, and no history of cardiovascular disease (CONTROL group). 20 patients with a history of a remote Q-wave myocardial infarction (3 women, 17 men, mean age 59±11 yrs) and no arrhythmias during one-year follow-up (MI group). 18 survivors of acute myocardial infarction (1 women, 17 men, mean age 55+12 yrs, 15 with CAD, 3 with DCMP) who presented with ventricular tachyarrhythmias reproducible during programmed electrical stimulation (VT group). Study groups did not differ significantly with respect to age and sex (K-W ANOVA nonparametric test, $p<0.05$). None of the study subjects had bundle branch block on baseline ECG.

2.2 *Body surface potential mapping*

All study subjects underwent BSPM using a commercial computerized system (Cardiag 112.2, METE Ltd., Prague, CR) A total number of 80 unipolar chest leads were simultaneously recorded in sitting position by means of a special lead array (5 rows, 16 columns). Signals were amplified, filtered and A/D converted (sampling frequency 500 Hz, 12 bit resolution, input range ±10mV).

2.3 *Data processing*

Both QRS onset and offset were determined for the complete set of 80 leads and further analysis was limited to QRS complex. Singular value decomposition (SVD), was applied for analysis of QRS maps [4, 5]. Of the resulting 80 signal components with increasing frequency and decreasing amplitude at each time sample and each leadpoint of matrix, only first 20 components were selected for subsequent analysis.. Root mean square was derived from all leads according to the formula:

$$RMS(t) = \sqrt{\sum_{i=1..80} V_i^2(t)} \qquad (1)$$

where t equals time sample, i means a number of leadpoint from 1 to 80, and Vi means value calculated by SVD (composed of the first 20 components) at the corresponding leadpoint. Root mean square signal was subsequently filtered at 40-250Hz and processed by standard time domain analysis same way as signal-averaged ECG. 5 variables were tested: unfiltered QRS duration derived from spatial amplitude curve in msec, filtered QRS duration in msec, total root mean square of filtered QRS in μVsec, root mean square of terminal 40 msec (RMS 40) in μVsec, duration of the terminal low amplitude signal under 40 μV (LAS) in msec.

2.4 *Statistical analysis.*

Average relative error was used for assessment of the reproducibility of individual parameters (48 measurements of subsequent QRS complexes). Stepwise discriminant analysis model was applied to select time domain variables that best discriminated among individual study groups. The classification output of discriminant analysis was used for calculations of sensitivity, specificity, and positive predictive values. Result were validated by simple resampling of .original groups into halfs and subsequent recomputing of classification for the second half using the a priori detemined classification functions from the first half of cases.

3 Results

Among 5 above mentioned variables, 2 that best discriminated study groups by 2 group discriminant model were selected. These were total filtered QRS duration, and QRS duration derived from spatial magnitude curve. These two variables were also the most reproducible with average relative error under 4%. Classification output of the discriminant analysis verified by simple resampling technique mentioned above is summarized in Table 1.

Table 1: Summary table of classification.

Group	VT vs CONTROL	CONTROL vs MI	VT vs MI
Sensitivity (%)	80	70	70
Specificity (%)	80	67	72
+ predictive accuracy	76	69	73
- predictive accuracy	81	69	72

4 Discussion

Mere multiplication of the ECG leads achieves more detailed analysis of signal-averaged ECGs [6]. Methods that derive spatial information about cardiac micropotentials offer advantages of abundant data reduction as well as frequency analysis and effective noise removal without signal averaging [7]. In this respect, analyses of both depolarization and repolarization phases have been attempted. Net QRST deflection area analysis has been suggested as a promising predictor of vulnerability to ventricular arrhythmias [8, 9]. Our approach is based on processing of QRS area only. This reflects experience that depolarization signal is more stable and reproducible in time as compared with the process of repolarization.

5 Conclusions

In this study, singular value decomposition of BSPM was demonstrated to be a potentially useful tool for detection of ventricular arrhythmogenic substrate. Predictive power of this method may better identify individual at risk of malignant ventricular arrhythmias than conventional signal averaging of ECG.

Acknowledgements

This study was supported by grant of the Grant Agency of the Czech Republic No. 406/95/0737

References

1. M.B. Simson in. *Cardiac electrophysiology: From the cell to the bedside,* eds. D.P Zipes, J Jalife (Saunders, US; 1995:1038).
2. P. Lander et al., *Circulation* **87,** 105 (1993).
3. N.C. Flowers and L.G. Horan. in: *Cardiac electrophysiology: From the cell to the bedside,* eds. D.P Zipes, J Jalife (Saunders, US; 1995:1049).
4. Z. Drska et al., *J.Electrocardiol.,* **28**(4), 340 (1985).
5. Z. Drska et al., *Physiol. Res.* **42,** 7 (1993).
6. D.S. Ho et al., *Circulation* **87**(3), 857 (1993).
7. G.J.H. Uijen, et al. *IEEE Trans Biomed Eng.,* **BME-31**:706 (1984).
8. J.A. Abildskov, et al., *Am J Physiol.* **239**:227 (1981).
9. C.L. Hubley-Kozey, et al., *Circulation.* **92**(7), 1825 (1995).

BODY SURFACE POTENTIAL MAP DATABASE DEVELOPED IN THE PROGRAM JUMP 2001

G. KOZMANN
KFKI Res. Inst. for Materials Science, Budapest, 1525 P.O. Box 49, Hungary

R.L. LUX,
Nora Eccles Harrison CVRTI, University of Utah, Salt Lake City, USA

M. TYSLER
Inst. of Measurement Science, SAS, Dubravska cesta 9, Bratislava 842/9, Slovakia

In the attempt reported, the users of the 32-electrode limited lead system in three countries (USA, Hungary, Slovakia) made an effort to pool their body surface potential map (BSPM) data, to achieve statistically considerable sample sizes in several clinical categories. For the database a common header and data structure was elaborated. Data before pooling into the databank were analyzed one-by-one for quality of the recording and for the completeness of supporting (EKG independent) medical documentation. Major clinical data were stored, retrospectively, using the original documentation. Until now, the BSPMs of 1678 subjects were considered.

1 Introduction

Elaborating reliable diagnostic criteria for BSPM classification is hampered by the lack of a large database of clinically validated maps taken from normal subjects and cardiac patients. Furthermore, according to the decision theory to each training sample size belongs an optimal dimensionality, too. Specifically, a limited training set size would allow only a low number of diagnostic parameters, to achieve the optimal reliability of the diagnostic criteria developed. According to an example published in a previous study a sample size of 30-75, 75-120, and > 120 is required for a reliable group representation when extracting 1, 2, 3 or more independent diagnostic parameters, respectively[1]. Unfortunately, until now, only few groups could achieve the adequate number of cases in statistical evaluations of BSPMs, consequently the clinical utility of BSPMs is still obscure.

The required sample sizes could be achieved in several decision categories by pooling data taken in different laboratories. However, the easy possibility of data exchange is rather limited due to the substantial differences in measuring point layouts and in the technical features of the acquisition systems used in the different centers.

In the attempt reported here, the users of the 32-electrode limited lead system[2] in three countries (Hungary, USA, Slovakia) made an effort to pool their BSPM data, to achieve the statistically reasonable sample sizes in classes of normal subjects and ischemic cardiac patients. The cooperation program was referred to as JUMP 2001 project[3].

This paper summarize the general principles of the databank development, the structure of the stored data, as well as the set of EKG independent evidences used to substantiate medical classification.

2 Method

Though the laboratories in the three cooperating countries follow a similar practice of data acquisition, still there are differences in some details. Consequently, the clarification of all these differences was required.

First of all, differences were found both in the form and content of the patient and measurement identification data. From this point of view the Slovakian protocol contained the most valuable details, therefore the header of the common database relies on their data, but in a reduced form.

Significant differences were found in the stored BSPM data as well. The data provided by the CVRTI, University of Utah, Salt Lake City represent the processed dominant heart cycles, in compressed form. In fact, the QRST segment is stored by the use of 216 coefficients of the truncated Karhunen-Loeve (K-L) expansion elaborated by Lux, Evans and their co-workers[4,5]. The Slovakian partner institutions store 2 sec of raw data of the 32 measured leads. The two Hungarian partners store either 7 sec of raw data of the 32 leads and/or the 216 K-L coefficients. In Salt Lake City and in Budapest the K-L coefficients are computed from an averaged beat. Sampling rates and AD converter resolutions are similar (1 kHz and 12 bit, respectively) in all the institutions.

The quality of the data was reviewed visually, and the exchange of the headers was carried out in order to transform the data in an identical form. For all the patients the 216 K-L coefficients were computed if those data were not provided by the co-operating laboratory. In all the cases, if the raw data were available, the P-QRS-T interval of the dominant electrical heart cycle was stored as well.

Beyond the technical requirements, a special attention was paid to the collection of the relevant clinical evidences supporting the medical classification. Consequently, before assigning a clinical classification to the data available, all the documents suitable for validation were reviewed in accordance with the requirements of the Common Standards for Electrocardiology (CSE) project in the field of the conventional 12 lead EKG.

Currently in the database the primary attention has been paid for the collection of the maps of normal subjects and coronary heart disease patients. The large group of normal subjects was provided by the CVRTI, University of Utah. This group was strictly validated as described in[6].
Tables 1. and 2. summarize the content of BSPM data files and that of the clinical findings used for the validation of coronary artery disease assignements.

BSPM data file:

File type	File content
A	Raw data in 1 μV units: 8 integers (for measurement ID) + record length in samples x32x2byte, binary
B	Compressed data in 1μV units: 216 K-L coeff. (float) + QRSonset + QRSend + Tend = 876byte, binary
C	Time normalized 192 lead BSPM data, expanded from 216 K-L coeff. in 1μV units: 300x192x2byte, binary

Table 1. Possible types and contents of BSPM data files

Clinical data file:

Document type	Evidences of (possible) IHD revealed by the documents of:
History	MI
	PTCA
	By-pass surgery
	Aneurysmectomy
Prevalence data	Symptoms
	Risk factors (for asymptomatic subjects)
Clinical findings	Stenosed and/or occluded vessels (Coronarography findings)
	Pathological wall motion pattern (2D Echo and ventriculography measurements)
	Perfusion defect (Tl 201 scintigraphy)
	Pathological exercise induced potential field response (XEKG tests)

Table.2. Summary of the main information sources used for validating coronary heart disease assignements.

3 Results

Within this study, a new header and data structure was elaborated based on the critical review of the existing ones.

In course of data evaluation, until now the BSPMs of 1678 normal subjects and cardiac patients were considered, 997 was collected at the CVRTI, University of Utah, 19 measurements were provided by the Slovakian partners and 672 cases were received from one of the two Hungarian centers. About the half of the Hungarian coronary artery disease patients has both rest and exercise BSPM measurements (taken at the end of the supine submaximal bicycle ergometer test). The number of the Hungarian contribution refers to the number of the patients, the number of records should be about 50% higher.

Though the revision of the data available is not completed yet, according to our expectation the following groups will reach or surpass the aimed sample size threshold of 120: normal subjects, (separately for males and females in three age groups), anterior myocardial infarction, inferior myocardial infarction, and coronary artery disease cases. The sample size in the group of hypertrophic cardiomyopathy should end up between 75 and 120, the number of patients with increased arrhythmia vulnerability around 50. The sample sizes of groups like bundle branch blocks and WPW syndrome, etc. are expected to be around 30. A significant increase in the number of cases is expected from the additional contribution of the Slovakian institutions.

Acknowledgments

This study was partly supported by the grant No. T5544 of the National Research Found, Budapest, a grant from the National Committee for Technological Development to support the Hungarian contribution to EC BIOMED I NEMY project.

The majority of the BSPM data were recorded and validated in the co-operating centers under the supervision of L.S. Green, University of Utah, Salt Lake City, USA, and K. Szász, Dept. Cardiac Rehabilitation, County Hospital, Deszk.

References

1. Gy. Kozmann *et al., Computers and Biomed.Res.* **24**, 170 (1991).
2. R.L. Lux *et al., IEEE Trans.* **BME-25**, 270 (1978).
3. Gy. Kozmann *et al.,* in *Computers in Cardiology 1995,* eds. A. Murray, R. Arzbaecher, IEEE Inc. (1995).
4. R.L. Lux *et al., Circ.Res.* **49**, 186 (1981).
5. A.K. Evans *et al., Circ.Res.* **49**, 197 (1981).
6. L.S. Green *et al., Circulation* **71**, 244, (1985).

STATISTICAL VALIDATION OF THE LUX-TYPE LIMITED LEAD SYSTEM

N. NAGY
University of Veszprém, Dep. of Image Processing and Neurocomputing, Egyetem u. 10, 8200 Veszprém, Hungary

GY. KOZMANN , ZS. CSERJÉS
KFKI Research Inst. for Materials Science, Budapest, 1525 Pf. 49, Hungary

The paper gives detailed data on the results of the study carried out to validate the 32 electrode limited lead system suggested by RL Lux et al. The experimental data of the study were taken by the 219 lead system elaborated at the University of Parma. Althogether 50 records were used (20 normal, 15 with myocardial ischemia and 15 with anterior myocardial infarction). In the Lux system from the 32 measured leads the potential values in the additional 160 locations are estimated by an optimal procedure. According to this study the average amplitude error in the estimated leads was 41,1 μV. The pattern similarity of the reference and the estimated maps was 0.97 in the interval of the QRS complex.

1. Introduction

Theoretically, for an accurate body surface potential field measurement, several hundreds of electrodes should be used. Fortunatelly, due to the high correlation between certain leads, the lead array of the measurements can be simplified considerably. The lead system introduced by RL Lux and associates is one of the limited lead systems, derived from a regular 192 lead system with a procedure reminiscent of the Gram-Schmidt ortogonalisation procedure, method relying on the covariance matrix of the sample population[1]. According to the authors, by selecting 30 suitable leads, the rest of the signals can be recovered with an average amplitude error of 32 μV, while the correlation between the original and the estimated maps was 0.983 in average. (Later the system referred to was completed by two additional electrodes, actually our study carries out the validation of this modified 32 electrode version of the limited lead system.)

The clinical validation of the system was carried out by Green et al. Their study demonstrated, that the known significant patterns of the maps were preserved by the simplified system[2]. This study is about a more extensive and quantitative validation procedure. In this approach based on experimental data both the amplitude and pattern errors were quantified throughout the QRS interval.

2. Methods

Experimental data were provided by the University of Parma. The body surface maps of 50 subjects were taken by the 219 lead, non-equidistant array. 20 of the 50 subjects were healthy (N), 15 had myocardial ischemia (I), 15 had anterior myocardial infarction (AMI).

In the first step of our procedure from the 219 lead system 192 lead maps were computed, by the use of bilinear transformation. These maps were used as reference maps in the analysis. Subsequently, the 32 leads of the limited system were selected and by the use of the transfer matrix of the Lux system, the potential values in the 160 non-measured electrode sites were estimated. The comparison of these data with the reference maps gives the basis of the validation analysis. To facilitate the comparison of the maps of different individuals,the length of the QRS interval of each patient was normalized.

For the sake of the statistical evaluation, the following error measures were used: average of the estimation error for a decile map (h_i), lead by lead average error for the whole QRS interval(h_j), and the global average of these for the QRS interval (g). The average errors in the estimated leads were visualized in map form. For the quantitative comparison of the reference and the estimated map patterns the correlation coefficients were used.

The error definitons are given below:

a./decile map by map average error (computed for N patients):

$$h_i = \frac{1}{N} \sum_{(N)} \sqrt{\frac{\sum_{j=1}^{160} \varepsilon_{ij}^2}{160}} \qquad (1)$$

b./lead by lead average error (computed for N patients):

$$h_j = \frac{1}{N} \sum_{(N)} \sum_{i=1}^{10} \varepsilon_{ij}^2 \qquad (2)$$

c./global average:

$$g = \frac{1}{160} \sum_{j=1}^{160} h_j \qquad (3)$$

where: ε_{ij} :error of lead j (j: 1, ..., 160) in decile i (i: 1, ..., 10)

N :patient number in the homogeneous clinical class

All these computations were carried out for the subsets of the different clinical classes, and the class dependent differences were evaluated. In this study representative samples of our results are shown in the figures.

3. Results

Typical results obtained for the AMI group are shown in Fig. 1. In this graph the average estimation error, the signal-to-noise ratio and the pattern correlation coefficients are plotted vs. the deciles of the QRS. In the other classes similar results were obtained. The average error for all groups and for all deciles yielded 40.1 uV. In this context we have to referr to the original paper, which considered 20μV RMS as a typical value for the sum of the electrical and biological noise, i.e. the estimation error doubled the inherent average noise of the measurements.

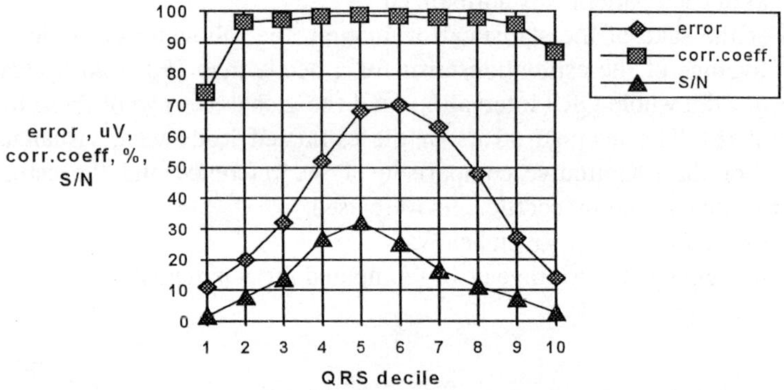

Fig. 1. Average estimation error, pattern correlation coefficients and signal-to-noise ratio versa deciles of QRS for the AMI group

The spatial distribution of the largest error leads are shown in Fig. 2.

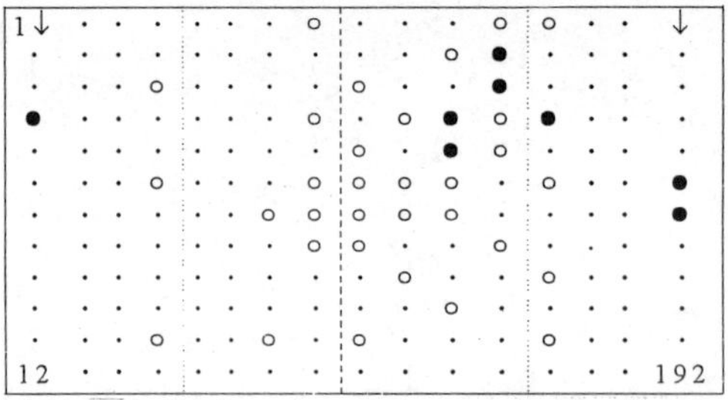

Fig. 2. 8 leads (black dots) with the largest average error for the N group (average error > mean+2*standard deviation) . 32 open circles represent the lead arrangement of Lux-type limited lead system.

4. Discussion

Our findings could be directly compared with the results of the original paper only in terms of the „global error" and the average map pattern correlation coefficients. Considering the first feature, our 40.1 uV average error is slightly higher than the 32 μV value,gained on the training set, but according to our interpretation these figures are largely compatible. Likewise, our mean map pattern correlation is slightly below the result published by Lux et al, still the difference looks negligible.

The amplitude errors are largely proportional with the signal levels, still in deciles from 3 to 8, the signal-to-noise ratio is in the range of 15 to 32. But in the early and late deciles the ratio decreases to a low level. Though it was not substantiated above, we have to stress that in all the groups considered, the estimation error was 3 to 4 times lower than the within group variability, i.e. one should expect only minor diagnostic performance decrease due to the estimation error term.

The lead-by-lead average errors show similar patterns in the 3 groups considered. This suggests, that the estimation error is not effected significantly by the pathology. As a by-product of our analysis 8 lead sites were identified, where the estimation error was large. By the use of additional electrodes at these locations, the quality of the map recordings could be improved significantly.

Acknowledgements

This study was partly supported by a grant from the National Committee for Technological Development to substantiate the cooperation in the EC BIOMED 1 project, NEMY (Non-invasive Evaluation of the Myocardium).The authors express their gratitude for Prof. E. Musso, director of the Institute for General Physiology, University of Parma, for providing 219 lead map data.

References

[1] Lux, R.L., Smith, C.R., Wyatt, R.F., Abildskov, J.A.: Limited lead selection for estimation of body surface potential maps in electrocardiography. IEEE Trans. BME-25:270-276, 1978

[2] Green, L.S., Lux, R.L., Stilli, D., Haws, C.W., Taccardi, B.: Fine detail in body surface potential maps: Accuracy of maps using a limited lead array and spatial and temporal data representation. J.Electrocardiol., 20(1), 21-26, 1987.

COMPARISON STUDY FOR EXAMINATION OF THE INFORMATION EQUIVALENCY OF THE SAVARD-63 AND THE LUX-192 LEAD SYSTEMS

GY. SÁNDOR, GY. KOZMANN, ZS. CSERJÉS
KFKI, Research Institute for Materials Science, P.O.Box 49. Budapest, 1525, Hungary
E-mail: sandor@r1.atki.kfki.hu

I. PRÉDA, A. PINTÉR, M. MEDVEGY
Haynal Imre University of Health Sciences Szabolcs u. 35. Budapest,1135, Hungary

Based on a specific application of the Laplacian type inter-electrode set transformation method some important limitations of the approach was demonstrated. The paper includes results that show the differences between the information content of the BSPMs measured by the 63 lead system suggested by P. Savard and the 192 lead system suggested by R.L. Lux. Laplacian interpolation method was applied in order to produce 63 lead BSPMs. The error analysis was accomplished for normal subjects, patients with ischemic disorders and patients with myocardial infarcts. The mean value of the error was found to 138 μV that corresponds a 54% relative error and mean correlation value was found 0,87. For presentation the spatial information distortion we calculated the deviations for each single lead. The error distribution of the three patient groups did not show significant differences.

1 Introduction

Our laboratory is involved in creating a large (more than 2000 items) body surface potential map (BSPM) data bank of normal subjects and cardiac patients[1]. Currently as the data bank is increasing we recruit BSPM records that were taken by different kind of lead systems. The large part of the files are recorded by the Lux-32 type lead system[2]. Also we have files from the Hopital du Sacre-Coeur of Montreal recorded by the Savard-63 system[3]. The highest resolution records come from the Laboratory of the University of Parma which consists of 219 lead[4]. Taking into consideration of the incompatibility of the files recorded by different lead systems the comparison of their information content by the currently used transformation methods and verifying the transformation errors has great importance. In our data base the final goal is to convert all the files in the Lux-192 type form.

In this study we present results on the validity of the transformation from the Savard-63 form into Lux-192 BSPMs. To this end the Laplacian interpolation suggested by Oostendorp *et al.* was used[5].

2 Materials and Methods

Five hundred maps of 50 subjects were used for the analysis. All measurements were taken by the 219 lead Parma system. The population we studied consists of 20 normal subjects and 15-15 patients with ischemic disorders and anterior myocardial infarcts, respectively. Lux-192 type reference maps were produced from the 219 lead maps by accomplishing a bilinear transformation. A similar procedure was used for producing Montreal-63 lead maps. Subsequently the estimation process was executed, i.e. 192 lead maps were estimated from the simulated input data, using the Laplacian transformation method. The point of the algorithm is to apply a constrain in order to obtain a smooth potential distribution. From this condition comes the demand to minimize the second order gradient (Laplacian) of the BSPM. At an arbitrary node of a rectangular grid the potential value, ϕ can be approximated by means of the Taylor expansion using a measured potential ϕ_0 and the distance h between the unknown and measured sites:

$$\phi(x+h,y)=\phi_0+h\left.\frac{\partial\phi}{\partial x}\right|_{x0}+\frac{1}{2}h^2\left.\frac{\partial^2\phi}{\partial x^2}\right|_{x0} \qquad (1)$$

Writing Eq.1 in a two dimension form that is expressing the four adjacent potential values, the Laplacian at each time instant can be expressed by the means of the equations without knowledge of the gradients.

Our examination focused and was confined to the QRS segment, the most dynamically alternating part of the electrical heart-cycle. In order to the statistical evaluation we normalized the length of the QRS interval. We checked both the spatial and the temporal distribution of the amplitude error and also the Pearson's correlation values. The statistical parameters we calculated for characterization of the transformation method are detailed elsewhere in this volume[6].

3 Results

Figure 1. shows the average amplitude errors for the normal group and the average standard deviation of the error. For the better representation we also demonstrate the RMS values of the reference maps. It is shown that the Laplacian interpolation yields 247 μV maximal error at the 5th decile of the QRS. Large within-map variance can be also observed that is the average standard deviation is 77 μV. Comparing the overall (for the whole QRS) mean errors and expressing their ratio to the RMS values of cardiac signals 138,5 μV and 54%, were found respectively. The highest correlation value at a single BSPM can achieve the value of 0,95 while the overall mean value is 0,86. Our study proved, that the values of the errors depend marginally on the clinical classification of the patients (see Figure 1/B). The lead dependency of the transformation error was also investigated. Figure 2. shows the spatial properties of the global transformation error distribution.

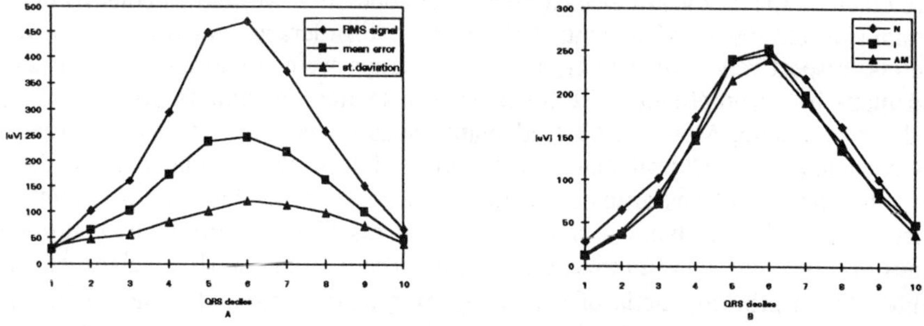

Figure 1: The cardiac RMS signal, the mean error and the standard deviation of the errors within the analyzed normal group with regard to the single deciles (A). The average errors of the normal, ischemic and infarction groups (B).

4 Discussion

The estimated error values coming from this study confirms some recently published results[7]. Our examination focused on the QRS segment as the most rapid changing part of the ECG. The segmentation of the QRS wave makes unambiguous the large deviation of the error from the average. This observation supports that both the absolute and the relative transformation error depends strongly on the deciles in question. The significant changes of the relative error with respect to the RMS values clearly manifests from Figure 1. Furthermore the course of the correlation between the reference and the transformed maps shows stability.

Our study revealed, that in our specific transformation problem, the Laplacian transformation is going with significant error. According to our interpretation behind this phenomenon, the inadequacy of the basic assumption of the Laplacian transformation stands. Quite probably, at the inter-electrode distance of the 63 lead Savard system, the 3 term truncated assumption of the potential estimation (Eq. 1) fails. A further difficulty may steam from the use of a standardized geometry instead of the real ones. Additional source of inaccuracy is coming from the minimization technique of the two dimensional Laplacian.

5 Conclusion

As the correlation coefficients seem to be more promising than the amplitude errors, we may expect clinical utility of the method only when robust parameters are computed from the transformed maps. Though the utility of the Laplacian method was demonstrated in recent papers, some further studies on its applicability seems to be justified.

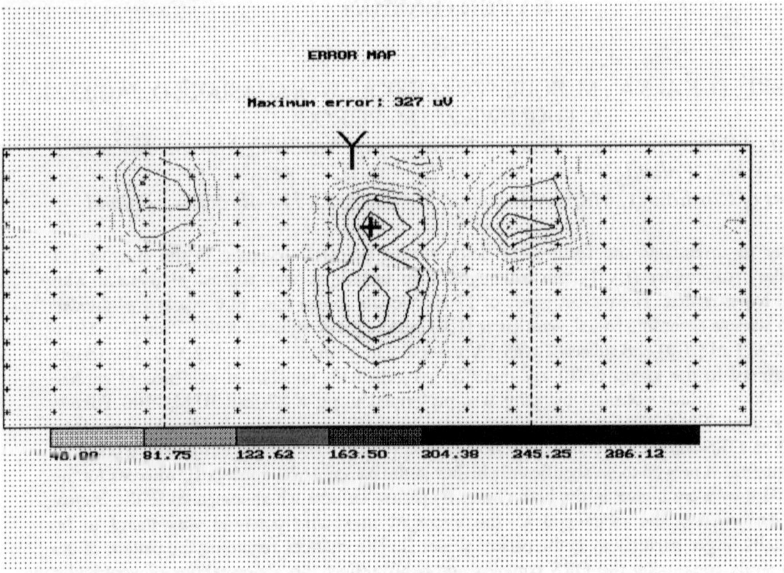

Figure 2. The spatial error distribution.

Acknowledgments

The authors express the grace to Prof. Musso for the experimental lead maps and to R. Hoekema for the transformation matrix data. The project was supported in part by the National Research Fund under grant no. F21247.

References

1. Gy. Kozmann *et al,* Comp. in Card.'94 409-411, IEEE, Washington, (1994).
2. Lux *et al,* Circulation 59, 356 (1979).
3. P. Savard *et al,* J of Electrocardiol., 18 (3), (1985).
4. D. Stilli *et al,* J of Electrocardiol., 21 (1), (1988).
5. T.F. Oostendorp *et al,* J. of Computational Physics. 80, 331-343 (1989).
6. N. Nagy, *et al,* in this volume.
7. R. Hoekema *et al,* IEEE EMB, Amsterdam, (1996).

ASSESSMENT OF LEFT VENTRICULAR HYPERTROPHY BY QRS ISOINTEGRAL MAPS IN PATIENTS WITH ESSENTIAL HYPERTENSION

J. JAGIELSKI[1], D. KAŁKA[2], M. SOBIESZCZAŃSKA[1], W. BANASIAK[2], D. JAGIELSKI[1], A. FUGLEWICZ[2], M. PIERÓG[2]

[1]*Department of Pathophysiology, Wroclaw University of Medicine, Marcinkowskiego 1, 50-368 Wroclaw, Poland*

[2]*Department of Cardiology, Military Hospital, Weigla 4, 53-114 Wroclaw, Poland*

In order to investigate the features of body surface potential mapping in the case of left ventricular hypertrophy (LVH), the isointegral map technique was applied in patients with essential hypertension. The patient group of 27 individuals (mean age: 48.6 years) was divided into two subsets according to left ventricular (LV) muscle mass: subset I with LV mass < 230 g (mean: 209.3 ±11.1 g) and subset II with LV mass > 230 g (mean: 253.2 ±12.3 g). The results were referred to the group of 30 age-matched subjects with no clinical evidence of cardiac disease. Body surface potential mapping was performed using a 87-lead HPM 7100 Fukuda Denshi system. The following group-mean isointegral maps were constructed for the three time intervals of QRS complex: A (QRS), B (QR-S) and C (Q-RS). The values of maximum potential for the integral A proved to be significantly higher in the patients of the subset II, whereas for the integral B they were higher in the both (I and II) patient subsets when compared to the control group. As concerns the isointegral C, the averaged maximum potential was found to be substantially larger exclusively in the patient subset II. The changes regarding the pattern of the time integrals comprising the QRS complex probably reflect the abnormalities of ventricular repolarization properties dependent on the advance of LVH. The results seem to justify the conclusion that body surface isointegral mapping can be considered as the useful tool in diagnosing left ventrticular hypertrophy.

Introduction

A method of body surface potential mapping (BSPM) is considered to be a non-invasive and an unique approach for exploring the cardiac electric field. A predominance of this method, with regards to the conventional 12-lead electrocardiogram, is determined by the fact that body surface mapping permits detection of precious physiologic and diagnostic information, acquired on the basis of a huge amount of electrocardiographic signals collected from many sites spread over the entire thorax. The advantage of the surface maps is a direct association of the zones of positive and negative surface potentials with major waveforms and electric events of the heart. Furthermore, BSPM gives emphasis to the location-intensity interrelation providing a spatial resolution not offered by the other electrocardiographic method that stress the time-intensity interaction. Surface mapping was also found to be characterized by a higher degree of accuracy as compared with the standard ECG testing. Evidence is still being accumulated that

BSPM might be of great value in detecting as well as in predicting various conditions which are not clinically apparent [1,2,3]. Among many others, the attempts have been made to verify the anticipation that surface mapping could prove to be a reliable tool for evaluating left ventricular hypertrophy in diagnosing of which the criteria of conventional ECG are often insufficient and misleading.

The present study was undertaken to assess the usefulness of body surface potential mapping in detecting left ventricular hypertrophy following arterial essential hypertension by using the time integral technique.

Material

A study population consisted of 27 consecutive patients (18 males and 9 females) whose age ranged from 29 to 56 years, with the mean age of 48.6 ±5.7 years. All of them demonstrated clinically defined arterial essential hypertension (blood pressure >160/90 mmHg) in the course of which left ventricular hypertrophy (LVH) occurred. On the echocardiographic examination performed in each patient LVH was determined as the concentric one, i.e., with increased left ventricular mass accompanying by increased relative wall thickness [4] Patients enrolled in this study were divided into two subsets according to left ventricular muscle mass evaluated echocardiographically. Subset I comprised 12 patients (mean age: 41.6 years) with LV mass less than 230 g (mean mass: 209.3± 11.1 g), whereas subset II included 15 patients (mean age: 55.1 years) with LV mass > 230 g (mean mass: 253.2± 12.3 g). Patients with previous myocardial infarction, angina pectoris, cardiac valvular disease or abnormalities of serum electrolyte (K, Na, Ca, Cl) were excluded from the study. A group of 30 age-matched subjects (23 males and 7 females), showing no clinically documented impairments of cardiovascular system, served as the control.

Methods

Body surface mapping procedure was performed with the use of the HPM 7100 Fukuda Denshi system. Digitized electrocardiographic signals were recorded simultaneously from 87 leads covering the torso (59 placed on the anterior thorax and 28 on the back), with Wilson's central terminal as a reference, and sampled with a frequency of 1000 samples/sec/channel. A subject of interest were isointegral maps constructed for QRS complex which was divided into the three following time intervals: A = QRS, B = QR-S and C = Q-RS. The mentioned isointegrals, expressed in microvolt-seconds, were calculated for each lead as the algebraic sum of all positive and negative potentials from the appriopriate time instants of onset and offset, multiplied by the sampling interval. The time instants of every interval onset and offset were identified manually from superimposed Frank X, Y and Z leads.

Left ventricular mass was determined on the basis of echocardiographic measurements according to the formula reported by Devereaux and Reichek:

$$\text{LV mass [g]} = 1.04\,[(\text{LVID} + \text{VST} + \text{PWT})^3 - (\text{LVID})^3 - 13.6;$$

where LVID = end-diastolic left ventricular internal dimension, VST = interventricular septal thickness, PWT = posterior wall thickness [5].

Statistical analysis was performed using the Student's test considering p value < 0.01 as statistically significant.

Results

In the consequence of the statistical analysis performed, the group-mean QRS, QR-S and Q-RS isointegral maps for the subset I and II of patients demonstrating left ventricual hypertrophy, likewise for the control subjects were constructed. As the discriminating factor, reflecting a characteristic of the successive A, B and C time integrals, the maximum value of surface potential was established. The findings revealed that the maximum values calculated for the A integral were significantly higher in patients of the subset II in comparison with the values obtained for the control group. As concerns the B integral, the maximum potential proved to be larger for either (I and II) patient subset when referred to that in normal subjects. The maximum values of potential established for the integral C were significantly higher exclusively in the patient subset II when compared to those in controls.

Discussion

The preliminary findings obtained in the present study showed that a condition of left ventricular hypertrophy, developing as the adaptive mechanism in the course of arterial systemic hypertension, have an appreciable effect on the pattern of isointegral maps constructed for the successive time intervals of QRS complex. There was a statistically significant increase of the maximum values of body surface potential observed in patients demonstrating echocardiographically recognized left ventricular hypertrophy in comparison with the data collected from the control subjects. In this regards, our observations are in the general accordance with the outcomes described by the other authors [3,6,7].

The considered alterations in the isointegral body surface potential characteristics are probably to reflect the abnormalities regarding intrinsic repolarization properties ongoing within the hypertrophed left ventricle muscle. It is noteworthy that in the patients with a moderate stage of LVH the changes of the maximum potential values occurred only in the A isointegral map comprising the initial phase of QRS complex, which corresponds to interventricular septum activation. On the other hand, in the patients demonstrating a severe LVH the increase of the maximum potential was found in the all isointegral maps covering every time intervals of QRS complex.

The conclusion can be drawn that the abnormalities of the QRS isointegral maps are correlated with the extent of LVH advance. Therefore, isointegral body surface mapping seems to be a promising and valuable technique in detecting left ventricular hypertrophy, but its full clinical reliability remains to establish through the further investigations.

References

1. D.M. Mirvis, *Circulation*, 75, 684 (1987)
2. L.B. Mitchell et al., *Circulation*, 86, 383 (1992).
3. M. Yamaki et al., *Circulation*, 79, 312 (1989).
4. H.M. Krumholz et al., *JACC*, 25, 879 (1995).
5. J. Tingleff et al., *Eur. Heart J.*, 17, 143 (1996).
6. H. Igarashi et al., *Jpn. Circ. J.*, 51, 284 (1987).
7. H. Hoshi et al., *Jpn. Heart J.*, 28, 829 (1987).

DIAGNOSIS OF NON-Q WAVE MYOCARDIAL INFARCTION BY ISOAREA DEPARTURE MAPS USING DIFFERENT TIME PERIODS

M. MEDVEGY, I. PRÉDA, A. PINTÉR
Cardiovasc. Center, Imre Haynal Univ., Budapest, Hungary-1135, Szabolcs 35.

R.A. NADEAU, P. SAVARD, G. TREMBLAY, J. NASMITH, D. PALISAITIS
Montréal Univ., Research Centre, Montréal, Canada, 5400 Gouin ouest H4J 1C5

GY. SÁNDOR
Research Institute for Materials Science, Budapest, Hungary-1525, P.O.B. 49.

The known 0-1/3 QRS, 0-QRS and 0-QRST isoarea departure maps give only an approximate localization of potential losses of different heart regions. The new, specific isoarea departure maps which involve only 10 ms time periods detect the electrical events related to the different activation time of the different heart regions. There are no statistical differences between the different types of isoarea departure maps in detecting potential losses. However, the selective isoarea departure maps are more favourable in the discrimination of multiple potential losses.

1. Introduction

The diagnosis of acute non-Q wave myocardial infarction (NQMI) is generally based on clinical observations, laboratory test results and ST-T changes on the ECG.[1] However, these diagnostic signs are missing when chronic NQMI is being considered. Therefore, attempts have been made to diagnose chronic NQMI by different non-invasive methods, like body surface potential mapping (BSPM).[2,3,4,5]

BSPM methods may detect electric abnormalities - such as potential losses during depolarisation, which could develop due to NQMI but are insufficient to cause a Q wave. The QRST, entire QRS and first 1/3 QRS isoarea departure maps that are used in the literature gave only an approximate diagnosis of NQMI.[2,3] Previous studies indicated that changes due to potential losses are usually present only during a limited time period at a characteristic time point of the depolarisation.[6,7]

The aim of the current retrospective study was to analyse selective body surface isoarea departure maps drawn at 0-8, 10-18, 20-28, 30-38, 40-48 ms after the QRS onset in clinically proven NQMI in the chronic phase of the disease and to compare them to the less selective isoarea maps (first 1/3 QRS, QRS, QRST).

2. Methods

45 patients (pts) (32 m, 13 f, 61 /41-75/ yrs) with proven non-Q MI were examined by BSPM. 21 healthy adults (14 m, 7 f, 31 /17-38/ yrs) constituted the control group to calculate the departure maps. No study patient had a cardiac disorder other than ischemic heart disease. Exclusion ECG criteria were atrial fibrillation, intraventricular conduction disturbances and signs of left ventricular hypertrophy or strain.

BSPM were recorded by 63 unipolar leads using the Montréal configuration.[8] The ECG signals were amplified, sampled at 500 sample/sec and converted to a 10 bit digital format by a custom made system (Cordic). To improve the signal-to-noise ratio, signal averaging was performed for periods of 52 sec. After baseline correction, five "selective" and three "conventional" isoarea maps were constructed with the torso surface represented by a rolled-out cylinder cut along the right midaxillary line. Finally, departure maps were generated to the mean ± 2 S.D. of the maps of 21 normal subjects at each lead for all periods (5+3 departure maps for each pts). On the departure maps, the potential difference is indicated if it exceeded the 2 S.D.

To localize the potential losses, the body surface projection area of the heart regions[9] and the cardiac activation sequence[10] were taken into account. Similar changes in two consecutive selective maps were required to determine the location of the potential loss on the basis of the selective maps. The localization of the potential losses were verified by the coronary artery status, wall motion abnormalities on ventriculography, fixed perfusion defect on exercise thallium[201] test and localization of the repolarisation changes of the acute phase ECG.

3. Results

Characteristic signs on selective isoarea departure maps are shown in Figure 1.

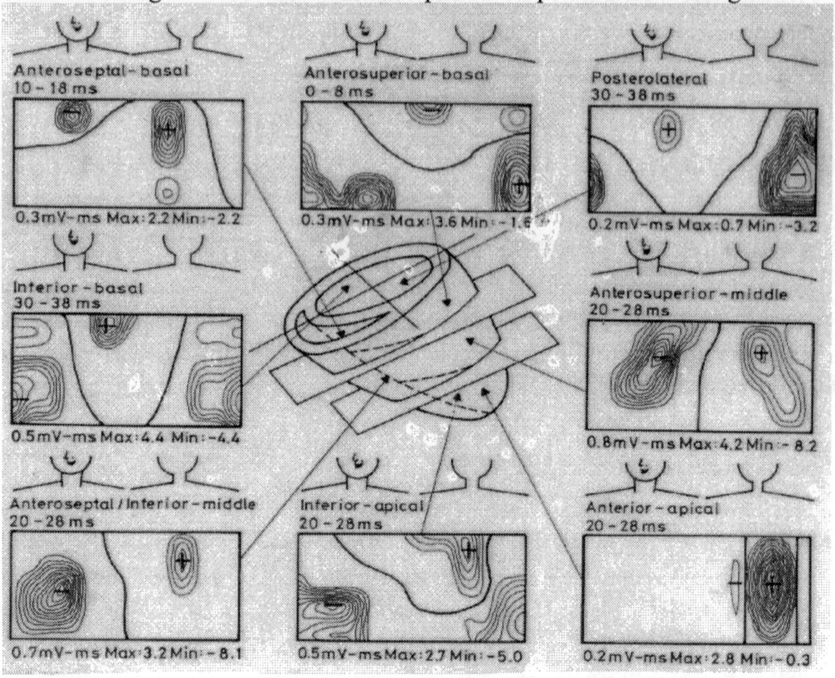

Figure 1: Characteristic changes of selective isoarea departure maps for different localization of potential losses. Difference between two lines, the maximum and minimum values are given.

The initial anterior-superior middle or anterior-superior left sided abnormal negativities indicate anteroseptal-basal or anterosuperior-basal potential losses referring directly to the necrosis site. Abnormal negativitiy on the right side at about 10-24 ms indicates anteroseptal/inferior-middle changes. An abnormal positivity on the back indicating anterior-apical potential loss is a reciprocal change due to a well localized frontal-apical potential loss which does not produce an anterior negativity because of the neighbouring high positive areas. This second positivity is present at about 16-46 ms. Inferior negativity at about 20-24 ms indicates inferior apical potential loss. Anterior left sided negativity at about 24-42 ms indicates anterosuperior middle potential loss. Abnormal negativity on the back at about 30-40 ms indicates posterolateral (basal or middle) potential losses. Potential loss of the inferior-basal region can result in an abnormal negativity in the right upper frontal part of the chest because in this time period (34-40ms) the anterior regions are already depolarised but its negativity results in a less negative value.

Sensitivity, specificity and the ratio of the verified localizations are displayed in Table 1. There were no significant changes, but the tendency in the specificity and the ratio of verified localizations is more favourable in the cases of selective isoarea departure maps.

Table 1: Differences between selective and non-selective isoarea departure maps

Isoarea departure maps	**Sensitivity**	**Specificity**	**Ratio of verified localization**
Selective maps	**82 %**	**71 %**	**86 %**
First 1/3 QRS	88 %	57 %	84 %
Entire QRS	88 %	62 %	76 %
QRST	91 %	52 %	67 %

The main advantage of the selective maps is that the short time periods can help us in the discrimination of multiple potential losses by the different activation time of the different regions (Fig. 2)

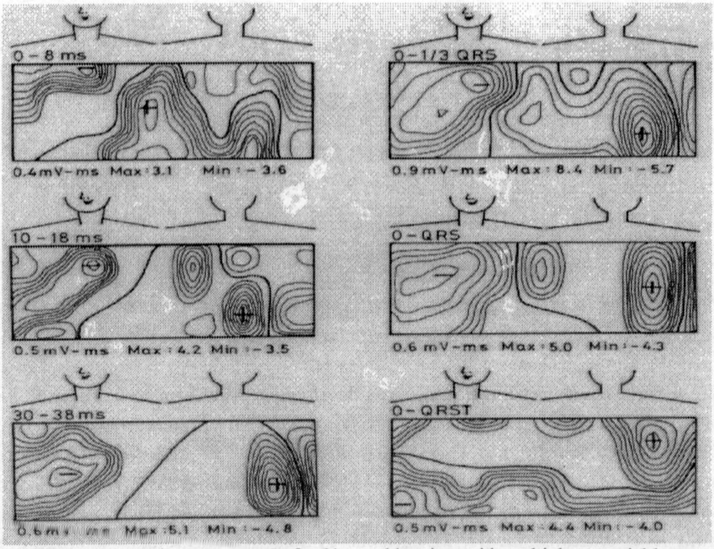

Figure 2: Different isoarea departure maps of a 64 yrs old patient with multiple potential losses: anteroseptal-basal, -middle and -apical. 0-8 ms selective map showed the minimum according to the anteroseptal-basal potential loss. 10-18 ms selective map indicated a septal-middle potential loss. 30-38 ms selective map revealed indirect reciprocal sign of the anterior-apical potential loss. 0-1/3 QRS and 0-QRS departure maps only suggested these potential losses while 0-QRST map did not give any information on the location. Difference between two lines, the maximum and minimum values are given.

Acknowledgements

Supported by grant „Foundation for Hungarian Higher Education and Research" and by a grant from the Medical Research Council of Canada. The authors would like to thank Dr András Paksy for his statistical advices.

References

1. RH Selvester et al. in *Comprehensive electrocardiology*, ed. PW Macfarlane et al. (Pergamon, New York pp:565-629, 1989)
2. L Ambroggi, *J Electrocardiol.* **19:**225-234 (1986)
3. L Ambroggi et al. *J Electrocardiol.* **21:**321-329 (1988)
4. J Osugi et al. *J Electrocardiol.* **17:**55-62 (1984)
5. M Hirai et al. *Am Heart J.* **108:**975-982 (1984)
6. M Medvegy et al. *Circ. Suppl.* **94:**I-731 (1996)
7. Zs Cserjés et al. *Jap.Heart J. Suppl.* **35:**93-94 (1994)
8. P Savard et al. *J Electrocardiol.* **18:**211-222 (1985)
9. NC Flowers and LG Horan, in: *Cardiac electrophysiology. From cell to bedside*, ed. DP Zipes and J Jalife (Saunders Comp, Philadelphia. pp:1049-1067, 1995)
10. D Durrer et al. *Circ.* **41:**899-912 (1970)

ANTIDEPRESSANT DRUGS AND ECG BODY SURFACE MAPS

I. PACLT
Department of Psychiatry, First Faculty of Medicine, Charles University, Prague, Czech Republic

O. KITTNAR, J. SLAVÍČEK
Department of Physiology, First Faculty of Medicine, Charles University, Prague, Czech Republic

Some antidepressant drugs have cardiovascular side effects (antimuscarinic, antihistaminic and quinidine-like effect). To compare the ECG effects of antidepressant drugs, the electrocardiogram, vectorcardiogram (VCG) and body surface maps (BSM) were recorded in 1) psychiatric patients without cardiovascular diseases, both sexes, treated by a) tricyclic antidepressants (TCA) amitriptyline, dosulepin, 150–300 mg daily dose, 22 patients, b) lithium, serum level 0.6±0.08 meq/l, 21 patients, c) selective serotonine reuptake inhibitor (SSRI) citalopram, daily doses 20-60 mg, 30 patients, and in 2) controls, 23 patients, of the same age (40± 5 years). In TCA patients the heart rate was increased, QT and RR intervals shortened ($p<0.01$, antimuscarinic effect) which was not observed in lithium and SSRI patients. All antidepressants decreased the absolute value of maximum (extremum) of depolarization isointegral maps, Li and TCA the initial and citalopram the later phase of depolarization. Citalopram decreased the amplitude of R wave and changed the location of minimum in repolarization isointegral maps and the location of Q and S wave amplitude. The results confirm the antimuscarinic effects of TCA in therapeutic doses and precise the intraventricular effects of antidepressants.

Tricyclic antidepressant drugs (TCA) display some cardiovascular side effects: 1) antimuscarinic, 2) antihistaminic and 3) quinidine-like effects [1]. The antimuscarinic effect (atropine-like effect) is represented by tachycardia, mydriasis, memory defects and obstipation. The antihistaminic effect is expressed by the increase of body weight due to the water retention. The quinidine-like effect consists of the decreased intraventricular conduction. The antimuscarinic effect is most pronounced [2]. TCA have a restrictive effect on the membrane Na-K pump manifested by the prolongation of the action potential duration, QRS duration, of the refractory period and of the QT interval (quinidine-like effect) [3].

Selective serotonine reuptake inhibitors (SSRI) have lower affinity to noradrenergic muscarinic and histamine receptors than TCA have. The heart rate is unchanged or slightly reduced. It is not entirely known, if SSRI increase the tone of parasympathetic, or decrease the tone of sympathetic nervous system [4]. The side effect of lithium on cardiovascular apparatus was described as the isoelectricity of T wave with bundle branch blocks and presence of U wave [5].

The purpose of the present work was a comparison of electrocardiographic parameters in depressive patients treated with TCA (amitriptyline, dosulepin), SSRI citalopram, and lithium in prophylactic use recording ECG, body surface maps (BSM) for a more detailed analysis. BSM Taccardi [6] technique permits-due to a high number and density of leads in the precordial area-to extract almost all accessible ECG informations.

Three groups of patients, both sexes and those aged 30–45 years from the Department of Psychiatry, Prague were studied (Table 1).

Table 1
Characteristics of examined groups

	Controls	TCA	Lithium	Citalopram
Number	21	22	21	30
Age	40.81±9.2	42.54±16.76	45.86±10.92	41.20±14.74
Men	12	5	13	6
Women	9	17	8	24
Serum level (meq/l)			0.66±0.08	
Daily dose (mg)		75–300		20–60
Duration of therapy		4–5 weeks	11–22 years	4–5 weeks

Mean ± S.E.M. (age)

ECG, VCG and BSM [6] were recorded using the diagnostic system Cardiag [7,8]. Thirty two parameters of heart electric field have been measured [9,10]: ECG: heart rate, duration PQ, QRS, QT, QTc, RR. VCG: P, QRS, T loop direction, shape, in frontal, transversal and left sagittal planes, QRS-STT space angle, QRS axis deviation in frontal plane. Mapping: isopotential, depolarization and repolarization (DIPM, RIPM) maps, their maximum and minimum (uV). Isointegral depolarization (DIIM), repolarization (RIIM), total (DRIIM) maps, their maximum and minimum (absolute values, uVs). Isoarea depolarization (DIAM 30, DIAM 40) and repolarization (RIAM 35, RIAM 80) maps, their maximum and minimum (uVs), isopotential maps of asynchronnous maximum R wave (IPMAM-R, uV). Isopotential maps of asynchronnous minimum Q and S wave (IPMAM-QS, uV) [9,10].

For the statistical evaluation the analysis ANOVA and T-test was used.

The results are summarized in Table 2.

Table 2
Effects of antidepressant drugs on some ECG parameters in patients and controls.

Parameter Number	Controls 21	TCA 22	Lithium 21	Citalopram 30
Heart rate	71.91±8.69	90.96±16.66 ***	74.91±13.01	75.57±13.66
QT (ms)	371.05±21.50	342.55±37.86 *	401.62±131.25	375.00±33.77
RR (ms)	845.62±101.28	682.55±131.62 **	827.33±171.95	821.07±151.97
DIIM max (uVs)	39.50±17.80	31.94±14.36 *	32.25±13.59	27.87±11.75
RIIM max (uVs)	67.19±22.28	50.50±18.80	62.50±27.41	43.38±24.41 *
DIAM max 30 (uVs)	5.65±1.98	4.21±1.32 *	4.61±1.18 *	4.43±1.70
IPMAM-R (mV)	1.91±0.70	1.59±0.50	1.69±0.70	1.39±0.45 *

DIIM - max - maximum (extremum) of depolarization isointegral mapRIIM - max - maximum (extremum) of repolarization isointegral mapDIAM - max - maximum (extremum) of depolarization isoarea map (isointegral map from the beginning of QRS to 30t ms of depolarization) IPMAM-R - maximum amplitude of waveMean ± S.E.M. * $p<0.05$, ** $p<0.01$, *** $p<0.001$ *in comparison with controls.*

In TCA patients the most pronounced tachycardia was observed with the shortening of QT and RR intervals (anticholinergic effect). In TCA and lithium patients the parameter DIAM max 30 (absolute value of maximum, extremum in the initial phase of depolarization) was significantly decreased (quinidine-like effect). In citalopram patients the DIIM max and

RIIM max (absolute value of maximum, extremum in the later phase of depolarization and repolarization) was decreased (delay of intraventricular activation and repolarization). Furthermore, the maximum amplitude of R wave (IPMAM-R) was lower than in controls (Tab. 2).

The minimum (extremum) of repolarization isointegral map (RIIM min) in controls is localized both on the right precordium and on the back thorax but in the lateral wall of thorax there are the positive values. On the other hand. The QS-IPMAM (the most negative amplitude of Q and S wave) is localized in the front right precordium only and in upper part of thorax. Both parameters were placed one intercostal space lower in SSRI patients, than in controls; $p<0.05$). The location of the other parameters was not significantly different.

In cellular level clomipramine, amitriptyline and maprotiline significantly decreased the calcium current during AP in rat heart ventricle myocytes studied by patch clamp method [11]. These agents and SSRI citalopram decreased the peak amplitude of Ca current. Lithium substitutes the Na in the membrane of heart cells [12], respectively decreases the i_{NaCa} current [13].

The decrease of maximum (extremum) in all groups of our patients in isointegral and isoarea maps probably depends on the decrease of calcium current (quinidine-like effect). From the clinical point of view in our patients TCA ambulatory doses provoked both anticholinergic effect (tachycardia) and small quinidine-like effect, while the other antidepressants showed only small quinidine-like effect, detectable also by signal averaged ECG [14].

References

1. AH Glassman and JT Biggert, Arch. Gen. Psych. 38, 815 (1981).
2. MT Boehnert and FH Lowejoy, Jr., New Engl. J. Med. 313, 474 (1985).
3. FM Weld and JT Biggert, Circ. Res. 46, 167 (1980).
4. AH Glassman et al, Nord. J. Psychiatry Suppl. 30, 41 (1993).
5. JE Mitchell and TB Mackenzie, J. Clin. Psychiatry 43, 47 (1982).
6. B Taccardi, Circ. Res. 12, 341 (1963).
7. M Stojan et al, Physiol. Res. 42, 85 (1993).
8. O Kittnar et al, Physiol. Res. 42, 123 (1993).
9. J Slavíček et al, Cor et Vasa 27, 212 (1995).
10. I Paclt et al, Homeostasis 36, 223 (1995).
11. I Minarovič et al, J. Mol. Cell. Cardiol. 27, 130 (1995).
12. EE Carmeliet, J. Gen. Physiol. 47, 501 (1964).
13. NC Janvier and MR Boyett, Cardiovasc. Res. 32, 69 (1996).
14. B. Mladosevicova et al., Int. J. Cardiol. 54, 27 (1996).

THE INITIAL QRS LEFT IN SEVERE VENTRICULAR PRESSURE OVERLOADING: A BODY SURFACE POTENTIAL MAPPING STUDY

J. LIEBMAN

Case Western Reserve University, Rainbow Babies and Childrens Hospital, 11100 Euclid Avenue, Suite 380, Cleveland, OH 44106-6011, USA

Body Surface Potential Mapping with 180 electrodes was performed in 31 children with severe pressure overloading, including 19 with severe aortic stenosis and 12 with severe pulmonic stenosis. The BSPM's were very different. In aortic stenosis, the major change from normal is that the maximum is very abnormally to the left and posterior from normal while in pulmonic stenosis the major change from normal is that the maximum is only a little left of normal, but the peak negative potential is more superior than average and near the spine.

1 Introduction

It is known that the initial QRS of the electrocardiogram may be directed to the left in various cardiac abnormalities including severe pressure overload of the right or left ventricles[1]. In previous studies of aortic stenosis[2] and in pulmonic stenosis[3] we have shown that the more severe the stenosis the more likely is the initial QRS to the left. Although the mechanisms are not known, body surface potential mapping may provide important insights into those mechanisms.

In this study we present 12 patients with severe pulmonic stenosis and initial QRS to the left and 19 patients with severe aortic stenosis and initial QRS to the left.

2 Material and Methods

Each of the 31 patients was examined by one of us (JL), had a standard electrocardiogram using either the Siemens-Elema Mingograph 61 or the Marquette - 15 with six channels recorded simultaneously and had a Frank System vectorcardiogram using either an Instrument for Cardiac Research device (Instant VCG) or the Marguette (MAC15). The standard ECG and Frank VCG were recorded just before recording of the body surface potential maps (BSPM).

The BSPM potentials were recorded, processed and displayed as previously described [4-8]. The acquisition system utilizes 180 Ag-AgCl passive electrodes with active cable along with sheilding and high impact impedance of the amplifiers. Thus, no electrode paste is necessary. The electrodes are enclosed in a semi elastic soft plastic vest secured with velcro. A selection of vest sizes is used to accommodate variations in size and body habitus. The electrodes extend from the level of the clavicle to just above the umbilicus. The majority of the patients used a vest with 135 electrodes anterior and 45 electrodes posterior. The ECG signals are conducted through coaxial cables to very high input resistance sample and hold amplifiers, where each electrode is referenced to the Wilson central terminal. Details of the instrumentation and design were described by Kavuru at al.[7] and pseudocolor display by Thomas and Lee[6], Lee at al[8] and Huebner et al.[9].

3 Patient Material

There were 19 patients (average age 15 years) with severe valvular aortic stenosis and initial QRS to the left on the standard ECG and Frank system about to have cardiac surgery. Of the 19, 11 were catheterized and the average left ventricular systolic pressure was 218 mmHg. There were 12 patients with severe pulmonic stenosis with initial QRS to the left on the standard ECG and Frank system VCG about to have cardiac surgery or balloon valvuloplasty. The average age was 8 years; all 12 were catheterized and the average RV systolic pressure was 117 mmHg.

On the Frank system VCG in the 19 patients with AS, the initial QRS was anterior left and in 2/19 posterior and left. On the Frank system VCG and the 12 patients with PS, the initial QRS was anterior left or straight anterior in all. In none was the initial QRS to the right.

In the BSPM of normal children, at the onset of ventricular activation there is invariably a maximum (the peak positive potential) over the sternum or slightly to the left, and usually superior. The peak negative potential (minimum) is more variable but is usually left anterior or slightly posterior and inferior to the maximum.

In all 19 patients with severe AS, the initial maximum was well to the left, near the left axillary line, with two posterior to that line. The early minima were more variable but invariably the overall early negative potentials were to the right of the overall peak positive potential.

In all 12 patients with severe PS the maximum was only a little left of the sternum and in 3 cases more inferior than average. The minimum was very variable but in 8/12 was more superior than average and in 11/12 was near or over the spine (more to the right of the maximum).

Thus, the BSPM's clearly show very different early QRS findings in severe AS and PS. In severe AS the changes in the initial maxima and minima indicate that the "vector" of initial activation is to the left and posterior consistent with marked hypertrophy of the free posterior wall of the left ventricle. On the other hand, in severe PS the initial maxima and minima indicate that the "vector" of initial activation is to the left anterior inferior, consistent with the hypothesis of marked hypertrophy of the left anterior inferior portion of the right ventricular anterior wall below the septum, plus possibly the influence of right septal hypertrophy. Proximity effects may play a role.

It is useful to look hypothetically at the vector of the initial QRS. There are five areas of the ventricle initially activated at or near the same time. Normally, the largest contribution is the rightward anterior vector from stimulation of the left posterior side of the septum half to two-thirds down, by the left posterior branch of the left bundle. (Fig. 1a) This branch also stimulates activation of the left ventricular (LV) posterior free wall resulting in a left posterior vector. (Fig. 1b) Since the septum at that level has a greater muscle mass than does the LV posterior free wall, the septal vector is larger than the free posterior wall vector. At close to the same time the anterior branch of the left bundle stimulates the septum to cause activation up the septum, resulting in a vector which is superior and slightly to the right posterior. (Fig. 1e) The right bundle courses down the right side of the septum to go through the moderator band. From here it give a small right septal branch causing activation of what is believed to be the right ventricular portion of the septum[11]. The result is a small vector to the left and posterior. (Fig. 1c) The right bundle, on going through the moderator band then stimulates the endocardium which, according to Myerberg[11,12] very rapidly causes stimulation of the entire right ventricular endocardium. The result is a prominent anterior vector which should be to the right. (Fig. 1d) Therefore, adding the five vectors that make up initial activation results in a normal initial QRS to the right, anterior and superior (Fig. 1).

Fig. 2 is the hypothetical summation of initial QRS vectors when there is severe hypertrophy of the free left ventricular posterior wall (Fig. 2b). The large vector to the left and posterior changes the vector from all five areas from right and anterior to left and anterior. In Fig. 3 is the hypothetical summation of initial QRS vectors and there is severe hypertrophy of the left anterior inferior wall (Fig. 3d). The large vector to the left and anterior inferior changes the vector from all five areas from right anterior superior to left anterior inferior. (The inferior aspects are not delineated in the figure).

Obviously the concept as to mechanisms described above have to remain hypothetical without more proof. The imminent successful solution to the inverse problem would help, as would firm data as to specific changes in activation sequence in various pathologies including severe hypertrophy. The data of Ruttkay-Nedecky et al[13] is also consistent with the above in that the greater the echographic mass in patients with aortic stenosis and coarctation of the aorta, the smaller the initial QRS vectors. (If the QRS is to the left, the magnitude of the initial vector to the right is zero.)

That initial QRS left can be used as a clinical tool is without question, indicating severity, although the mechanism remains to be specifically delineated. Ruttkay-Nedecky suggests remodeling of the left ventricle, which would include hypertrophy of specific areas and could also include changes in activation

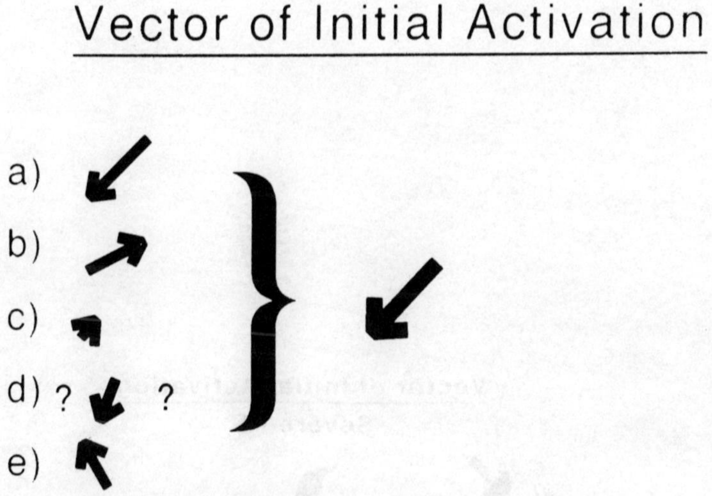
Vector of Initial Activation
a)
b)
c)
d) ? ?
e)

Fig. 1

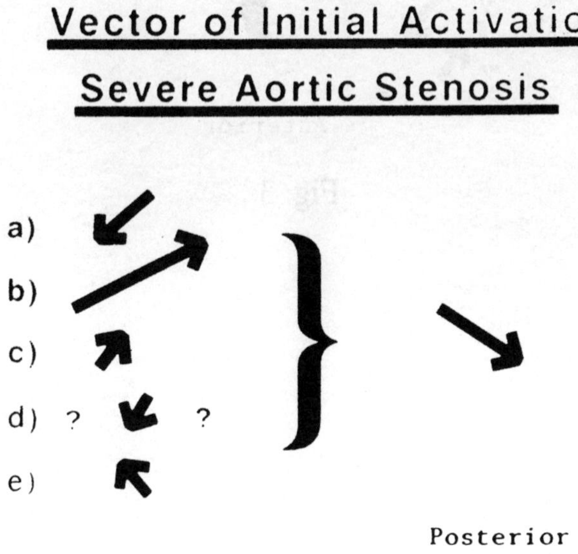
Vector of Initial Activation
Severe Aortic Stenosis
a)
b)
c)
d) ? ?
e)
Posterior

Fig. 2

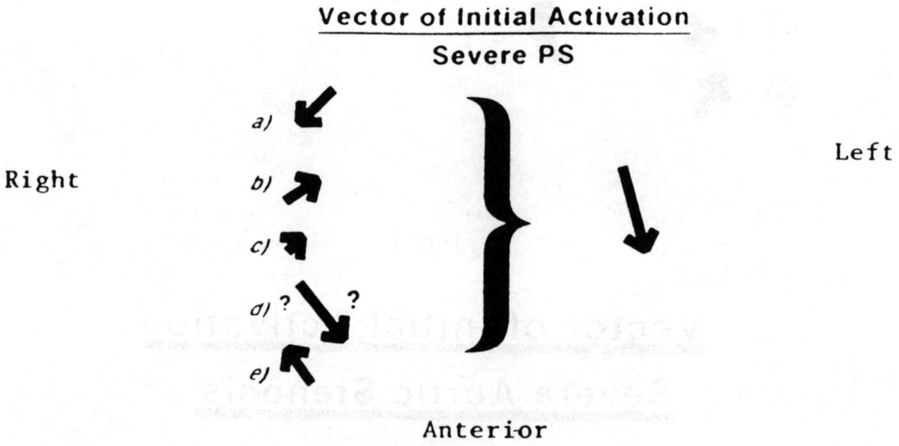
Vector of Initial Activation
Severe PS
Right
Left
a)
b)
c)
d) ?
?
e)
Anterior

Fig. 3

sequence. We believe that the former is evident from our data but present technology has not yet allowed knowledge of change in activation sequence.

References

1. Liebman, R. Plonsey, J.L. Ankeney, *Jap Ht J* **23 (Suppl),** 480 (1982)
2. Liebman, C.W. Thomas, Y. Rudy, R. Saltzberg in *Electrocardiology '92*, eds. P. Macfarlane and F. de Padua (World Scientific, Singapore, 1988)
3. J. Liebman, R. Saltzberg, C.W. Thomas in *Electrocardiology '93*, eds. P. Macfarlane and P. Rautaharju (World Scientific, Singapore, 1994)
4. C.W. Thomas, K. Laurita, G. Sun, J. Liebman, A. Waldo, *J Electrocardiol* **22 (Suppl)**, 64 (1990)
5. J. Liebman, C.W. Thomas, R. Fraenkel, Y. Rudy, R. Plonsey in *Pediatric and Fundamental Electrocardiography*, eds. J. Liebman, R. Plonsey, Y. Rudy (Martinus Nijhoff, The Netherlands 1987)
6. J. Liebman, C.W. Thomas, R. Fraenkel, Y. Rudy, J Electrocardiol 26, 25 (1993)
7. M.S. Kavuru, H. Vesselle, C.W. Thomas in *Pediatric and Fundamental Electrocardiography*, eds. J. Liebman, R. Plonsey, Y. Rudy (Martinus Nijhoff, The Netherlands 1987)
8. C.W. Thomas, D. Lee in *Pediatric and Fundamental Electrocardiography*, eds. J. Liebman, R. Plonsey, Y. Rudy (Martinus Nijhoff, The Netherlands 1987)
9. D. Lee, C.W. Thomas, Y. Rudy, J. Liebman, *Proc 13th Int Congress on Electrocardiology*, Washington DC, 17 (1986)
10. W. Huebner, C.W. Thomas, Y, Rudy, J. Liebman, *Proc 13th Int Congress on Electrocardiology*, Washington DC, 9 (1986)
11. R.J. Myerburg, K. Nilsson, H. Gelband, *Circ Res* **30**, 217, 1972
12. R.J. Myerburg, H. Gelband, K. Nilsson et al., *Circ Res* **42**, 27 (1978)
13. I. Ruttkay-Nedecky, E. Vanzurova, V. Szathmary, K. Kanalikova, R. Osvald, *J Electrocardiol* **27**, 201 (1994)

BODY SURFACE MAPPING EVALUATION OF REPERCUSSIONS OF THE REDUCTIVE VENTRICULECTOMY (BATISTA OPERATION) ON THE ELECTRICAL ACTIVATION OF THE HEART.

PASTORE,C.A;MOFFA,P.J.;TOBIAS,N.M.;MORAES,A,P.;KAISER,E.;
BACAL,F.;STOLF,N.;BOCCHI,E.;BELLOTTI,G.;PILEGGI,F. -
Heart Institute of HC FMUSP/UNIP - Al.Franca 797 -
CEP 01422 - 000 - São Paulo - Brazil

ABSTRACT

Body surface mapping aspects and its resulting departure areas of 15 patients, 13 male, aged between 38 and 68 years (average 49.7) were studied, all of which had been submitted to the reductive ventriculectomy surgery during the period January/95 to October/96. Each patient had a pre and post-operative BSM carried out, follow-up 45 days. Both positive and negative (± 2 standart deviations) Das were measured. Negative Das in the pre-op exams were highly significant with averages of 894.8 cm^2 for QRS and 440 cm^2 for ST-T. Average of positive Das were 658.8 cm^2 for QRS and 499 cm^2 for ST-T. QRST departure areas both negative and positive were of no statistical significance. Post-op exams had the negative Das of QRS with average of 466.2 cm^2 and ST-T with average of 253.8 cm^2. Positive DA's averges were 376.3 cm^2 for QRS and 174 cm^2 for ST-T. These findings evidenced a signifant)p< 0,05) reduction of the departure areas, both negative and positive, of QRS as well a of ST-T, which is in agreement with the voltage decrease found in all electrocardiographic and vectorcardiographic exams, and were compatible with the loss of myocardial lateral wall muscle resulting from the ventriculectomy. Four patients who died in the immediate and late post-operative had a dramatic reduction in the sizes of Das (p< 0,05) suggesting that an excessive or inadequate removal of wall tissue might have hindered a perfect remodeling of left ventricle chamber. Body surface mapping follow-up may contribute to improve this new surgical procedure.

INTRODUCTION

The partial ventriculectomy is a relatively simple surgery and consists in the resection of a large wedge of wall muscle from the lateral wall of the left ventricle, beginning at the apex, extending between the papillary muscles and ending proximal to the mitral annulus[1]. This surgery technique was designed by the Brazilian surgeon Dr. Randas Batista, as an interesting option for treatment of refractory heart failure in idiopathic dilated cardiomyopathies, since it can reverse some aspects of the cardiac remodeling like hypertrophy, dilation, change in left ventricular shape and augmented wall stress[2-5].

Anatomic and electric modifications of the heart activation which follow this type of surgery can be analysed through the classical non-invasive methods[6-7]. The purpose of this study is to analyse these repercussions using the Body Surface Mapping (BSM).

METHODS AND MATERIALS

Study Population

The study population consisted of 15 patients, 13 male, between 38 and 68 (average 49.7) years of age. These patients had been submitted to the partial ventriculectomy during the period ranging from January 1995 to October 1996. Each patient had a pre and a post operative BSM carried out, within a 45-day follow up. A clinical evaluation of patients was performed and all of them underwent ondomyocardial biopsy, echocardiography and coronary angiography to exclude myocarditis, ischemic cardiomyopathy and other forms of heart muscle disease.

Body Surface Mapping

BSM was performed using a HPM 7000 unit system (Fukuda Denshi Co.) in the preoperative and in the postoperative, within a 45-day follow-up. A departure area (DA) was obtained according to the potential distribution below and above the means normal range (- 2 SD and + 2 SD), which is determined by averaging the potential of normal control values in each lead point on the BSM. The DA of QRS, QRST and ST-T, both negative and positive ones, were calculated based on this method.

Statistical Analysis

Was performed using a chi-square test and Fischer`s exact test.Values less than 0.05 were considered to be significant.

RESULTS

Pre-op findings: the negative departure areas (DA) of QRS and ST-T averaged 894.8 cm^2 and 440 cm^2 respectively. The positive DA of QRS and ST-T averaged 658.8 cm^2 and 499 cm^2 respectively, and the QRST positive DA showed results similar to the negative ones.

Post-op findings: the negative DA of QRS and ST-T averaged 466.2 cm² and 253.8 cm² respectively. The positive DA of QRS and ST-T averaged 376.3 cm² and 174 cm² respectively. Both negative and positive DA of QRST figures were also of no statistical significance.(Table I)

TABLE I

cases	DA negatives cm^2		DA positives cm^2	
01 - 15	QRS	ST-T	QRS	ST-T
aver.pre	894.8	440.0	658.8	499.0
aver.post	466.2*	253.8*	376.3*	174.0*

p< 0,05

DISCUSSION

A significant reduction of DA (both negative and positive) of QRS and ST-T was obtained in the postoperative exams in all patients. This evidence is in agreement with the voltage decrease found in all ECG and VCG exams. The loss of lateral wall muscle itself brings about a reduction of the expression of electrical activity of the heart. In this way the DA are also expected to show a reduction, once they are highly sensitive to these modifications. Notwithstanding all the above effects, the reduction of left ventricular chamber and consequently of the volume of blood in it may contribute to decrease voltages and reduce the departure areas according to the description given before (Broddy's effect).

In the imediate postoperative one patient died (ventricular tachycardia) and 3 more patients died of progressive heart failure (26.6%) . In this group we observed a dramatic reduction in the size of DAs (p< 0.05), in the postoperative exam.(Table II). A possible cause of this findings could be that the removal of lateral wall muscle was inadequate to ensure a perfect remodelling of the left ventricule , perhaps because of either large loss of the lateral wall muscle or inappropriate location of the surgical area.

Table II

	DA negatives cm^2		DA positives cm^2	
	QRS	ST-T	QRS	ST-T
Case 4 - pre	266	227	343	420
post	23	0	476	30
Case 7 - pre	1035	386	331	240
post	280	0	0	25
Case 8 - pre	842	132	667	25
post	105	0	0	0
Case 10 - pre	730	363	603	403
post	66	0	0	0
aver - pre-op	718	277	496	270
aver - post- op	94*	0*	95*	11*

* $p < 0.05$

Fig 1.- ECG, VCG and BSM (Pre op , case 4)
DAs negative and positive of QRS and ST-T.

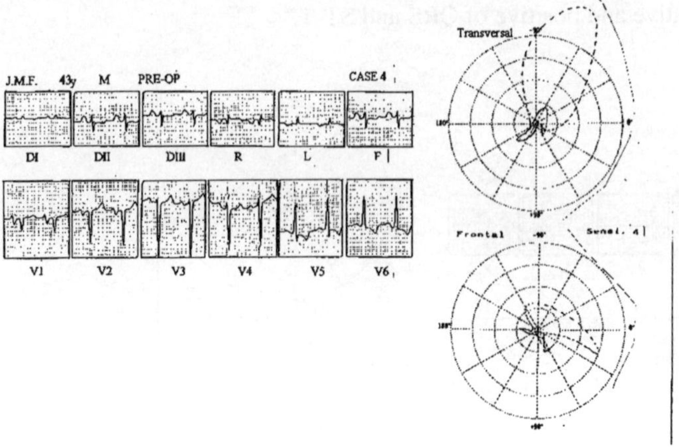

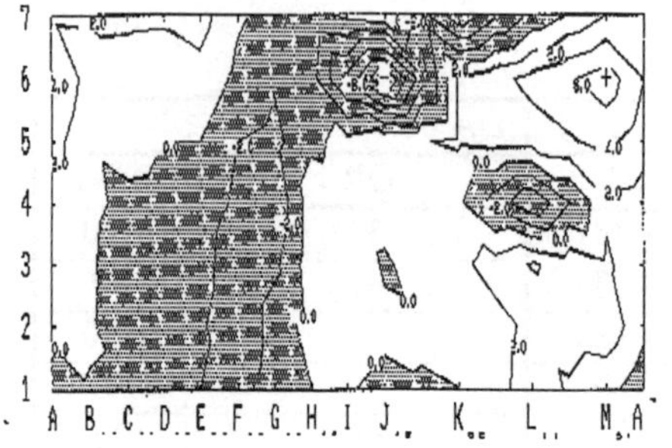

Fig 2.- ECG, VCG and BSM (Post-op , case 4)
DAs negative and positive of QRS and ST-T.

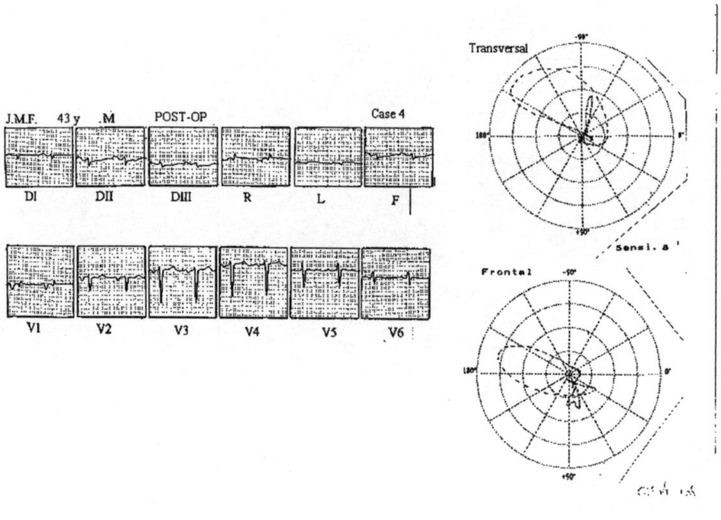

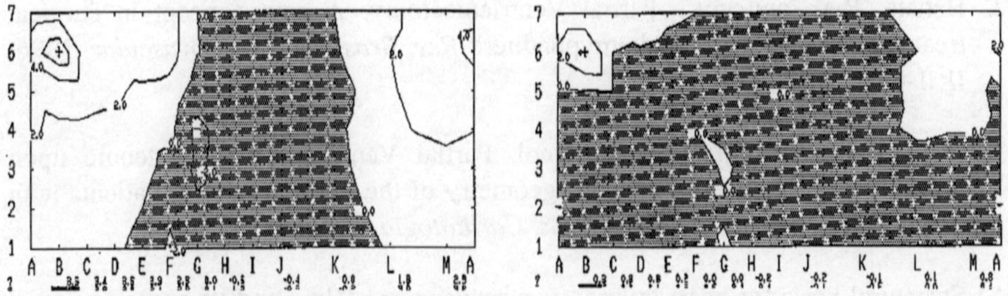

CONCLUSIONS

In the BSM it was evidenced that the most relevant factor to contribute to the reduction of DA sizes was the removal of the left ventricle lateral wall. Other factors like bundle branch blocks, left ventricle hypertrophy and myocardial infarction had a less significant role in these alterations.

The pre and post-operative follow-up of the Partial Ventriculectomy using the Body Surface Mapping may contribute to the improvement of this new surgical procedure.

REFERENCES

1. Bocchi, E.A.; Bellotti, G.; Moraes, A.P.; Bacal, F.; Moreira, L.F.; Esteves Filho, A.; Fukushima, T.; Guimarães, G.; Stolf, N.; Jatene, S.; Pileggi, F..Clinical outcome after left ventricular surgical remodeling in patients with idiopathic dilated cardiomyopathy referred to heart transplantation. Short term results. In publication *(Circulation).*

2. Batista, R.V. and col. Partial Ventriculectomy: A new concept in surgical treatment of end-stage cardiomyppathies. *Rev. Bras. Cir. Cardiovascular*. 1996; II: 1-6.

3. Bellotti, G.; Bocchi, E.A.; and col. Partial Ventriculectomy outcome upon mechanical properties, shape and geometry of the left ventricle in patients with dilated cardiomyopathies. *Arq. Bras. Cardiologia*. 1996; 67: 395-400.

4. Structural basis for heart failure: ventricular remodeling and its pharmaculogial inhibition.
Chon Jn Circulation 1995; 91: 1504-7.

5. Ventriculectomy - A direct apllication of Laplace's law. David A. Kass. Johs Hopkins School of Medicine. Arq. Bras. Cardiol. 1996; 67: 401-402.

6. Pastore, C.A.; Moffa, P.J.; Moraes, A.; Tobias, N.; Kaiser, E.; Bacal, F.; Moreira, L.F.; Stolf, N.; Bocchi, E.; Bellotti, G.; Pileggi, F. Pre and post-operative electrocardiographic aspects of patients submitted to the reductive ventriculectomy (Batista Operation). *XVIII Congress of the Cardiology Society of São Paulo. 1997; Abstract.*

7. Moffa, P.J.; Pastore, C.A.; Moraes, A.P.; Tobias, N.; Kaiser, E.; Bacal, F.; Moreira, L.F.; Stolf, N.; Bocchi, E.; Bellotti, G.; Pileggi, F. Analysis of pre and post-operative vectorcardiographic findings of patients submitted to the partial ventriculectomy (Batista Operation). *XVIII Congress of the Cardiology Society of São Paulo. 1997; Abstract.*

REFERENCE SAMPLE WITH APPROPRIATELY ADJUSTED CHARACTERISTICS IMPROVES THE DIAGNOSTIC ACCURACY OF DEPARTURE ISOINTEGRAL MAPS

Slavomira FILIPOVÁ
IVth Department of Internal Medicine, Faculty of Medicine, Comenius University, Bratislava, Slovak Republic
Milan TYŠLER, Mária TURZOVÁ, Vladimír ROSÍK, Peter KNEPPO
Institute of Measurement Science, Slovak Academy of Sciences, Bratislava, Slovak Republic

Previous clinical studies with departure isointegral body surface potential maps (DI-BSPM) have shown that strictly normal composition of the reference sample may lead to an unwanted amount of false positive findings, especially in the course of examination of patients with various degrees of CHD, arterial hypertension (with / without LVH). Then the patients with acute MIs, old MIs are correlated through the ideal reference sample in the course of DI-BSPM examination.
The aim of the study was to compare the effect of using reference samples with well defined pathologies in order to remove the confounding influence of complications (chronic CHD, arterial hypertension=AH) on the signs of acute and old local ischemic changes. The special programme of the DI-BSPM in the ECG device CARDIO PC was used to cumulate data from volunteers and patients with well defined pathologies and to create reference samples with following characteristics: (1) healthy subjects without any organic or functional cardiovascular disorders (n=76) ; (2) AH-patients without CHD (n=83); (3) normotensive patients with clinical signs of CHD, without AMI / old MI (n=104); (4) patients with AH with chronic / stabile forms of CHD, but without old MI (n=72) . The above reference samples were used for construction of DI-BSPMs for individual patients with well documented cardiovascular pathologies (LVH, AMI, old MI respectively). The highest incidence of false positive signs of myocardial injury was observed if AH patients with LVH were compared with either the reference sample (1) or (3). We have proposed to use the different reference samples for DI-BSPMs, adequate to the clinical characteristics of the patient examinated.

1. Introduction

The standard departure mapping studies have used the "ideal healthy" population for the construction of the group data for the departure mapping reference samples. The aim of presented study is to answer on the following questions : /1/ Has the reference sample characteristics the influence on the departure isointegral QRS and ST-T mapping results? /2/ Is the "healthy" reference sample the cause of higher rate of the false positive results of myocardial injury according to DI-BSPMs ? /3/ How the arterial hypertension (AH) and left ventricular hypertrophy (LVH) and coronary heart disease (CHD) influence on the assessment of electro-cardiographic abnormalities in DI-BSPMs?

2. Material and Methods

The study population consisted of 335 subjects. For the purpose of the reference samples we have created four groups:

Group I :	*the healthy persons*	*(n = 76)*	*text abbreviation : "NORM"*
Group II:	*patients with AH, without CHD*	*(n = 83)*	*"AH"*

Group III: normotensive patients with CHD, without MI (n = 104) "CHD"
Group IV: patients with AH + CHD, without MI (n = 72) "AH & CHD"

Cardio PC, the device developed in the Institute of Measurement Science (Slovak Acad. Sci., Bratislava) for 12-lead ECG, Frank VCG and body surface mapping measurement and processing is used. The system enables simultaneous measurement and following processing of up to 64 ECG signals from body surface *[1]*. For practical clinical use 3 limited arrays are implemented to system (Barr-24, Lux-32 and NEKTAL-32). Measuring program also enables ECG measurement in 63-lead full grid system according to Savard. For following clinical study was realized with the limited body surface lead array Lux-32.

The software for BSPM is a menu driven modular package. It includes a resident organizer, programs for ECG measurement and processing, for instantaneous and isointegral potential mapping and for departure isointegral and isochrone mapping. Sampling frequency 1, 2 or 4 msec and record length of 5 to 20 sec can be selected. Program for integral mapping computes maps over time intervals defined by standard instants (e.g. P wave, QRS complex, ST-T period, P-QRS-T period) or any selected interval defined in milliseconds can be given. The departure isointegral mapping (DI-BSPM) program enables to cumulate the reference sample maps and to compute patient's departure maps from selected reference sample (***Figure 1***).

DG: AH, LVH, without CHD **Pt : N499 - P.S. / M , 36 yrs. /**
Departure isointegral map / reference sample: "NORM" /

J Te / J point - offset of the T wave /

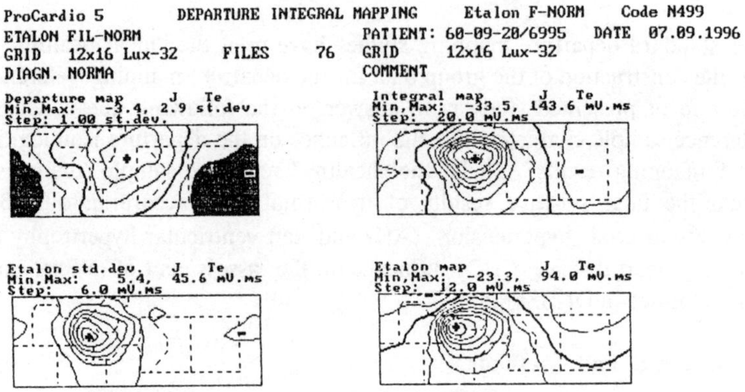

Figure 1: The method for departure isointegral maps.
The patient's individual isointegral map or repolarization interval JTe (from J point to the end of T wave) is calculated with reference sample averaged JTe map "NORM" (reference map is situated in the right and below). The final result (map in the left side above) shows the departure map with the area more than minus 2 st. dev. (black area).

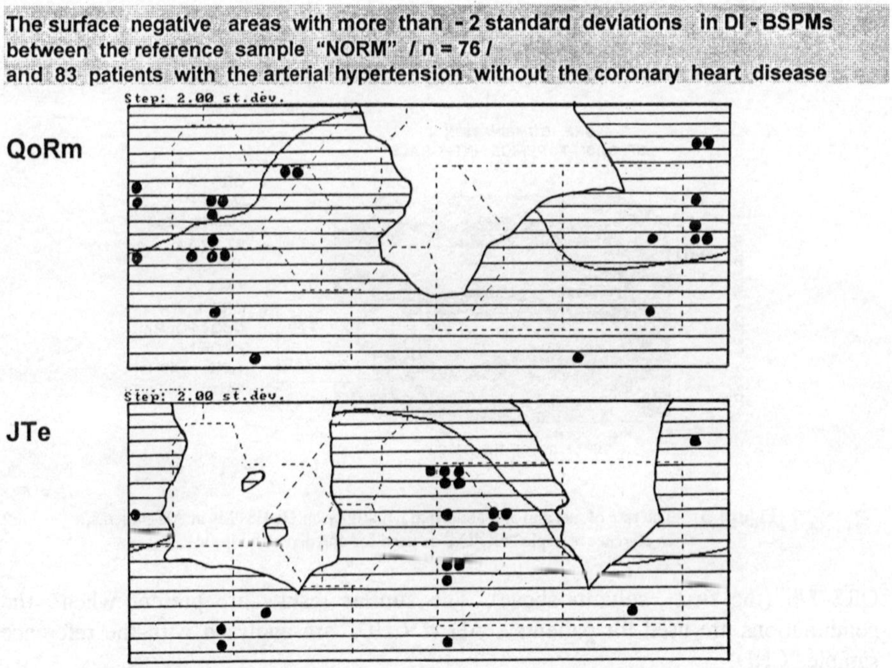

Figure 2 : The surface areas with more than - 2 st.dev. for 83 patients with AH, without CHD, when "NORM" reference sample was used for DI-BSPM.

3. Results

The individual QRS and ST-T departure maps were constructed for AH patients without CHD using the "ideal" reference sample "NORM"(like is depicted in Fig.1).

Figure 2 summarized the place of the areas more than minus 2 st.dev. for 83 AH patients without CHD. Only limited regions for QRS annd ST-T intervals are free of the significant influence of hypertensive myocardium. The same situation exists for 72 "AH & CHD" patients when the reference sample "CHD" was used.

When the integration QRS and ST-T intervals are longer, the frequency of false negative abnormal DI-maps is lower (for example, for 30 milliseconds interval during QRS complex false negative DI-maps are in 45% cases, for whole QRS interval in 20%).

If the combination more (from 3 to 6) QRS-T integration intervals is used (***Figure 3***), that can suppress the false negative results on 12 % or 0 % (0 % for combination of 6 QRS-T isointegral intervals). In Fig. 3 is shown, that all 83 AH patients have the signs of hypertensive myocardium on DI-maps in the combination

THE RATE OF NORMAL [<- 2SD] AND ABNORMAL [>- 2SD] NEGATIVITY ON DI-BSPMs IN 83 HT- PTS WITHOUT CHD, WHEN THE REFERENCE SAMPLE IS REPRESENTED WITH THE GROUP I ("NORM") QRS-T periods (combination)

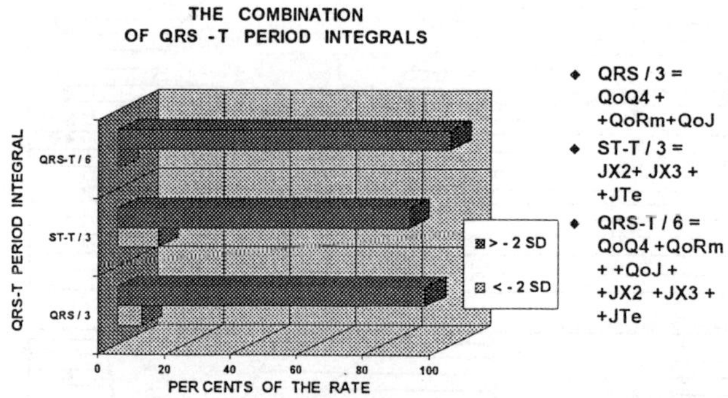

Figure 3: The rate of normal and abnormal negativity on DI-BSPMs in AH-patients, when eference sample "NORM" is used for the departure procedure.

QRS-T/6 (the first column above). The similar results are present when the combinations are used for patients "AH & CHD" are analyzed with the reference sample "CHD".

4. Conclusions

Presence of the high incidence of false positive signs of myocardial injury (the false body surface mapping result of MI-damage, ...) was observed in hypertensive patients without or with LV hypertrophy and without or with coronary heart disease.

Our results suggest the proposal : to use the different reference samples for departure isointegral BSPMs, adequate to the clinical characteristics of the patient examinated (presence of arterial hypertension, LVH, CHD, etc...).

It is necessary to enlarge the reference samples and to specify more exactly their clinical characteristics according to complementary methods (e.g. echo-cardiographically, invasively).

5. References

1. S. Filipová et al. The role of the norm definition for the correct using of the integral departure mapping. In, *Body Surface Mapping and High Resolution ECG* (Yasui S, Abildskov JA, Yamada K, Harumi K, Eds) . Life Medicom Co., Ltd. Nagoya 1995, pp. 109-123.

THE INFLUENCE OF THROMBOLYTIC THERAPY ON THE EVOLUTION OF ST-T DEPARTURE ISOINTEGRAL BSPMs IN PATIENTS WITH ACUTE MYOCARDIAL INFARCTION

Slavomíra FILIPOVÁ, Stanislav CAGÁŇ
IVth Department of Internal Medicine, Faculty of Medicine, Comenius University, Bratislava, Slovak Republic

The aim of the study was to analyze the evolution of the departure integral body surface potential maps of the repolarization period (ST-T) in the patients with AMI (with and without thrombolysis -TL) and then after the period of 6-30 months. The study group consisted of 145 patients (1st examination) and of 121 patients (2nd examination) fulfilling the clinical criteria of the first AMI. 27% of them underwent the selective coronarography. The reference groups (n=335) served for construction of the departure maps.
Results: (1) The evolution of the pattern of DI-BSPMs were correlated to the success of TL therapy and of eventual revascularization invasive procedures (CABG, PTCA). (2) In the group of patients without TL, the differences between the 1st and 2nd examination depended on the success of invasive revascularization. (3) The signs of resting silent residual ischemia on DI-BSPMs of the 2nd examination were accompanied by other ECG signs of ischemia (late ventricular potentials), without reflection in patient's clinical status.

1. Introduction

According to controlled studies the successful TL is followed by early reperfusion in 50-70% patients compared with the spontaneous reperfusion rate 30%, and reduces the extent of ventricular damage and the early and 1-year mortality rates associated with the acute myocardial infarction (AMI). The aim of the study was to analyse the evolution of the departure integral body surface potential maps (DI-BSPM) of the repolarization period (ST-T) in the patients with AMI (with and without TL administration) and then after the follow-up period of 6-30 months.

The main question was asked from the electrocardiographic point of view: Is the long-time evolution of repolarization (ST-T) period changes according to the DI-BSPMs in the patients with AMI the marker of the successful i.v. thrombolytic therapy and presence or absence of significant residual myocardial ischemia ?

2. Material and Methods

The first examination was realized in 145 patiens from 6 to 21 days after acute onset of the first attack of AMI. The common non-invasive clinical criteria for the success of TL were used.

Group 1	*n = 40 (27,6 %)*	*patients with successful TL*
Group 2	*n = 19 (13,1 %)*	*patients with failed TL*
Group 3	*n = 86 (59,3 %)*	*patients without TL administration*

The examination was repeated for the same patients after the period of 6-30 months. We examined 121 (83,5 %) patients from the first study population (group 1: n = 32, group 2: n = 17, group 3: n = 72). 27% of them underwent the selective coronary angiography. The reference groups I-IV served for construction of the departure maps. At all, currently the reference groups involve 335 subjects.

Separately the reference maps for normotensive and hypertensive patients without acute or old MI were used. *[1].*

A device Cardio PC developed in the Institute of Measurement Science (Slovak Acad. Sci.) for clinical ECG, VCG and BSPM measurement and processing is used. The system enables simultaneous measurement and following processing of up to 64 ECG signals from body surface *[2].* For presented clinical study the limited body surface lead array Lux-32 was used *[3].* The program for integral mapping computes isointegral maps over time intervals defined by standard instants. The departure integral mapping enables to integrate the cumulated reference groups into the processing of DI-maps. In all patients the complete repolarization intervals (from J point to offset of T wave) were used for integration.

3. Results

3.1. DI-BSPMs After Successful TL

According to our results, the evolution of the pattern of DI-BSPMs were correlated to the success of TL therapy and of eventual revascularization invasive procedures (CABG, PTCA). On the ***Fig. 1*** is shown the evolution of negative potential abnormal area during the repolarization (more than minus 2 stand. dev.) early after successful TL (Fig. 1A), which was persisted 5 weeks after TL (Fig. 1B) and significantly diminished during the examination realized 3 week after PTCA (Fig. 1C).

3.2. DI-BSPMs After Failed TL or Without TL Treatment

In the group of patients without TL, the differences between the 1st and 2nd examination depended on the success of invasive revascularization. ***Fig. 2*** shows the significant large (with the departure integral values more than minus 5 stand. dev.) repolarization abnormalities in DI-BSPMs during the JTe and QoTe periods immediately after the failed TL (Fig. 2A) and apparent regression of abnormal areas after the revascularization procedure (Fig. 2B).

The change in the values of normalized peak negativities, comparing the 1st and 2nd recording, were best correlated with results of revascularization interventions.

3.3. The Clinical Relationships (Table 1)

In the follow-up period 3 from 4 cases of re-infarctions were happened in the non-revascularized subgroups (***Tab. 1***, subgroups 1A , and 3B). The abnormal late potentials had the highest frequency in the non-revascularized subgroups (B) and predominantly were present in the group 2 (patients with failed TL) ant in the group 3 (patients without TL). All 10 sudden cardiac deaths have occurred in the subgroups B. The patients from the group 1 was without deaths. We found the combination of sudden cardiac death plus positive late potentials in 6 patients, all from subgroups without revascularization (2B and 3B).

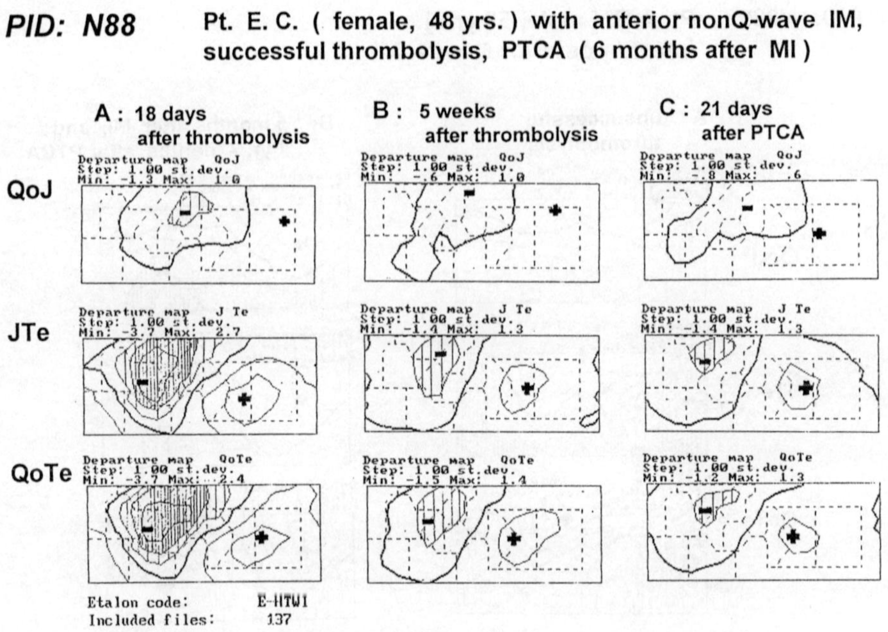

Figure 1 : DI-BSPMs after successful TL in patient with the anterior non-Q wave AMI.
Fig. 1A: in acute phase , 1B: 5 weeks after TL, 1C: 3 weeks after PTCA.

	GR. 1	1-A	1-B	GR. 2	2-A	2-B	GR. 3	3-A	3-B
n	32 24,4%	4	28	17 13,0%	5	12	72 55,0%	15	57
reMI	1	0	1	0	0	0	3	1	2
abnor. LVP	9	1	8	7	1	6	26	3	23
exits	0	0	0	3	0	3	7	0	7
exits + LVP	0	0	0	2	0	2	4	0	4

Table 1 : The follow-up clinical and ECG parameters of the groups 1, 2 and 3.
Abbreviations in table: **reIM** = re-infarction, **abnor. LVP** = abnormal ventricular late potentials, **exits** = sudden cardiac deaths
A = after the revascularization therapy (PTCA, CABG). **B** = without the revascularization therapy

PID: N280 **Pt. A.B. [male, 58 yrs.]**
inferio-posterior Q-waveMI

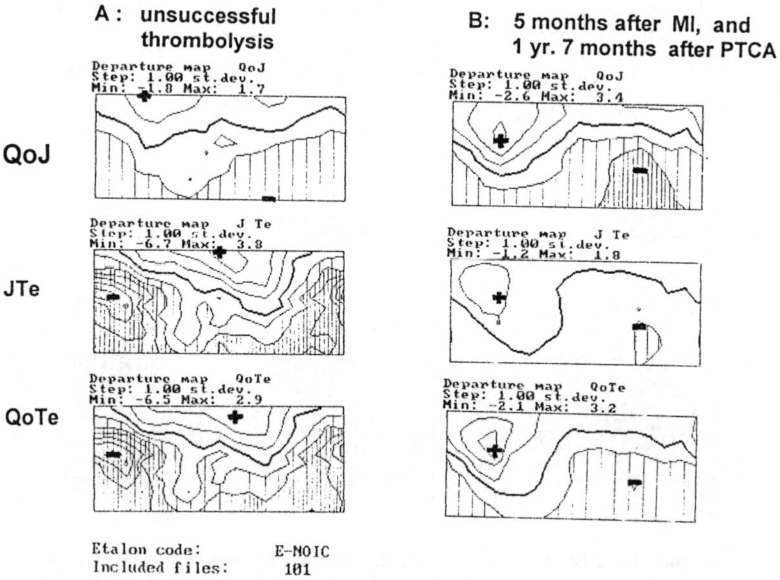

Figure 2 : DI-BSPMs after failed TL in patient with the inferior-posterior Q wave AMI.
Fig. 2A: in acute phase , 2B: after successful PTCA

4. Conclusions

The evolution of patterns of ST-T period DI-BSPMs correlates to the success of thrombolysis and to the invasive opening of infarction-related artery. The signs of residual ischemia on DI-BSPMs of the 2nd examination weree accompanied by other ecg signs of ischemia (abnormal late potentials) without reflection in patient's subjective clinical status. The highest benefit from the revascularization have the patients after the failed TL and patients without TL therapy. All 10 sudden cardiac deathes in our follow-up study were present in non-revascularized patients and 6 of 10 had the abnormal ventricular late potentials before.

5. References

6. S. Filipová, M. Tyšler, et al. : Reference sample with appropriately adjusted characteristics improves the diagnostic accuracy of departure isointegral maps. In, *Electrocardiology'97* (in press)

2. S. Filipová et al. The role of the norm definition for the correct using of the integral departure mapping. In, *Body Surface Mapping and High Resolution ECG* (Yasui S, Abildskov JA, Yamada K, Harumi K, Eds) . Life Medicom Co., Ltd. Nagoya 1995, pp. 109-123.

3. R. Lux et al. *IEEE Trans.Biomed.Engn.*25:270-276, (1978).

ELECTROCARDIOGRAPHIC ESTIMATION OF LEFT VENTRICULAR HYPERTROPHY REGRESSION BY VERAPAMIL. A LONGITUDINAL FOLLOW-UP.

K. KOZLÍKOVÁ, I. HULÍN
Institute of Pathophysiology, Medical Faculty, Comenius University, Sasinkova 2, 811 08 Bratislava, Slovak Republic
E-mail: kozlikova@fmed.uniba.sk

J. MURÍN, J. BULAS
1st Medical Department, Faculty Hospital, Mickiewiczova 13, 813 69 Bratislava, Slovak Republic

A clinical, echocardiographic and electrocardiographic body surface mapping longitudinal follow-up of a 58 years old male patient with hypertension complicated by left ventricular hypertrophy was performed. Normalization of blood pressure was achieved during the course of treatment with verapamil (13 months). Regression of left ventricular mass from 372 g to 279 g (75%) was found. This was in agreement with decreasing trend of maxima in QRS isointegral maps (72%) as well as in QRS isopotential maps (78%) where also a decrease of primary minimum was found (78%).

1 Introduction

Hypertension with left ventricular (LV) hypertrophy is much more serious disease than without it. Therefore, regression of LV hypertrophy during the antihypertensive treatment is very helpful.

Hypertrophy is established by echocardiographic methods in clinical practice. Results have been often correlated with electrocardiographic (ECG) methods[1], mostly 12 lead electrocardiography or vectorcardiography. Only a very limited number of papers deals with hypertrophy and ECG body surface mapping[2] (BSM). Therefore, we have focused our attention to the estimation of the LV hypertrophy regression by ECG BSM and echocardiographic methods and their mutual correlation during a 13-month treatment with verapamil (Isoptin).

2 Methods

We have repeatedly examined a male patient, 58 years old. He had suffered from hypertension HT II (WHO) detected in 1987 and had been treated with Corinfar during 3 years. At the beginning of this treatment, asymetric LV septal hypertrophy with normal systolic function was detected. The patient had also mild ischaemia and obesity (weight / height = 102 kg / 183 cm). He was ex-smoker.

In February 1994, concentric hypertrophy was detected and the treatment with verapamil (Isoptin) began. It lasted for 13 months under strong supervision but control examinations have continued.

During our study, the M-mode echocardiography was performed 4 times. The thickness of interventricular septum (IVS) and the LV posterior wall (LVPW) and the LV internal diameter (LVID) during diastole were measured. LV mass (LVM) was calculated after Devereux[3]

$$LVM\ [g] = 1.04 \times [(IVS+LVID+LVPW)^3 - LVID^3] - 13.6 \quad .$$

ECG BSM examinations were performed 7 times. The first 2 done within 1 week were taken as control state. Last measurement was done 35 months after beginning of the treatment.

BSM were registered with the microcomputer-based mapping system ProCardio[4,5] which includes a limited 24-electrode system after Barr. Two to 3 successive records of duration 4 to 4.4 s were made at each session from which 8 to 15 beats were analysed. The onset and the offset of the QRS complex was established from root mean square signal. Isopotential maps (IPM) and isointegral maps (IIM) of the whole QRS complex were constructed. We have looked for the highest and the lowest amplitudes in IPM during the whole duration of QRS complex and analysed their values, positions and time of appearance. Values and positions of absolute extrema in IIM QRS were analysed. Peak-to-peak values were calculated in both types of maps.

3 Results

Normalization of blood pressure was achieved during the course of treatment with verapamil and was confirmed by ambulatory blood pressure measurements with normal findings at the end of the study.

Regression of LV mass from 372 g to 279 g (75%) was found at the end of treatment (13 months). It was due to decreased thickness of interventricular septum from 18 mm to 13 mm (72%) and left ventricular posterior wall from 13 mm to 9 mm (69%), although the cavity dimension slightly increased from 47 mm to 52 mm (115%). After a short interruption of the treatment the LV mass slightly increased to 295 g (79%).

We found decreasing trends in both maxima of IIM QRS (72% - Fig. 1) and in maxima of IPM QRS (78% - Fig. 2) at the end of the supervised treatment (13 months). There was also a decrease of primary minimum absolute value (78%) while the secondary minimum remained almost unchanged (97%), but it dominated over the primary one (Fig. 2).

The peak-to-peak values of IIM QRS as parameters of the heart electric power decreased to 77% (Fig. 1). The peak-to-peak values of IPM QRS calculated for primary and secondary minimum decreased to 79% and 83%, respectively (Fig. 2). Later increase of all evaluated values is probably due to the interrruption of treatment which was later continued again.

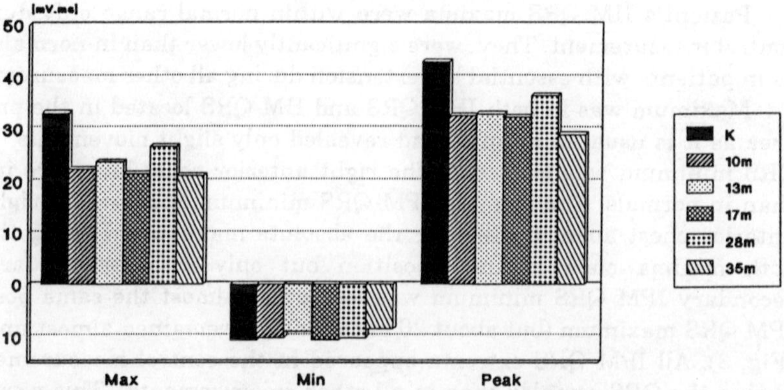

Figure 1: Amplitudes of the IIM QRS absolute extrema during the study.

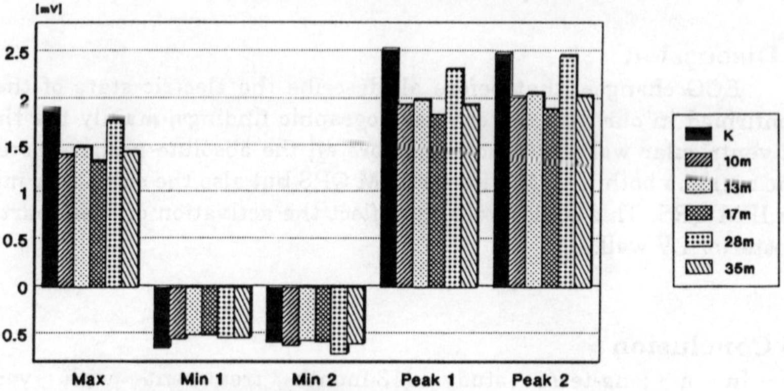

Figure 2: Amplitudes of the IPM QRS absolute extrema during the study.

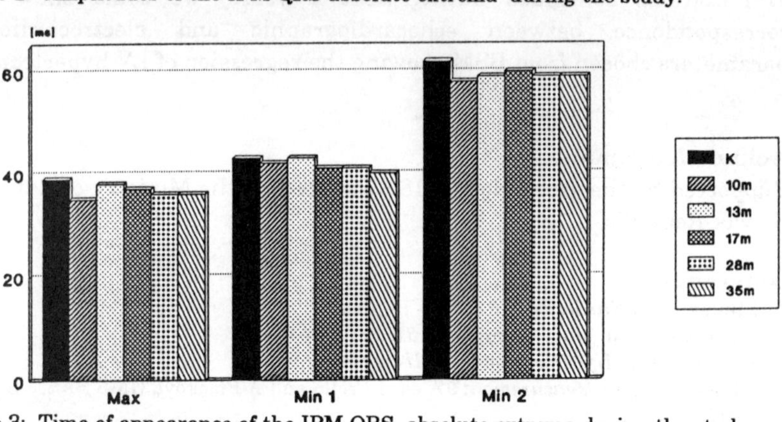

Figure 3: Time of appearance of the IPM QRS absolute extrema during the study.

Patient's IIM QRS maxima were within normal range only during the control measurement. They were significantly lower than in normals as well as in patients with essential hypertension during all other measurements [2].

Maximum was in both IPM QRS and IIM QRS located in the precordial area as it is usual in normals and revealed only slight movements. The IIM QRS minimum was located at the right anterior chest but more inferiorly than in normals. The primary IPM QRS minimum appeared at right upper anterior chest about 5 ms after the absolute maximum. During the study both minima changed their position but only in restricted area. The secondary IPM QRS minimum was located at almost the same position as IPM QRS maximum (but about 20 ms later) and remained almost unchanged (Fig. 3). All IPM QRS extrema appeared in the control measurement later during the QRS complex than in all other measurements. This was not due to any prolongation of QRS duration.

4 Discussion

ECG changes, that before all describe the electric state of the heart, confirmed in our case the echocardiographic findings, mainly the thickness of ventricular walls. It concerns before all the absolute positive potentials - the maxima both in IPM QRS and IIM QRS but also the secondary minimum in IPM QRS. This could probably reflect the activation of basal parts of the posterior LV wall.

5 Conclusion

In a long-term study (13-month treatment with verapamil, examinations continued during next 2 years) we could show a good correspondence between echocardiographic and electrocardiographic parameters chosen from BSM showing the regression of LV hypertrophy.

Acknowledgement

Supported by the grant No 1/4118/97 offered by the Ministry of Education of Slovak Republic.

References

1. J Bulas et al, *Kardiológia 6 (1997 - in press)*
2. H Igarashi et al, *Jap. Circulat. J. 51, 284 (1987)*
3. R B Devereux, *Hypertension 9/II, II-19 (1987)*
4. V Rosík et al, in *Measurement'97,* ed. I Frollo and A Plačková (IMS SAS, Bratislava, 1997)
5. K Kozlíková et al, in *Measurement'97,* ed. I Frollo and A Plačková (IMS SAS, Bratislava, 1997)

SOLUTION OF DIRECT AND INVERSE PROBLEMS OF ELECTROCARDIOGRAPHY USING A MULTIDIPOLE MODEL

G.GELMANAS, V.JURKONIS, L.GARGASAS
Institute of Cardiology, Kaunas Medical Academy,Sukileliu 17, Kaunas, Lithuania
E-mail: vytmi@kma.lt

This paper deals with the "direct" and "inverse" ECG problem. The investigation is based on a multidipolar concept of the equivalent generator of the heart and body conceived as a homogeneous rectangular parallelepiped. Data from 100 synchronous Wilson leads and 12 ECG leads have been used. The model have been applied for diagnostication of right ventricular hypertrophy (sensitivity 69%, specificity - 98%).

1 Introduction

For solution of direct ECG problems a phenomenological multidipole model of the genesis of QRS complex has been proposed. It consists of 20 dipoles representing different parts or segments of the heart ventricles. Taking into account the electric anisotropy of myocardial tissue the dipoles in this model are seted not perpendicular to the heart surface but at some inclination to the direction of tissues. In order to solve the border task an original method for counting up derivation vectors has been proposed using the mirror principle of description the human body as mass of rectangular parallelepiped [1]. The proposed model creates possibility to solve the direct task by changing the parameters of dipoles according to physiological indices for obtaining some electrocardiographic facts of myocardial pathology. Using this model in a way of imitation modelling the myocardial infarct of various localizations have been detected [2]. On the basis of multidipole model, a special phenomenological model for localization of Kent bundle has been created.

For solution of inverse ECG problem, an algorithm of multidipole analysis, based on 100 leads surface ECG, has been proposed. The method is easy for realization, diagnostic statements established by using electrophysiologic knowledge are comprehensive for practising physicians.

In order to decrease a degree of instability of the solution of the inverse problem solution (according to Liapunov) a modification of the model has been made. Only 14 dipoles (three in the septum, nine in the left and two in the right ventricles) have been used. The algorithm makes it possible to establish ischemic, infarctional, fibrotic and hypertrophic changes in cases when those changes cannot be detected by 12 leads ECG. This algorithm is a part of the multilead ECG analysis system, which is used in the Cardiological clinic of Kaunas Medical Academy. This system was applied for analysis of 100 leads ECG of 832 patients. The sensitivity of the algorithm was 79%, specificity - 84%, positive predictive value - 85% and diagnostic effectiveness - 81%.

Further investigation revealed some shortcomings of the proposed method, such as insufficient specificity and difficulties in applying for clinical practice due complexity of 100 leads ECG recording device. We attempted to increase the specificity of this method without considerable reducing of sensitivity and for this purpose entirely another way have been chosen. The main point of chosen method was reduction of number of free parameters (dipoles) according to the concrete diagnostic task i.e. creation of specialized phenomenological models which permits to solve the inverse problem of electrocardiology. In our opinion such method is more perspective than inverse task solution with purpose to obtain anyone diagnostic statement in general. Therefore the goal of this study was to demonstrate the possibilities of proposed method for detection of right ventricular hypertrophy - the most complicated case in ECG diagnostic.

2 Methods and materials

According to this concrete task we created the phenomenological model which consists of four dipoles. The first dipole represents right ventricle and oriented horizontally from left to right. The second dipole represents the left ventricle and oriented in the opposite direction. Since in forming of the apex the importance of right ventricle is undoubted two additional dipoles have been incorporated into model. The third dipole represents the right part of apex and oriented from left to right with elevation of 45^0 and fourth represents the left part of apex and oriented in the opposite direction but with the same elevation.

Basing on anatomical data we supposed that the modulus of the dipoles representing the right ventricle are three times smaller than others. Since the number of dipoles decreased significantly in further investigation we could use the standard 12 leads ECG. Basing on these presumptions and using the geometric model of the heart the lead vectors corresponding this model have been calculated. While the lead vectors have been computed the inverse task of electrocardiology we solved by using the method which was presented in literature [3].The final result of investigation were values of four dipole moments which have been used for diagnostication of right ventricular hypertrophy. The study cohort consisted of 509 patients: 270 patients have been included to learning and 239 patients to control set. The learning set consisted of 50 young healthy persons that anamnestic data excluded pulmonary and other diseases which could cause the overload of right ventricle, 120 patients that the echoscopic measurements were in normal limits and 100 patients that echoscopy revealed right ventricle enlargement. The control cohort consisted of 122 patients that echoscopy excluded right ventricle hypertrophy, 37 patients that echoscopy revealed right ventricle enlargement and 80 patients with chronic pulmonary disease.

3 Results and discussion

It could be supposed that in case of right ventricle enlargement the values of dipoles representing the right part of heart must be increased. According to this presumption at the first stage of study the searching of diagnostic features have been performed. But during study became clear that such presumption is not of full value because the chosen method of solving of inverse task (calculation of inverse matrix) is very sensitive for input data and causes the high degree scattering of solution values. Standard methods of statistics (calculation of mean values and dispersion) were sufficiently sensitive but not specific and for this reason for right ventricle enlargement detection we used not only absolute values of dipole moments but ratios between various dipole moments too:

- 1 and 2 dipoles ratio;
- 3 and 4 dipoles ratio;
- 1+3 and 2+4 dipoles ratio.

In addition for diagnostic algorithm we used not only absolute values of ratio but also investigated its distribution in the following spaces of two measurements:

- in x axis 1 and 2 dipoles ratio was put , in y axis - ratio of 3 and 4 dipoles moments;
- in x axis ratio of 1+3 and 2+4 dipole moments was put and in y axis - ratio of 3 and 4 dipoles moments.

In these spaces the areas of cases with (or without) right ventricle enlargement were determined. By using learning set the diagnostic algorithm consisting of 21 rules have been developed. Those 21 rules are based on assessment the absolute and relative values of the dipoles. The diagnostic efficacy of algorithm for detection of right ventricle enlargement was investigated in 239 patients (control set): the sensitivity was 69% (81 true positives from 117 cases), specificity - 98% (120 true negatives from 122 cases), positive predictive value - 98%, negative predictive value - 77%, diagnostic effectiveness - 84%. Having in mind the fact that sensitivity of computerized standard ECG analysis methods for detection of right ventricle hypertrophy is relatively low (20-55% for various ECG computer programs), we could affirm that presented algorithm is more sensitive than others [4] and its specificity is comparatively high.

4 Conclusions

Solution of inverse problem based on the phenomenological multidipole model and calculation of inverse matrix of lead vectors for multilead ECG is sensitive but not well enough specific method in sense of the electrocardiographic diagnosis.

In order to increase the specificity of ECG biophysical analysis we propose for concrete electrocardiographic task create physiologically determined specialized model with aim to reduce number of free parameters and to provide purposeful searching for changes of diagnostic parameters.

Basing on this premise the method of biophysical analysis for right ventricle hypertrophy detection have been developed. The sensitivity and specificity of this method was 69% and 98% respectively.

References

1. V.Jurkonis et al, in Building Bridges in Electrocardiology, ed. A. van Oosterom (Nijmegen, 180,1995).
2. G. Gelmanas, V. Jurkonis et al., Med. Biol. Engineer. Comput., D34, Suppl. 1, Part 2, 51(1996).
3. G. Gelmanas, V. Jurkonis, in Building Bridges in Electrocardiology, ed. A. van Oosterom, (Nijmegen, 174,1995).
4. Common Standards for Quantitative Electrocardiology. CSE 9th Progres report, ed. L.Willems, (1989).

V. Computer Assisted Electrocardiography

COMPUTERIZED ANALYSIS OF THE SPATIAL VELOCITY CURVE OF THE T LOOP : A NEW DIAGNOSTIC APPROACH

P. ARNAUD, M.C. FORLINI
INSERM, U. 121 . Hôpital Cardiologique
BP Lyon Montchat, 69394 Lyon, France

As the dynamics of the repolarization phase on the surface ECG is not well known, we propose to study the velocity curve of the vectorcardiographic T loop as a function of time.
We performed a program in order to compute this curve and to determine its 5 fiducial points : onset, first peak, nadir, second peak, offset. In a total population of 7364 subjects, partitioned into 10 normal and abnormal groups, the velocity values and the time intervals were calculated. Significant intergroup differences were observed, allowing to characterize and quantify the particular dynamics of T in each diagnostic group.

Introduction

The dynamics of the intra-QRS potentials is currently analyzed from the surface ECG using several methods. It is not the case for T potentials.

The concept of spatial velocity of the surface ECG was introduced by Hellerstein and Hamlin in 1960 [1]. Some few studies of the velocity curve were published from the sixties, most of them concerning QRS [2]. The spatial velocity of T was initially investigated by Mori [3] and by Sano [4] and recently by Sasaki [5].

For fifteen years, the QRS velocity curve as a function of time was routinely displayed by our vectorcardiographic system (Lyon program) [6] and proved to bring additional information for diagnosis. It was also used in research protocols to assess the electrophysiological properties of antiarrhythmic drugs [7]. Our program has now been completed with the spatial velocity curve of T (Figure 1).

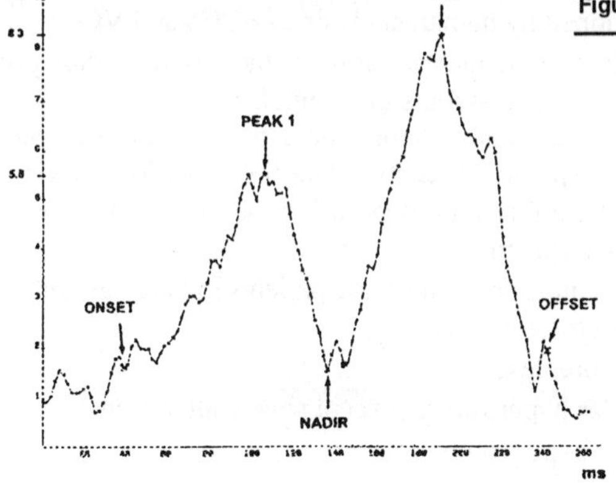

Figure 1 : **A normal velocity curve of T loop in function of time from a healthy woman, 30 years old**

Methods

The Frank vectorcardiograms, defined in a tri-orthogonal X, Y, Z frame of reference, were recorded at rest and many spatial parameters of QRS and T were computed using the Lyon system [6]. A complementary filtering of T was performed.
The spatial velocity between two consecutive sampling points was expressed as :

$$\text{linear velocity } (\mu V/ms) = \sqrt{((x_i - x_{i-1})^2 + (y_i - y_{i-1})^2 + (z_i - z_{i-1})^2)}.\ SR/1000$$

where x_{i-1}, x_i, y_{i-1}, y_i.....are the coordinates of two consecutive spatial vectors occuring at times i-1 and i, and SR the sampling rate per second.
The velocity curve of T as a function of time had a characteristic bimodal shape in most cases, displaying two peaks (PEAK1 and PEAK2) and a nadir point (NAD) of minimal speed between them (Figure 1). In a few cases the first peak was absent.
Automated analysis : Using 5 fiducial points previously processed - onset (ONS) and offset (OFF) of T, time occurrence of the T maximal, half-area and half-time vectors - we have elaborated an algorithm, proceeding by 6 steps, allowing to determine the precise localization of NAD, PEAK1 and PEAK2. If PEAK1-NAD or NAD-PEAK2 intervals are inferior to 6 ms this case is eliminated.

This algorithm was assessed in a test population (n = 125, of whom 11 were normal). The automated recognition of PEAK1, NAD and PEAK2 was correct in 113 cases (90.4%) by comparison with visual analysis by one observer.
Fourteen parameters were calculated :

- velocity values of the peaks and PEAK2/PEAK1 ratio,
- time intervals : ONS-PEAK1, PEAK1-NAD, ONS-NAD, NAD-PEAK2, PEAK2-OFF, NAD-OFF, PEAK1-PEAK2, T duration and ratios NAD-PEAK2/PEAK1-NAD, NAD-OFF/ONS-NAD, PEAK1-PEAK2/T duration.

Populations

The study was performed on a retrospective data base of 7547 subjects. Out of them, 183 (2.4%) were eliminated by the procedure above-mentioned of the program. The remaining 7364 cases were partitioned by human analysis of ECGs and VCGs:

- firstly into 4 groups according to the interpretation of the *repolarization phase*:

NOR H (n = 2316) : normal T wave from patients in hospital,
NOR Y (n = 1157) : normal T wave from ambulatory subjects, 19 to 21 years old,
REP A (n = 3669) : non ischemic repolarization abnormalities of various origin,
ISCH (n = 222) : ischemic T alterations recorded during the first weeks after an acute coronary episode.

- secondly into 6 groups originating from the same patients in hospital, but partitioned according to *QRS classification* :

N QRS (n = 428) : normal QRS complex,
RVH (n = 245) : right ventricular hypertrophy (except severe alterations),
LVH (n = 823) : left ventricular hypertrophy,

AI (n = 212) : anterior or-septal or- lateral infarction,
PII (n = 308) : postero-inferior infarction,
WPW (n = 60) : ventricular preexcitation.

Results

Description of normal velocity curves :

- Velocity values in the NOR H group (mean ± SD and 95 % C.I.) :
  PEAK1 : 5.4 ± 2.8. C.I. : 5.3 - 5.6
  PEAK2 : 8.2 ± 3.9. C.I. : 8.1 - 8.4
  PEAK2/PEAK1 : 1.55 ± 0.45. C.I. : 1.53 - 1.57 (asymmetric limbs of T wave).

Correlation between PEAK1 and PEAK2 : r = 0.71. Correlation between the maximal spatial amplitude of T and the velocity of PEAK1 : r = 0.70, of PEAK 2 : r = 0.89. Similar correlations were observed in the other groups.

- Velocity values in the NOR Y group : higher values of PEAK1 (7.6) and PEAK2 (12.6) in relation with higher amplitude of T (0.64 vs 0.35 mV).
- Time intervals in the NOR H group :
  ONS-PEAK1 : 47.2 ± 25.2. C.I. : 46.2 - 48.3
  PEAK1-NAD : 35.1 ± 14.8. C.I. : 34.5 - 35.7
  NAD-PEAK2 : 37.4 ± 15.4. C.I. : 36.8 - 38.0
  PEAK2-OFF : 40.7 ± 18.4. C.I. : 39.9 - 41.4
  NAD-OFF/ONS-NAD : 1.02 ± 0.39. C.I. : 1.00 - 1.03
  NAD-PEAK2/PEAK1-NAD : 1.35 ± 1.13. C.I. : 1.30 - 1.39
  PEAK1-PEAK2/T dur : 0.47 ± 0.13. C.I. : 0.46 - 0.47

The time intervals are independent from each other and from velocity values.

- Time intervals in the NOR Y group : since PEAK1-PEAK2 interval is slightly increased (74.0 vs 72.5 in the NOR H group, P = 0.03), ONS-PEAK1 and PEAK2-OFF are much more increased (77.0 and 61.8 respectively).

Bi-group comparisons : significant differences of mean values (P<0.05) were observed in the following groups by comparison with the NOR H group :

- Velocity values :

REP A : ↗ PEAK1 (5.6 vs 5.4), ↗ PEAK2 (8.8 vs 8.2),
↗ PEAK2/PEAK1 (1.61 vs 1.55).
LVH : ↗ PEAK1 (6.2), ↗ PEAK2 (10.3), ↗ PEAK2/PEAK1 (1.72).
Note that RVH values were nearly normal.
ISCH : ↘ PEAK2 (7.4).
PII : ↘ PEAK2 (7.7).
AI : ↘ PEAK1 (4.7), ↘ PEAK2 (6.2), ↘ PEAK2/PEAK1 (1.44).
WPW : ↗ PEAK2 (9.4).

- Time intervals :

REP A :	↘ PEAK1-NAD (33.8 vs 35.1)	⇒ premature NAD
	↗ NAD-PEAK2 (39.0 vs 37.4) and	
	↗ PEAK2-OFF (46.4 vs 40.7)	⇒ delayed OFF
	↗ T duration (166 vs 160).	
LVH :	↘ PEAK1-NAD (31.9 vs 35.1)	⇒ premature NAD
RVH :	↘ NAD-PEAK2 (35.0 vs 37.4)	⇒ premature PEAK 2
ISCH :	↘ ONS-PEAK1 (43.4 vs 47.2)	⇒ premature PEAK1
	↗ PEAK2-OFF (45.1 vs 40.7).	
AI :	↘ PEAK1-NAD (32.3 vs 35.1)	⇒ premature NAD
	↗ PEAK 2-OFF (45.2 vs 40.7)	⇒ delayed OFF
	↗ T duration (164 vs 160).	
PII :	↗ ONS -PEAK1 (52.7 vs 47.2)	⇒ delayed PEAK 1
	↗ PEAK1-NAD (37.2 vs 35.1)	⇒ delayed NAD
	↗ PEAK2-OFF (46.1 vs 40.7)	⇒ delayed OFF
	↗ T duration (174 vs 160).	
WPW :	↘ ONS-NAD (73.6 vs 82.3)	⇒ premature NAD

Conclusion

This descriptive study showed the *dynamics* of the T loop in normals and in different groups of patients. *Specific patterns* were observed : for instance, ischemic vs non - ischemic repolarization abnormalities result in a premature time of occurrence for the first peak and in a lower velocity value for the second peak.
This new method is expected to be useful in routine cardiology. To this end, our program allows to localize the fiducial points and to calculate the velocity and time intervals values.

References

1. H.K.Hellerstein and R. Hamlin, *Am J Cardiol.* 6, 1049 (1960).
2. K. Yano and H.V. Pipberger, *Circulation.* 29, 107 (1964).
3. H. Mori, T. Nagayama, T. Oda *et al*, *Jap Circulation J.* 32, 149 (1968).
4. T. Sano, T. Hiroki, H. Hazama *et al*, *Jap Circulation J.* 32, 1011 (1968).
5. A. Sasaki, A. Takimiya, T. Arai *et al, Jap Heart J.* 37, 879 (1996).
6. P. Arnaud, P. Rubel, D. Morlet *et al*, *Methods Inf Med.* 29, 393 (1990).
7. S. Fareh, P. Arnaud, J. Fayn *et al*, *Cardiology.* 87, 129 (1996).

COMPUTERISED EXERCISE ELECTROCARDIOGRAM ANALYSIS SYSTEM "KAUNAS-LOAD"

A.VAINORAS, L.GARGASAS, R.RUSECKAS, V.MISKINIS, R.JURKONIENE
Institute of Cardiology, Kaunas Medical Academy,Sukileliu str.17-106,3007 Kaunas, Lithuania
E-mail: vytmi@kma.lt

H.SCHWELA, U.J.BAUER
Erfurt Clinicum,Nordhauser str 74, 99089 Erfurt, Germany

Computerised ECG analysis system "Kaunas-Load" is described.The structure of software and measured parameters are discussed.By the mean of "Kaunas-Load",reaction of ABP during bicycle ergometry in relation to maximal power and heart rate is made.Practical recommendation for evaluation of these relations are being proposed.

1.Introduction

Electrocardiogram(ECG) registration and analysis system during a bicycle ergometry or any other functional test consists of hardware compatible with IBM PC computer and software adapted to it.Developed software allows to realise ECG monitoring during any functional test and record synchronously 12 lead ECG in desired time sequence.After a functional test the gathered ECG can be filtered and reconstructed baseline shift.Four programmes are working during ECG analysis:pattern recognition,measuring of parameters,diagnostic and representation of data.The main manager-special ruling program guides all programmes.Measuring program presents the following parameters for every cardiocycle in every lead:RR interval, duration of the P wave,PQ interval,duration of the QRS complex,R amplitude,S amplitude,ST dislocation in 40 ms distance after J point,maximal T wave amplitude,JT interval,JTa interval and JTc(corrected according Bazett)interval.All parameters in every lead are averaged and presented in tables as a mean for one lead or ECG.More complex parameters are also calculated-angle of maximal QRS vector,global QRS duration and others.On the basis of measured parameters diagnosis of arrhythmia is made for every registered ECG,paediatric ECG analysis is included as well.Data presentation program is one of the biggest working program in the system and all measured data are laid out in three levels by this program:1)initial data for every cardiocycle,for every lead,every ECG,2)the means of parameters for all leads of ECG,3)diagnosis and integrated data for the whole functional test.Changes of parameters are displayed with the help of two dimension trends(2D) or three dimension trends (3D). The system allows to present about 150 2D trends.All gathered ECG can be stored in special developed archive that allows to compress ECG data from 5 to 12 times without any error.The developed system is flexible and could be adapted to every type of ergometer and computer."Kaunas-Load" systems have been used for analysis of more than 3000 tests in Kaunas Medical Academy.The usage of such systems in 15 medical centres of our Republic confirmed the preference of computerised exercise ECG analysis against conventional methods.

In"Kaunas-Load" there are possibilities in any time to add arterial blood pressure(ABP) measured by hand,manually,or by any other mean.Measures of ABP are archivysed together with ECG records in computer's memory.Software display ABP data together with heart rate(HR) changes in 2D trend.Evaluation of ABP changes in relation to achieved power(N) and HR is made on the basis of data obtained in Erfurt Clinicum.

The aim of present study was to assess the quantitative characteristics of heart rate(HR) and load dependent BP response to exercise for healthy persons,patients with hypertonic disease and diabetes mellitus.

2.Patients and Methods

The study cohort comprised three groups of subjects.The first group consists of 34 healthy men(HV),the second - 20 men with hypertonic disease(AH) and the third-19 men with diabetes mellitus (DM).The group of pts with diabetes mellitus was included into the study because the hypertensive reactions are frequent for these patients.There was no age difference between AH and DM groups but HV subjects were younger($p \leq 0,01$).Body mass index was different in all the three groups and the largest was in AH group.The highest physical capacity was in HV group(192.1W),less-in AH(107.0W) and DM(78.7 W) groups.Usually with physical capacity linked parameter PWC170 was the largest in HV group,less in DM group and still less-in AH group(but not in DM group).

A veloergometric test was performed in supine posture.The exercise began with 65W,increasing by 30W every 6 minutes for patients and by 60W-for healthy subjects and stronger patients.The cessation of load was carried out according to standard recommendations.An exercise electrocardiogram was obtained by synchronous recording 12 lead ECG with computerised system "Kaunas-Load".BP was measured by a standard cuff sphygmomanometer on right brachial artery.The off-line input of BP measurement data was performed during the test or after it.After stress and recovery the collected ECG and BP parameters including HR,systolic and diastolic BP with achieved maximal capacity were assessed.

3.Results and Discussion

The parameters obtained during a veloergometric test are presented in the table.The achieved maximal capacity,increase of heart rate dHR and systolic blood pressure dSBP during the test one after another are given in the last three columns.HR in rest before stress was the lowest in HV group-69.9±1.8(M±SEM),in DM group it was 81.5±3.1 and in AH group-89.0±2.9.BP in rest before stress(SBPo-systolic,DBPo-diastolic) in HV group(table) was reliably($p<0.01$) different from BP in AH and DM(table) groups while the difference of BP in AH and DM groups was less reliable($p\leq 0.05$).

Table.The results of investigation of HV(n = 34),AH(n = 20),DM(n = 19) groups

Gr.	Parameter	10*ΔSBP / N	ΔSBP / ΔHR	SBPo	DBPo	SBP max	DBP max	N
HV	max	6.757	1.833	140	95	260	110	305
	min	3.265	.714	110	70	190	40	125
	μ	5.062	1.109	129.7	81.5	225.4	87.1	192.1
	sem	.141	.038	1.5	1.2	3.1	3.1	6.1
AH	max	13.846	6.636	180	110	270	150	185
	min	4.211	.656	150	80	200	80	65
	μ	7.672	1.816	162.5	97.3	237.5	115.3	107.0
	sem	.660	.204	2.80	1.9	4.74	3.193	8.54
DM	max	12.308	3.333	185	110	235	130	125
	min	4.0	.606	120	72	140	80	75
	μ	6.760	1.590	148.2	90.0	205.5	107.6	78.7
	sem	.557	.165	4.91	2.26	5.9	3.04	6.0

10*ΔSBP/N - PPI(explanation in text), ΔS/ΔHR - PRI (explanation in text), SBPo - systolic blood pressure at rest, DBPo - diastolic blood pressure at rest, SBPmax and DBPmax - blood pressure during maximal load, respectively systolic and diastolic, N - maximal load, ΔHR - increase in heart rate during stress test and ΔSBP - increase in SBP during stress test.

The differences of BP during maximal load have been observed also and the most reliable were between DM group on one side and AH, HV groups on the other side.The maximal increase of SBP in AH and HV groups was resembling.This fact can be related with requirements for patients' security during stress test(not exceed permissible maximal BP values) but not with possibilities to achieve that maximal values of BP.However, when during the test it is not possible to achieve maximal values of BP some straits araise in evaluation of BP increase as a reaction to load.Another kind of difficulties in ABP assessement during the exercise appear due to the lack of possibility to distinquish ABP increase conditioned by hypertensive reaction as well as by augmented sensitiveness of organism to inconsiderable influence.At present these situations cannot be separated yet. For analysis of ABP and HR during maximal load development(table) the ratio of SBP and HR increase(dSBP/dHR) as well as ratio of SBP increase and developed power(dSBP/N) has been used.The first parameter can be called as pressure-rate index(PRI) and the second-pressure-power index(PPI).In the table these parameters are presented in second and third columns but parameter PPI, in order to avoid operating with small values, was multiplied by 10(PPI=10 dSBP/N) and fluctuated from 1 to 10.In the table the mean values and SEM are presented.It can be seen that these two parameters in AH group were significantly different as compared with HV and DM groups.PRI didn't differ reliably between HV and AH groups but persistently higher values have been seen in the last one.By using the mean values PRI and PPI of HV group the normal limits of alterations to these parameters have been defined as $\mu\pm2\sigma$.

Then for parameter PRI normal limits would be PRI=1.109±2 x 0.222(lower limit PRImin=0.665, upper limit PRImax=1.553) and for parameter PPI=5.062 ± 2 x 0.823(lower limit PPImin=3.416, upper limit PRImax=6.708).Taking into account the presented limits the decreased,normal or increased SBP response to load could be defined.To a certain degree the hypertonia and hypertension are analogous terms although the term "hypertonia" however is related with ABP value which is established in the rest during a well-balanced state while the term "hypertension" is related with increased ABP changes during stress test.Then, according to assessed parameters, the hypertensive reaction to stress could be defined when the parameters are PRI > 1.553 and PPI > 6.708 and hypotensive - when PRI < 0.665 and PPI < 3.426. The situation when the increased SBP changes are accompanied by the increased HR changes can be named as hyperreactive response to load and it will be defined when PPI > 6.708 and PRI < 1.553. The last type of response could be related with hyperactivity of the sympathetic nervous system and related to, the so called "white coat hypertension".

4.Conclusions

1)Arterial blood pressure response to load could be defined as hypotensive, normotensive and hypertensive. The situation when systolic blood pressure increase in parallel to heart rate (PRI~ 1) could be named as hyperreactive reaction.
2)Two parameters - pressure-rate index (PRI) and pressure-power index (PPI) - were proposed for quantitative systolic blood pressure evaluation. These parameters were significantly different ($p \leq 0.01$) for patients with hypertonic disease as compared with the groups of patients with diabetes mellitus and healthy persons.
3)The normotensive reaction for men was defined when parameter PPI =10 dSBP/N was in limits 3.416 - 6.708($\mu \pm 2\sigma$) and parameter PRI= dSBP/dHR - in limits 0.666-1.552.

COMPUTERIZED SYSTEM FOR STANDARD ELECTROPHYSIOLOGY STUDIES AND ABLATION TREATMENT OF THE HEART

H.P. VÄNTTINEN, J.J. NOUSIAINEN, J.A. MALMIVUO
Ragnar Granit Institute, Tampere University of Technology,
P.O.Box 692, FIN-33101 Tampere, Finland

P. MÄKYNEN
Tampere University Hospital, Department of Cardiology,
FIN-33101 Tampere, Finland

A large amount of data is acquired during a standard electrophysiology (EP) study. For this reason a computerized data acquisition, analysis and archiving system for EP studies of the heart is a valuable aid for cardiologists in diagnosing arrhythmias and for researchers in collecting data for various purposes. We have developed a system for standard EP studies and ablation treatment running under Windows on a standard PC. The number of channels, temporal accuracy and amplitude precision of the system are sufficient for clinical use. The user-friendly nature of this software, its reliability and quick adaptation to rapidly changing situations during the EP study, are essential in minimising exposure times and discomfort to the patient. Our system supports the most common EP study methods such as the measurement of V-A conduction times to localise structures like accessory pathways supporting re-entrant arrhythmias. It can also be used during catheter RF-ablation treatment to monitor the ablation and its effects. The built-in ablation monitoring capability is a great advantage, enabling combined EP study and ablation treatment, thus reducing exposure times and the total time needed per patient. For clinical use, the software includes versatile tools for reducing the amount of data acquired (i.e. storing only interesting findings and deleting unnecessary data). For research purposes, the system allows long recordings containing, for example, long stimulation series. The system also has a number of automatic data analysis tools, including facilities to recognise pacing series, study anterograde and retrograde conduction and detect refractoriness. Our system is already in regular clinical use at Tampere University Hospital (TUH) and has been used successfully during standard EP studies and ablation treatments.

1 Introduction

Cardiac electrophysiology (EP) studies are a relatively new technique for diagnosing arrhythmias. The first His-potential measurement was performed by Scherlag et. al.[4] in 1969 and present-day standard EP studies are based on this successful experiment. The power of this invasive method is that the phenomena are recorded where they occur, i.e. on the endocardium. EP studies are especially effective in localising and studying mechanisms supporting re-entrant arrhythmias, which are often caused by inborn accessory pathways[1]. A great advantage of the catheter method is that once the structure supporting the arrhythmia has been localised, transcatheter RF-ablation treatment can be applied to destroy the structure. Despite the invasive nature of the EP study, it is a safe method to study and treat arrhythmias in those patients who are susceptible to life threatening arrhythmias and usually it does not lead to complications. Thus, only a short recovery time is required after the treatment.

Currently, similar systems for EP studies are quite expensive. Thus, a low-cost system with sufficient properties to test the electrophysiologic properties of the heart and to monitor RF-ablation would facilitate the more widespread use of these studies and ablation treatment.

2 System Description

The Electrophysiology Studies (EPS) for Windows software[3] was developed to meet the requirements of standard clinical EP studies. The goal was to make a very easy-to-use Windows application which could be run on inexpensive standard hardware and could be used to control the data acquisition processor and store the data acquired for subsequent analysis. Microsoft Windows® 3.1 (or higher) was chosen for the environment, because it is the most widespread operating system and Windows applications have many common features. Thus, it is quite easy to adopt the use of a new application if the most frequently required functions work in a familiar manner. An initial version of this software[2] was developed under DOS.

The system requirements adequate for standard clinical EP studies are real time data acquisition, storage and display of 16 channels with a sampling rate of at least 500 Hz and built-in basic data analysis functions. However, at the moment the software is capable of acquiring and storing the data from 24 channels and displaying 1 to 16 arbitrarily chosen signals in real time. The hardware consists of a standard 120 MHz Pentium PC with 32 MB RAM, 1.3 GB hard disk and high-performance video card with 2 MB VRAM using a 1024 × 768 pixel resolution and 256 colors. Data is acquired using a 16 channel data acquisition processor, DAP 1200/4, which performs the necessary A/D conversion and stores the data in an FIFO buffer, from where it is read into the computer's memory by the EPS for Windows software. The current system also includes an analog video splitter to divide the video signal so that multiple monitors can be used. In addition the software includes various tools for data analysis, management and archiving.

The EPS for Windows software has three main operating modes: analysis, monitoring and recording (Figure 1). In both monitoring and recording modes, data acquisition is enabled. The difference between these two modes is that in monitoring mode, the acquired data is stored only in memory in a loop of 60 seconds, while in recording mode the data is stored both in memory and on disk. The 60 s loop buffer allows interesting events that occurred during the last 60 seconds to be saved. In analysis mode, data acquisition does not take place and all the analysis, data management and printing functions are available. During data acquisition most of these functions are disabled, because using them would severely disturb the data acquisition process and some data could be lost.

The user can study individual recordings by scrolling the signals back and forth by small increments or screen-by-screen. The user can measure time intervals on the display, make annotations for printout, compare and group signals together, hide uninteresting signals temporarily, rename signals easily and change the amplification and/or horizontal time scale if necessary. The results of certain predefined measurements, selected from the menu, are automatically stored in the study report. Other results are copied onto the clipboard, so that they can be pasted into the desired field of the report editor. Additionally, the results and annotations are stored in a memory metafile, so they can also be shown in the printout.

EPS for Windows is also useful during transcatheter RF-ablation treatment. It can be used to monitor impedance and temperature during the ablation. There is also a separate operating mode for ablation treatment where all ablations are recorded automatically according to changes in impedance level. The software also automatically adds two seconds of pre- and post-ablation ECG in order to facilitate the study of ablation effect.

To facilitate the management of recordings, the software maintains a list of recordings in chronological order. Comments in the recordings can be edited and one or more recordings can be deleted by selecting them from the list and pressing a two key shortcut. All these data management functions are also available during data acquisition. Other functions available during data acquisition are heart rate monitoring and insertion of bookmarks. Analysis functions available after data acquisition include recognition of stimulation series, detection of refractoriness and automatic detection of anterograde and retrograde conduction. In analysis mode, the user can copy arbitrary sections and views from a recording and a 60 s buffer into a new recording which is then added to the list. Artefacts or peaks in the signals with large amplitudes that disturb other signals can be cut away by applying a clip function that removes peaks exceeding a user-defined threshold. The software allows very long continuous recordings by dividing them automatically into shorter recordings of 200 seconds' duration. This aids in data analysis and management.

EPS for Windows allows the user to customise and save system settings for various types of study, or according to personal preferences. Other tools include file preview, file conversion for importing raw binary data files into EPS for Windows and a bookmark manager for adding/removing bookmarks and attaching comments to them. There are several printing options for formatting printouts, including a running time scale and standard scales of 2.5 cm/s, 5 cm/s and 10 cm/s. The file format used by the software is very suitable for archiving the studies, for example on CD-R discs. All data, including recordings, bookmarks, current settings, the study report with patient and study information, are saved in a single binary file which can be compressed using routinely available compression applications, down to as little as 30% of the original size.

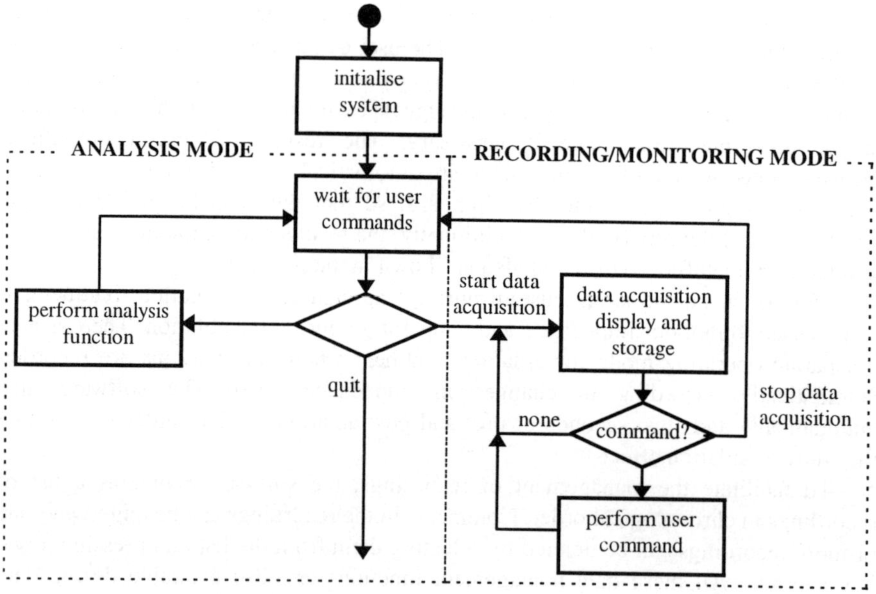

Figure 1: Flowchart showing the operating modes of EPS for Windows.

3 Results

The system has been developed in association with the Department of Cardiology at Tampere University Hospital. Between August 1996 and June 1997, an average of two EP studies/ablations per week have been performed at TUH using EPS for Windows. This system requires no exotic hardware or software. Thus, its operation and maintenance costs are low. The ability of the software to combine standard EP study methods and ablation monitoring can reduce exposure time and the total time needed per patient. This is also more comfortable for the patient.

References

1. R.N. Fogoros in *Electrophysiologic Testing* (Blackwell Scientific Publications, 1991).
2. J.J. Nousiainen in *Report No. 2/1994* (Ragnar Granit Institute, Tampere University of Technology, Tampere, 1994).
3. H.P. Vänttinen in *Interactive System for Electrophysiological Testing of the Heart* (Ragnar Granit Institute, Tampere University of Technology, Tampere, 1995).
4. B.J. Scherlag *et. al., Circulation*, B **39**, 13 (1969).

COMPUTER ASSISTED IDENTIFICATION OF ACCESSORY PATHWAYS FROM THE 12-LEAD ECG

STEPHANIE C. MCLAUGHLIN,

University Department of Medical Cardiology, Royal Infirmary, Glasgow, Scotland.

BRIAN DEVINE,

University Department of Medical Cardiology, Royal Infirmary, Glasgow, Scotland.

PETER W. MACFARLANE,

University Department of Medical Cardiology, Royal Infirmary, Glasgow, Scotland.

ABSTRACT.

Computer interpretation of the WPW pattern has tended until now to classify appearances as Type A or Type B. More recent data from electrophysiology investigations has allowed a more precise classification and this paper reports on the application of one such classification scheme to routine computer ECG analysis.

1. INTRODUCTION.

Computer analysis of the electrocardiogram has been in use for many years. However, interpretation of the WPW pattern(1) has essentially been confined to classification of the abnormality into Type A or Type B in keeping with the classification of Rosenbaum et al(2).

More recently, there have been a number of schemes introduced for determining the location of the accessory pathway. For example, Gallagher et al(3) described a scheme based on delta wave polarity in the 12-leads for describing 10 different anatomical locations of sites of epicardial pre-excitation. Yuan et al(4) compared 18 different sets of ECG criteria for localising the accessory pathway in the WPW syndrome.

In 1994, Fitzpatrick et al published a new algorithm for the localisation of accessory AV connections using the 12-lead ECG(5). These authors claimed that the technique was exceptionally sensitive and specific in localising 8 separate sites of accessory pathways. There were 3 left sided pathways around the mitral valve annulus, namely, left posteroseptal, posterolateral and anterolateral and 5 right sided pathways around the tricuspid annulus, viz. anteroseptal, midseptal, posteroseptal, posterolateral and anterolateral.

A diagnostic tree for localising accessory pathways was published in which the following criteria were used:

1. The QRS transition zone in the praecordial leads.
2. R - S < 1mV in Lead I.
3. R - S ≥ 1mV in Lead I.
4. The sum of the polarities of the delta waves in II, III and aVF.

5. Delta wave amplitude ≥ 1mV in Lead II.
6. Delta wave axis.
7. R - S > 0.8mV in Lead I.
8. R > 0 in Lead III.
9. S - R > 0mV in aVF.

This study reports on the methods used to include the above classification scheme in a program routinely used for 12-lead ECG analysis by computer.

2. MATERIALS AND METHODS.

The Glasgow Program for ECG analysis has been described previously(6). With respect to analysis of conduction defects, an average PQRST cycle is available from each of 12-leads. From this the various wave amplitudes and durations can be calculated. Of particular interest for the present study was the detection and measurement of the delta wave.

Within the Glasgow Program, there are routines for the detection of delta waves. Essentially, the logic assesses the slope of the first 30 milliseconds of the QRS complex and compares it with the slope of the remaining initial section of the QRS complex prior to the peak amplitude. In the absence of a delta wave, it is possible to calculate the intercept of the upper slope on the baseline. The further this intersection is from QRS onset, the higher the probability that a delta wave exists. Thus, the Glasgow Program basically calculates a confidence factor for the presence of a delta wave in each lead. The confidence factor of each of the 12-leads has a value between zero and 100%. In addition, an amplitude of the delta wave can be calculated as shown in Figure 1.

In order to enter the section of the program that determines the location of an accessory pathway, it is necessary to establish the presence of delta waves. This is done using the confidence factors as described above but in addition to this, other criteria are also utilised. The criteria utilised for detecting the presence of delta waves are as follows:

1. The sum of the confidence factors > 150.
2. QRS duration > 110 milliseconds.
3. PR interval < 160 ms.
4. 0 < P axis < 90.

If all of these criteria are met, then a delta wave is accepted as present. It was a study of 1,501 normal ECGs which had led to the critical values described above being selected. In a separate training set of 139 electrocardiograms showing anterior or inferior myocardial infarction, each of which had a QRS duration in excess of 100 milliseconds, the criteria were 98% specific.

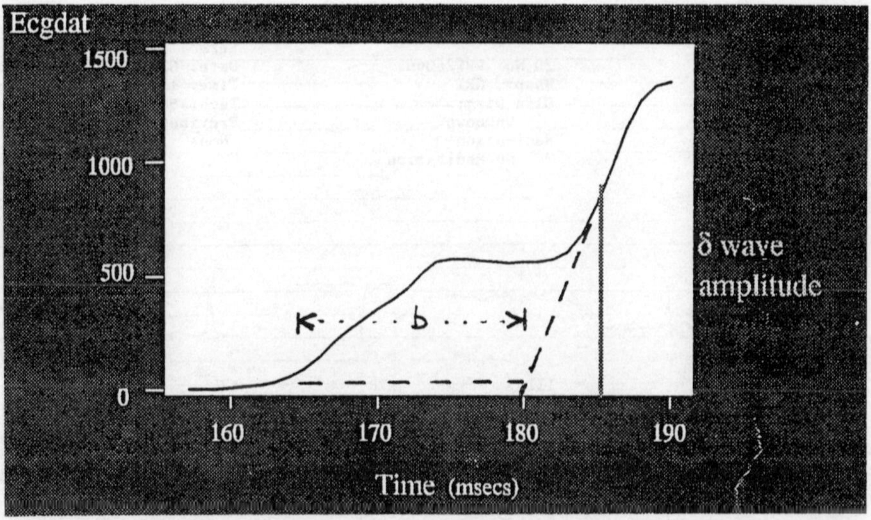

Figure 1: Calculation of the delta wave confidence factor which is related to the length of the base (b) of the delta wave.

Given that delta waves have been found and amplitudes obtained, it is possible to utilise the amplitudes of the delta wave in Leads I, II and III to calculate a delta wave axis as required by the classification scheme.

It is also a trivial matter to calculate the sum of the polarities of the delta wave in II, III and aVF as well as other amplitudes and the QRS transition zone in the praecordial leads.

The appropriate software was developed to implement the classification scheme. 8 new output statements were created for the program, e.g. WPW PATTERN - PROBABLE RIGHT ANTEROSEPTAL ACCESSORY PATHWAY. An example is shown in Figure 2.

3. RESULTS.

In 1,120 ECGs from the CSE Study(7), the program was 99.92% specific. This test set contained no ECGs with WPW pattern but included a wide variety of abnormal QRS pathologies and so was a useful test of specificity.

Todate, the sensitivity of the software has been assessed on a small group of 14 electrocardiograms with WPW pattern. The sensitivity for detecting WPW was 86%. Data from electrophysiological studies undertaken in these patients indicates 100% correspondence between the localisation of the pathway and the computer report.

GLASGOW ROYAL INFIRMARY
ECG REPORT

		Serno: 100004
Name:	ID No: WPW260661	Date: 02Dec94
Age: 32	Hosp: GRI	Time: 13:2:0
Sex: Male	Clin Diag:	Tech: 66 15
Race: Unknown	Unknown	Previous ECGs:
Loc:	Medication:	None
	No Medication	

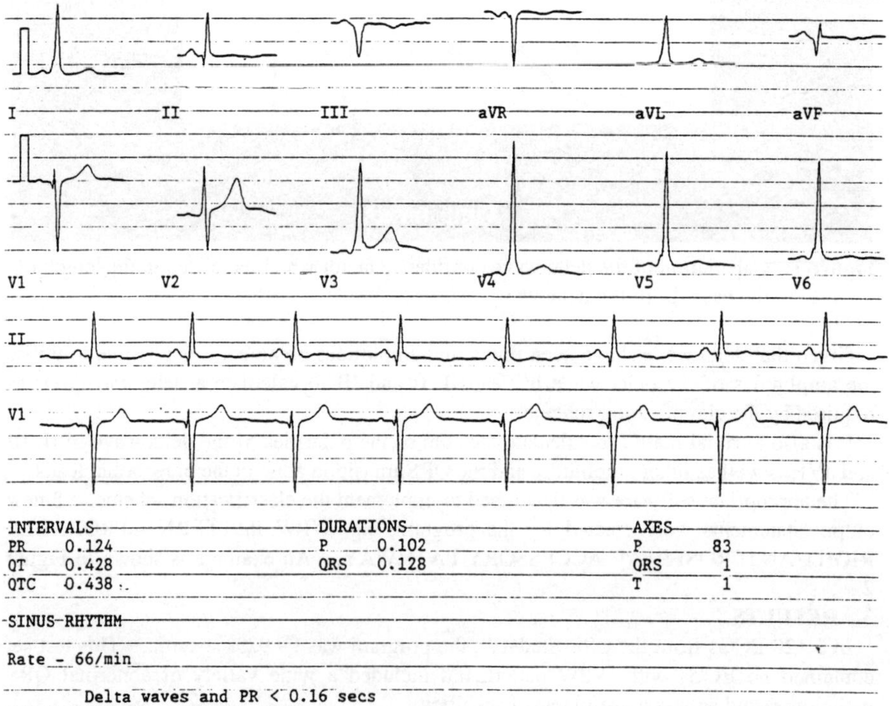

INTERVALS		DURATIONS		AXES	
PR	0.124	P	0.102	P	83
QT	0.428	QRS	0.128	QRS	1
QTC	0.438			T	1

SINUS RHYTHM

Rate - 66/min

Delta waves and PR < 0.16 secs
W.P.W. PATTERN - PROBABLE RIGHT
POSTEROSEPTAL ACCESSORY PATHWAY

Date : 16 Dec 1996

Summary - ABNORMAL   Signed -   Time : 14:52:58
Serial Comparison - ABNORMAL
with ECG of ********

Figure 2: An example of a computer assisted report of a WPW Pattern.

However, the series is much too small to suggest that the classification would always be correct.

4. DISCUSSION.

With the availability of cardiac electrophysiological studies, the importance of localising the accessory pathway in WPW pattern is of increasing importance. Although its location will ultimately be defined at EPS investigation prior to ablation in the usual circumstances, it is still nevertheless of value to have a preliminary indication of the location of the pathway. Fitzpatrick et al who introduced the classification system argued in their original paper(5) that their approach had many advantages over those of others and clearly these must translate into the automated approach. The only point of difficulty is in ensuring that the delta wave in the ECG is correctly detected. This can be difficult in certain situations particularly where there is an elevated QRS onset fused with a P wave.

Notwithstanding the above limitations, it is felt that the inclusion of a more specific location of accessory pathway into the Glasgow Program is a useful enhancement to the software.

REFERENCES.

1. L. Wolff, J. Parkinson, P. D. White, *Am. Heart J.* **5** (1930) 685-704.
2. F.F. Rosenbaum, H.H. Hecht, F.N.Wilson, F.D. Johnston, *Am. Heart J.* **29** (1930) 281-326.
3. J.J. Gallagher, E.L.C. Pritchett, W.C. Sealy, H.J. Kasell, A.G. Wallace, *Prog. Cardiovasc. Dis.* (1978) 285-327.
4. S. Yuan, T. Iwa, M. Tsubota, H. Bando, *Electrocardiol.* **25** (1992) 203-14.
5. A.P. Fitzpatrick, R.P. Gonzales, M.D. Lesh, G.W. Modin, R.J. Lee, M. Scheinman, *J.A.C.C.* **23** (1994) 107-16.
6. P.W. Macfarlane, B. Devine, S. Latif, S.C. McLaughlin, D.B Shoat, M.P.Watts, *Meth. Inform. Med.* **29** (1990) 354-61.
7. Willems et al, *New Eng. J. Med.* **325** (1991) 1767-73.

COMPARISON OF QRS ONSET LOCATION USING NEURAL NETWORKS AND CONVENTIONAL METHODS

PARVEEN CHISHTI
University Department of Medical Cardiology, Royal Infirmary, Glasgow, Scotland.

TOM C. AITCHISON
Department of Statistics, University of Glasgow, Glasgow, Scotland.

PETER W. MACFARLANE
University Department of Medical Cardiology, Royal Infirmary, Glasgow, Scotland.

ABSTRACT

Despite the fact that there are various computerised techniques available for measuring the fiducial points of ECG waveforms, there are still problems associated with the accuracy of these measurements particularly in the presence of noise. This study investigates the use of neural networks to locate the QRS onset and compares the results to those produced by an expert Electrocardiographer. Results from more conventional methods are also compared.

1. INTRODUCTION

There are many automated techniques available for measuring the fiducial points of an ECG signal, most of these being in the form of ECG analysis programs. However, since all measurement programs have their own philosophies with respect to optimum waveform analysis, this can lead to the problem of variations in the wave measurements. This problem was illustrated by Willems et al[1] who showed that in a combined data set of original and artificial ECG recordings, the difference in measurements between a group of 16 different programs varied widely. In an attempt to standardise such computerised measurements, the CSE reference library was established[2].

Inaccuracy of wave measurements is even more prevalent in cases where the ECG signal has been contaminated with noise. Whether through powerline interference or other artefacts, these inaccuracies can have the effect of producing false diagnoses and hamper the exchange of diagnostic criteria. An example of a noisy 12-lead ECG can be seen in Figure 1. ECGs such as this are a common problem faced by many medical staff and automated analysis systems, which usually have difficulty in interpreting the recording.

The aim of this present study, therefore, was to improve the accuracy and repeatability of detecting the QRS onset in the presence of noise using software based artificial neural networks. This method has already been investigated for identifying ST-T abnormalities[3] and in other diagnostic areas such as the diagnosis of Atrial Fibrillation and Myocardial Infarction[4].

2. MATERIALS AND METHOD

2.1. CSE Reference Library

The data used in this study was obtained from the CSE mutilead reference library. This library consisted of 250 ECGs, 26% being normal and the remainder abnormal.

Due to different ECG measurement programs having their own philosophies with respect to analysis, 125 artificial ECGs were created on the basis of a selected beat taken from the original recordings being reproduced to create a string of identical beats with stable RR intervals over 10 seconds for all 12 simultaneous leads. Every fifth ECG was then visually analysed by five expert CSE referees and all 125 ECGs were processed by 16 different ECG analysis programs. Individual onset and termination points were therefore produced by alignment of beats to a reference beat using methods of cross-correlation.

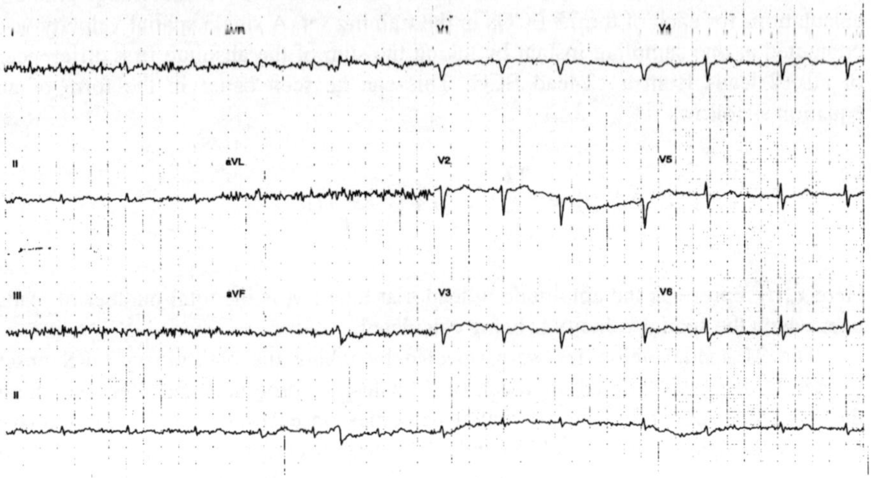

Figure 1 Example of a noisy 12-lead ECG

2.2. The Training and Test Set

A comparison of the results from this study to those of the CSE referees would require the alignment of beats reproduced for analysis purposes to the aforementioned reference beat. However as this was unavailable, it was necessary to produce a separate set of referee results to use as a 'Gold Standard' for this study. These new measurements were visually selected and recorded by an expert electrocardiographer who examined the spatial velocity and modal beat of each ECG and used the CSE QRS durations (offset minus onset) as a guide to maintain an exact correspondence between the two sets of results.

Since neural networks require to be trained with similar examples of the problem to be solved, in this case the networks had to be trained with QRS data for which the QRS onset was specified. The training set therefore consisted of 75 ECGs from the CSE library and the new referee QRS onsets were used to specify where the true onset would lie, as part of the training process. From these 75 ECGs, fifty were then randomly chosen to act as the test set with the addition of random 'white' noise. This is discussed later in more detail.

2.3. Training the Neural Network

The network investigated applied the feed-forward back propagation algorithm[5]. The idea behind this type of design is to minimise the mean square error between the actual output and the desired output of each neuron in a multi-layer network. The software for this type of network was already available in the department[6].

The input data comprised of 21 spatial velocities and 42 individual gradient calculations for each of the 75 ECGs in the training set. A single spatial velocity was computed at one sampling instant by taking the sum of the absolute first differences of all 12 leads from a 12-lead ECG. This can be seen better in the form of an equation as follows :

$$S.V.(t) = \sum_{n=1}^{12} |x_n(t+1) - x_n(t)| \tag{1}$$

Here $x_n(t)$ represents the amplitude in lead n at time t, n is the total number of leads over which the spatial velocity is being calculated.

The 21 spatial velocities were selected by taking the preliminary QRS onset located by the conventional approach of the Glasgow program[7] and then extracting the preceding and following 10 spatial velocities on each side of this preliminary point, each separated by 2 milliseconds. This was necessary since the idea was to create a window for the neural network in which the QRS onset would be located. The window would preferably be fairly small so that the time to train a specific network could be kept to a minimum. There would be no point in utilising a technique whose eventual run time far exceeded its practical use. For each of the 21 spatial velocities, two gradients were calculated on either side of these measurements, using methods of linear regression. This can be explained better using the following graph :

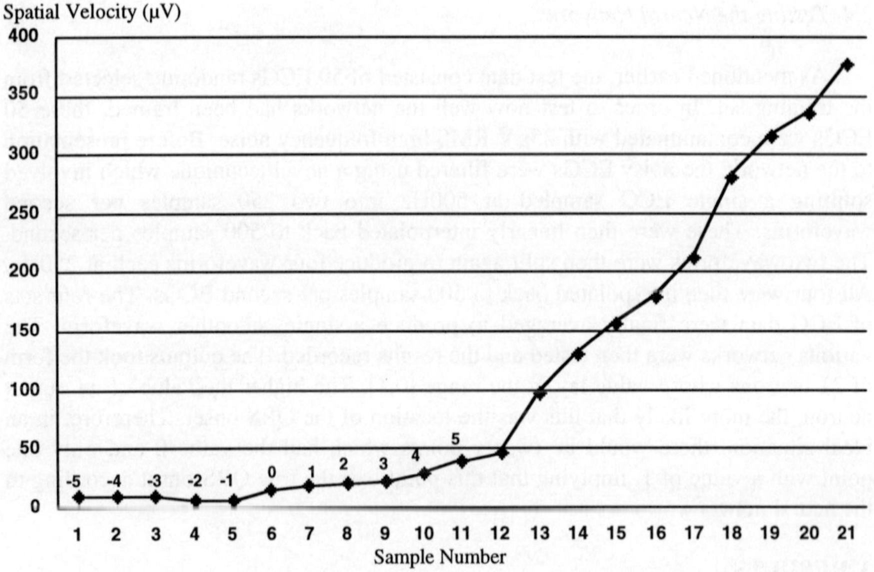

Figure 2 Illustration to show calculation of slope estimates

In Fig. 2 a sample of 21 input spatial velocities has been plotted. Consider the point marked 0 as being the current spatial velocity of interest. To calculate the gradient to the left of this point, the equally spaced five time points preceding the current spatial velocity were numbered -1 to -5. The corresponding spatial velocity measurements were then regressed onto these time points (0 to -5), to produce a regression equation from which the slope estimate could be extracted. Similarly, to compute a slope estimate to the right of the current spatial velocity, the five points following this spatial velocity were numbered 1 to 5 and the same process of linear regression was carried out, as before. This was done for all 21 points producing a total of 42 gradient estimates. This provided additional information to the network in terms of how the data was changing with time and therefore allowed the network to identify any common patterns in the data.

Various network configurations were investigated. Presentation of the input data was varied by training networks with the spatial velocities as the only inputs, the 42 gradients as the only inputs or a combination of the two. Also, networks with one or more hidden layers were trained in the hope that the addition of an extra layer would increase the capacity of the network to learn and store associations and therefore improve its overall effectiveness. Throughout the training process, the networks had knowledge of where the onset lay in the output field. This previous knowledge came from the actual referee onset estimates. The number of output neurons remained constant throughout at 21.

2.4. Testing the Neural Network

As mentioned earlier, the test data consisted of 50 ECGs randomly selected from the training set. In order to test how well the networks had been trained, these 50 ECGs were contaminated with 25μV RMS high frequency noise. Before presentation to the network, the noisy ECGs were filtered using a novel technique which involved splitting a single ECG sampled at 500Hz into two 250 samples per second waveforms. These were then linearly interpolated back to 500 samples per second. The two waveforms were then split again to produce four waveforms each at 250Hz. All four were then interpolated back to 500 samples per second ECGs. The four sets of ECG data were finally averaged to produce a single, smoother waveform. The various networks were then tested and the results recorded. The outputs took the form of 21 neurons whose value lay in the range [0,1]. The higher the value of an output neuron, the more likely that this was the location of the QRS onset. Therefore, in an ideal situation, there would be twenty points which had the value 0 and only one point with a value of 1, implying that this point was the true QRS onset according to the neural network.

3. RESULTS

Two of the networks tested performed best. These were (i) Network 63-50-21 which represented a fully connected network with 63 inputs (21 spatial velocities and 42 gradients), 50 hidden neurons (1 hidden layer) and 21 output neurons, and (ii) Network 63-63-21 which represented a fully connected network with 63 inputs, 63 hidden neurons (1 hidden layer) and 21 output neurons. Table 1 shows the overall result produced by these networks. Results from the conventional Glasgow Program (G.P.) as well as those produced by introducing the filter into the Glasgow program (F. & G.P.) have also been included. A score of 1 was awarded to a QRS onset which deviated from the referee result (Ref) by one sample and a score of 2 for that which deviated by 2 samples etc. A final score was thus formed. It can be seen from the final score that the filtering technique very significantly enhanced the conventional program. This was enhanced further by the addition of neural networks. The number of exact QRS onset locations was improved by 50-60% when compared to those of the filter alone. However, closer inspection of the results showed that when the filter was applied to the Glasgow program, the maximum number of sample points by which a particular QRS onset deviated from its 'Gold Standard' was five, whereas for the two neural networks combined, there were five cases in total which deviated by six samples from their true onset. So although the number of onsets correctly located improved, there was also an increase in the amount of deviation between the corresponding referee and neural network estimates for certain ECGs. Therefore it seemed that overall, the addition of neural networks did not prove to be significantly beneficial since the filtering method alone seemed to improve the accuracy of QRS onset location vastly.

Table 1 Comparison of the Glasgow Program (G.P.), the new filtering technique & Glasgow Program (F.&G.P.) and the filtering technique (& Glasgow Program) & neural networks.

lActual-Refl	G.P.	F. & G.P.	F. & 63-50-21	F. & 63-63-21
0	2	10	16	15
1	18	19	17	17
2	15	13	11	12
>=3	15	8	6	6
Score	162	74	67	70

4. DISCUSSION

Although the above results may not have demonstrated any benefit in the use of neural networks, it should however be noted that all the neural networks were trained and tested with an extremely small sample size. Ideally a much larger training set would be used with corresponding referee onsets, something which is difficult to achieve since this would require two or more experienced cardiologists willing to set aside time to go through the tedious task of picking out wave onsets by eye. It has been shown that with the introduction of the new filter alone, the amount of deviation between the actual and the true onset decreases vastly.

Although this study concentrated on QRS onset location, the main aim had been eventually to apply the technique of neural networks to locate the fiducial points of the P-wave. However since the method did not prove successful for the most dominant of the waveforms, the QRS wave, it seemed a pointless exercise to study the accuracy of P-wave onset location using the time consuming methods of neural networks.

REFERENCES

1. J. L. Willems, P. Arnaud, J. H. van Bemmel et al., *J.A.C.C.* **10**, 1313 (1987).
2. J. L. Willems, P. Arnaud, J. H. van Bemmel et al., *J. Electrocardiology, Supplemental Issue* **20**, 56 (1987).
3. B. Devine, P. W. Macfarlane, *Med. & Biol. Eng. and Comput.* **31**, 343 (1993).
4. T. F. Yang, PhD Thesis (Glasgow University) 1995.
5. R. P. Lippman, *IEEE ASSP Magazine,* 4 (1987).
6. B. Devine, MSc Dissertation (Glasgow University) 1990
7. P. W. Macfarlane, B. Devine, S. Latif, S. McLaughlin, D.B. Shoat, M. P. Watts, *Methods of Information in Medicine* **29**, 354 (1990).

POSSIBILITIES OF EVALUATION OF HEART FUNCTIONAL STATE IN DISABLED PATIENTS WITH COMPUTERIZED ECG ANALYSIS SYSTEM

S. KORSAKAS, A. VAINORAS, L. GARGASAS, V. MIŠKINIS
Institute of Cardiology, Kaunas Medical Academy,Sukileliu 17, Kaunas, Lithuania
E-mail: stakor@medi.lt

The problems of methods of evaluation of heart functional state in health and disabled patients using exercise tests are discussed. The results of comparing of the two methods are being presented: bicycle ergometer (B) and "concept" type ergometer(C). The results showed that while different muscle groups were working (B and C tests), the reaction of regulation systems of organism were different, even if the developed power and the stage intervals were just the same. The evaluation of heart functional state of disabled patients at present is not correct enough, because the model of describing the organism reaction is insufficient in comparison with different exercise tests.

1. Introduction

Various exercise tests are widely used for evaluation of functional capacity of the patient's organism in the clinical trials. The exercise tests permit to evaluate the adaptation of patients organism to maximal physical load and the diagnostic performance of the exercise ECG influences on detection of coronary artery disease. These methods are very useful for evaluation of functional state and compensation functions of organism in disabled patients. For motorically disabled persons it is complicated to use one of the most popular method - the bicycle ergometry. The "concept" type ergometer or gymnastic exercises methods are recommended to use in this case. The main problem is to evaluate the testing results of different methods. For comparison results of different methods of exercise tests it is recommended to use the same protocol. Is it enough for evaluation of the reaction of the whole organism? The objective of this study was to try to answer to this question.

2. Methods

The exercise tests are not enough standardised and the comparison of various methods are not discussed in literature. During exercise test the whole reaction of patients organism can be defined as a sum of: 1) the developed work power of muscles, 2) the influence of regulation system, and 3) the function of cardiovascular system. At present the most detailed analysis is done only on the first part. The evaluation of regulation system is limited to variables of heart rate (HR) or systolic blood pressure (BP). The analysis of ST interval is used only for evaluation of the cardiovascular system. In clinical practice the exercise protocol is used where the magnitudes of developed work power (bicycle or "concept" type ergometers), the speed and incline (treadmill) are standardised [1]. These parameters reflect only the function of muscles but it is not enough to evaluate the whole system of organism. For evaluation of regulation and cardiovascular systems it is necessaryed to standardise the time interval of stage (TIS). In the work [2] we suggested to divide the exercise protocols into three groups: 1) provocative, where TIS $\leq$ 1 min., 2) adaptive, where TIS $\leq$ 3 min., working, where TIS $\leq$ 6 min.

For accomplishment of this study we used a computerized ECG analysis system "Kaunas-Load" [3,4]. During any exercise test the program presents on the screen ECGs, the values of HR, ST changes and records synchronously 12 lead ECGs (10 s interval) in every stage and the desired time sequence. After an exercise test a computer analyses ECGs and presents the results on a screen or prints in three levels: 1) tables of parameters (11 averaged amplitudes and durations in every lead), 2) changes of parameters of two dimension trends (2D), and 3) three dimension integrative trends (3D) for each parameter for all test.

We tested some patients according to the standardised method using a provocative exercise protocol, where the initial workload was 50 W, increment of 25 W every one minute. Exercise tests were sign-or symptom - limited maximal tests using recommended criteria of termination [5]. Each person was tested in two methods: using the bicycle ergometer (B), and after one week, using "concept" type ergometer (C), which modelates the single sculler moves. In the first case during exercise test only the muscle of legs worked and in the second case muscles of arms, legs, and trunk worked. Both methods involve the different quantity of muscles which worked but the developed workload and time intervals of stage were the same.

3. Results and discussion

Methods were tested in Kaunas Medical Academy on four healthy students, whose mean age was 21 year, height - 1,68 m, weight - 59,2 kg, body mass index (BMI) - 20,85 kg/m^2. The initial data of investigated persons are presented in Table 1.

The changes of main parameters using bicycle (B) and "concept" type (C) ergometers are presented in Table 2.

Table 1: Initial data of investigated persons

N	Age (yr)	Height (m)	Weight (kg)	BMI (kg/ m^2)
1	21	1,72	65	22
2	21	1,67	61	21,9
3	21	1,71	59	20,2
4	21	1,64	52	19,3

Where BMI - body mass index

Table 2: Changes of parameters during B and C exercise tests

N	Test	HR_{max}	PWC_{170}	DP_{max}	JT_0	JT_{max}	ST_0	ST_{max}	Sys_{max}	$Dias_{max}$
1	B	179	.954	286.4	.29	.18	.34	-.20	160	95
	C	173	1.798	311,4	.29	.16	.23	-.60	180	80
2	B	211	.934	263.7	.23	.17	.34	-.20	125	80
	C	180	1.295	225.6	.26	.17	.55	-.53	120	70
3	B	199	1.898	318.4	.23	.17	.30	.25	160	90
	C	186	2.017	316.2	.24	.16	.69	.10	170	70
4	B	188	1.462	244.4	.24	.16	.44	.41	130	65
	C	191	1.481	286.5	.22	.16	.34	.41	150	80

Where: N - numbers of persons (the same as in Table 1.), Test - type of exercise: B - bicycle ergometer, C - "concept" type ergometer, W_{max} - maximal developed power, HR_{max} - heart rate during maximal workload, PWC_{170} - parameter for evaluation of HR and workload changes, DP_{max} - duple product ($HR x Sys_{max}$), JT_0 - mean of JT interval for 12 leads before test, JT_{max} - JT interval (mean) during maximal workload, ST_0 - sum of ST amplitude in 12 leads 40 ms after J point before test, ST_{max} - sum of ST amplitude in maximal workload, Sys_{max} - systolic blood pressure (BP) during maximal workload, Dias $_{max}$ - diastolic BP during maximal workload.

In both tests the maximal developed power W_{max} was the same. Parameters HR_{max}, PWC_{170}, DP_{max} reflecting the regulation system of organism show high variability (especially PWC_{170}, which connects heart rate, developed power and body mass) in B and C cases. Parameters ST_0 and ST_{max}, Sys_{max} and $Dias_{max}$ describing cardiovascular function do not show systematic changes in B and C tests. But in the C case the parameter Sys_{max} was bigger than in the B case.
The results of these investigations showed that working of different muscle groups (B and C tests), the reaction of regulation systems of organism had been different, even if the developed power and stage intervals were just the same. For corroboration of this conclusion we performed the next experiment with bicycle ergometer. The investigated person at first worked with both legs (T), after that -

only with the right (R) and the left (L) leg. The maximal workload was 100 W in all cases. The results of this experiment are presented in Table 3.

Table 3: Reaction of regulation system during B test, performed with both legs (T), only right (R), and only left (L) leg

Test	HR_{max}	PWC_{170}	DP_{max}	JT_0	JT_{max}	ST_0	ST_{max}	Sys_{max}	$Dias_{max}$
T	127	2.649	152.4	.30	.21	.50	.26	180	60
R	167	1.715	283.9	.28	.17	.44	-.21	170	80
L	166	1.615	298.8	.25	.17	.52	-.10	180	70

Abbreviations - just the same as in Table 2.

The comparison results of the experiment in all three cases showed the different values of parameters JT, ST, Sys_{max}, $Dias_{max}$, though the workload was just the same. The results indicate that, in general, for standardisation exercise's tests it has not been enough to standardise the workload and time interval of stage.

In conclusion, the evaluation of heart functional state for disabled patients at present is not sufficiently enough correct, because the model of describing the organism reaction is insufficient in comparison with different exercise tests.

References

1. G.F. Fletcher, G. Balady, V.F. Frolicher et al., "Exercise Standards. A Statement for Healthcare Professionals from the American Heart Association". Circulation 199I, 91, p. 580.
2. S. Korsakas, A. Vainoras, R. Ruseckas, V. Miskinis. "Standardization of Exercise Tests in Computerized ECG Analysis System". Medical & Biological Engineering & Computing, 1996,V.34, Suppl.1, part 2, P.49-50.
3. J. U. Bauer, H. Schwela, A. Vainoras, R. Ruseckas, S. Korsakas. "Computerized ECG Recording I Functional tests". Medical & Biological Engineering & Computing, 1996,V.34, Suppl.1, part 1, P.415-416.
4. A. Vainoras, L. Gargasas, R. Ruseckas, V. Miskinis, R. Jurkoniene, H. Schwela, U. J Bauer. "Computerized Exercise Electrocardiogram Analysis System "Kaunas-Load". In this issue.
5. B. Chaitman. "Exercise Stress Testing". In: Heart Disease. W. B. Saunders company, 1996; P.153-176.,

VI. Clinical Electrocardiogrpahy, Vectorcardiography, and Dipolar Electrocardiotopography

FACTORS AFFECTING THE SPATIAL ANGLE BETWEEN INTEGRAL QRS AND T VECTORS.

ANDRÁSYOVÁ D., ČIŽMÁROVÁ E. *, RUTTKAY-NEDECKÝ I.: Institute of Normal & Pathological Physiology, Slovak Academy of Sciences, Bratislava, Slovak Republic, *Pediatric Clinic Staré Mesto, Bratislava, Slovak Republic
E-mail: andrasy@unpf.savba.sk

It has been repeatedly shown that the spatial angle between integral vectors of depolarization and repolarization increases with deep inspiration. The aim of this study was to seek relationship of this variable with other cardiovascular parameters. The study consisted of two subgroups: 135 normal subjects without subjective and objective signs of cardiac pathology, aged 10-68 yrs (mean 37, SD 13) and 56 subjects with labile blood pressure (BP), aged 10-31 yrs (mean 18, SD 4). Standard ECGs, Frank lead scalar tracings and VCGs loops were obtained from a selected single beat, using the CARDIAG 128.1 (Veltech Prague) PC based electrocardiologic recording system. Recordings were made on seated subjects in end-tidal and in held deep inspiratory chest position, avoiding the Valsalva maneuver. Deep inspiration led to a significant increase of the spatial angle by 27.5 % ($p<0.01$) in normal subjects and by 36 % ($p<0.001$) in subjects with labile BP.

Initial values of the spatial angle were negatively correlated to their reactive values in healthy persons. The magnitude of the QRS-T angle and its deep inspiratory reaction were in significant relation to age ($p<0.001$). There were also a significant differences of heart rate (HR) according to age ($p<0.05$). In 10 (18 %) subjects with labile BP we found a decrease of the spatial angle during deep inspiration and the basal HR of these persons was significantly higher than of those who reacted by increment of the spatial angle (102±18 vs. 83±17 bt/min, $p<0.003$).

Introduction

The magnitude of the spatial angle between integral vectors of ventricular depolarization and repolarization (AQRS-AT) is a parameter independent on cardiac anatomic position, indicating inhomohenity of cardiac recovery.

Normal values for this and related variables were published earlier by Simonson et al.[1], by Ball and Pipberger [2], by Beswick and Jordan [3], and later by Riekkinen and Rautaharju [4].

Since there is still lack of data on the nature and sources of physiological variability of this characteristic, our study was undertaken to evaluate the influence of gender, age, heart rate (HR), respiratory chest movements and blood pressure variability in subjects without cardiac pathology.

Subjects and Methods

Our study group consisted of two subgroups: 135 normal subjects and 56 adolescents with labile blood pressure (BP). Characteristics of both subgroups are given on table 1.

Recordings were made in seated persons, in mid-respiratory chest position and immediately (cca 5 - 10 s) after held maximum inspiration. ECG, Frank lead VCG and 80 electrodes body surface maps were recorded by means of the Cardiag PC based electrocardiologic system (VELTECH, Prague). In this study, only the value of the spatial angle between integral QRS and ST-T vectors, evaluated by the computer, was taken into consideration.

The 24 hrs BP and HR were monitored in the subgroup of 56 adolescent with labile BP, by means of the apparatus Accutracer II (Suntech).

Data were analyzed by STATGRAPHICS, version 5, microcomputer software package (Statistical Graphics Corporation, Rockwille, Maryland, USA). Differences between mean values were evaluated by one and two-tailed t-tests. The effect of gender, age, HR on the spatial angle was assessed by the multifactor analysis of variance. Data are expressed as mean values and standard deviation (SD) or standard error (SE) of the mean. If not stated otherwise, $p<0.05$ was considered statistically significant.

Results

In the subgroup of normal subjects there were no significant gender related differences of the spatial angle AQRS-AT.

There was a statistically significant correlation between the magnitude of the spatial angle and age in the whole group ($r=0.324$, $p<0.001$).

Age related significant differences of the magnitude of the AQRS-AT angle were found only in men if soubgroup of younger and older than 35 years were compared (Fig. 1)

Already Simonson and his colegues [1] in 1957 reported a significant increase of the angle between QRS and T vectors in maximal inspiration (by 5 degrees). They supposed that this phenomenon cannot be explained sufficiently solely by the anatomic respiratory changes. However, in two of the above mentioned studies [3,4] the inspiratory changes were not significant.

In our study, held deep inspiration led, in agreement with Simonson et al.[1], in average to a significant increase of the AQRS-AT angle in normal subjects by 15 degrees ($p<0.001$) (Fig.2). It is interesting that in adolescents

Tab. 1 Characteristics of study subgroups

Normal subjects	N=135
Female	43
Male	92
Age ± SD	36.9 ± 16 yrs
Range	10 - 68 yrs
Subjects with labile blood pressure	N= 56
Female	12
Male	46
Age ± SD	18.3 ± 4 yrs
Range	10 - 31 yrs

criterion: at least 3 ambulatory measurements above 140/90 mm Hg

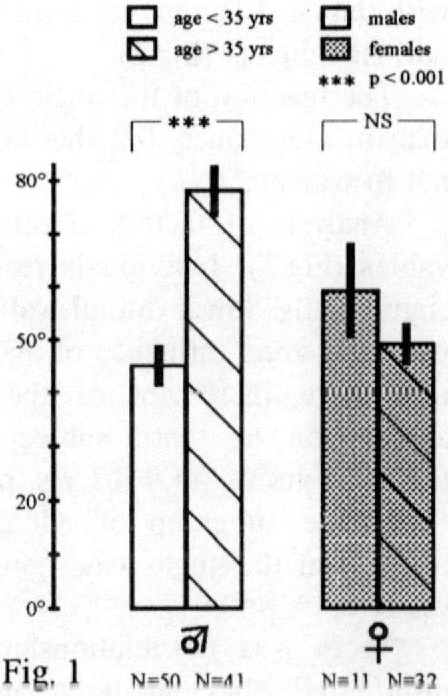

Fig. 1

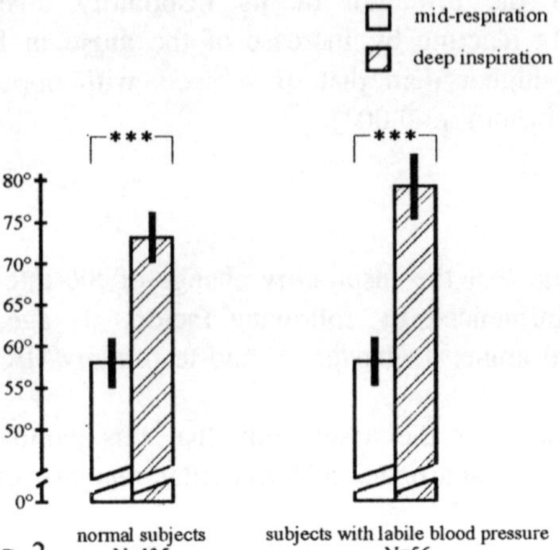

Fig. 2

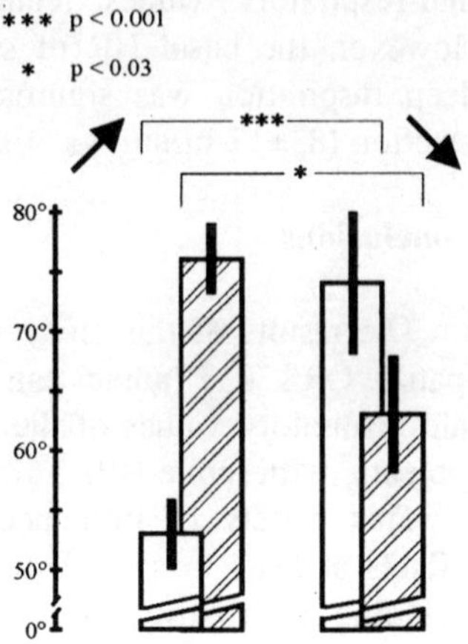

Fig. 3

Figure. 1 Mid-respiratory values of the spatial AQRS-AT angle (ordinate) in males and females aged under or over 35 years

Figure. 2 Effect of deep inspiration on the spatial angle AQRS-AT in the subgroups of healthy subjects (left panel) and in the subgroup with labile BP (right panel), values of the angle on the ordinate

Figure. 3 Comparison of values of AQRS-AT angle (ordinate) in mid-respiration and in deep inspiration between subjects reacting with an inspiratory increase of the angle (left panel) and subjects reacting with an inspiratory decrease of the angle (right panel)

with labile BP this reaction was greater (by 21 degrees, $p<0.001$) than in normal subjects (Fig.2).

The reaction of the angle in deep inspiration was greater in younger persons than in older ones, but this difference was statisticaly significant only in men, not in women.

Analysis of factors affecting this reaction has shown the effect of initial values (Fig.3). Individuals reacting with respiratory increase of the angle had significantly lower initial values than subjects reacting with decrease. There was also some influence of age, since the average age of those individuals with inspiratory increment of the AQRS-AT angle was significantly lower in comparison to those subjects with inspiratory decrement of this variable (34.8±14 yrs vs. 44.9±17 yrs, $p<0.003$).

In the subgroup of adolescents with labile BP the average inspiratory increase of the angle was significantly greater in males than in females (24±21° vs. 10±11°, $p<0.04$).

There was no relationship between 24 hrs BP values and the type of inspiratory behaviour of the angle in subjects with labile BP. Neither were the mid-respiratory values related to the direction of its inspiratory change. However, the basal HR of subjects reacting by increase of the angle in held deep inspiration was significantly higher than that of subjects with opposite reaction (83±17 bt/min vs. 102±18 bt/min, $p<0.003$).

Conclusions

The results of this study indicate that the inspiratory change of the integral spatial QRS - T angle can be influenced by following factors: 1. age, 2. mid-respiratory values of the spatial angle, 3. gender, 4. mid-respiratory HR (in subjects with labile BP).

This variety of influences speaks for the assumption that this parameter reflects at least to same extent the characteristics of ventricular repolarization, including its disparity.

References

1. E. Simonson, K. Nakagawa, O. Schmnitt, Am. Heart J. **54**, (6),919-939 (1957)
2. M.F. Ball and H.V. Pipberger, Am. Heart J. **56**, (4), 611-615 (1958)
3. F.W. Beswick and R.C. Jordan, Am Heart J. **62**, (3), 379-390 (1961)
4. H. Riekkinen and P. Rautaharju, Circulation, **53,** (1), 40-45 (1976)

ANALYSIS OF PRE AND POST-OPERATIVE ELECTROCARDIOGRAPHIC FINDINGS OF PATIENTS SUBMITTED TO THE REDUCTIVE VENTRICULECTOMY (BATISTA OPERATION)

PASTORE,C.A; MOFFA,P.J.; MORAES,A,P.; TOBIAS,N.; KAISER,E.; BACAL,F.; MOREIRA,L.F.; STOLF,N.; BOCCHI,E.; BELLOTTI,G.; PILEGGI,F.

Heart Institute of HC FMUSP /UNIP, Al.Franca 797 - CEP 01422 - 000 - São Paulo - Brazil

ABSTRACT

With the purpose of analysing electrocardiographic findings, 15 patiens have been studied, 13 male, aged between 38 and 68 years old (average 49.7), who had been submitted to the reductive ventriculectomy surgery during the period ranging from January 1995 to October 1996, at the Heart Institute,University of São Paulo Medical School.Each patient had a pre and postoperative ECG carried out, follow-up 45 days. For most of the patients both the pre and post-op ECGs showed a sinus rhythm and the QRS duration did not change (0.133 sec). The figures relating to the presence of left atrial enlargement (86.6%) and to left ventricular hypertrophy (100%) were the same in the pre and post ECGS. Bundle Branch Blocks were constantly found ,being the Left bundle branch block the most present (53.3%). Electrical findings of myocardial infarction in the pre-op ECGs were seen in 4 cases ,two of them with inferior, one lateral and one inferior plus anterior. Our attention was also called, both in pre and post-op ECGs to: a important presence of left ventricular hypertrophy, no modifications in QRS duration and important lowered voltage of QRS in all cases in the post-op ECGs. In what refers to aspects of myocardial infarction seen in pre-op exams, comparison with the post-op showed two cases with pre-op inferior myocardial infarction extended to the lateral wall ; the case with anterior and inferior and the case with lateral , both suffered extension to the lateral wall. Six cases whose pre-op exams showed no signs of myocardial infarction had this developed in the lateral wall after surgery. All these cases amount to a total of 10 patients (66,6%) with aspects of myocardial infarction in the post-op. ECG findings are giving therefore evidence of the repercussion of this new surgery technique, which modifies the heart's anatomy, electrical activations and the cardiac function itself.

INTRODUCTION

The Partial Ventriculectomy has been reported by Dr. Randas Batista since 1994 as a new surgery technique[1]. It can be considered an alternative method for treating patients with severe cardiomyopathies of the dilated type, with serious ventricular dysfunction (NYHA IV).

Some of these patients, waiting for a donor for a heart transplant, have been submitted to this palliative operation, which consists in resection of a large wedge of wall muscle from the left ventricle lateral wall. The reduction of left ventricular diameters after the surgery with increase in wall thickness to chamber radius ratio, could determine a decrease in wall stress valve regurgitation, fiber slippage and myocardial oxygen demand, with consequent improvement in ventricular performance and work efficiency[2-5].

Groups of surgeons in Brazil and abroad have started to establish protocols to study the clinical-surgical evolution of patients operated on with this technique. The anatomic modifications of the heart bring about electrical repercussions that can be evaluated through diagnostic exams to measure the cardiac electrical activation, such as the Electrocardiography (ECG), Vectorcardiography (VCG) and Body Surface Mapping (BSPM)[6-7]. This study has the purpose of discussing the electrical patterns of such modifications by employing the ECG, in an attempt to contribute to the development of this new technique.

METHODS AND MATERIAL

Study Population

The study population consisted of 15 patients, 13 male, from 38 to 68 (average 49.7) years of age. These patients had been submitted to the Reductive Ventriculectomy during the period ranging from January 1995 to October 1996 at the Heart Institute ,University of São Paulo (Brazil) Medical School. Each patient had a pre and a post-operative ECG carried out, within a 45 days follow-up.A clinical evaluation of the patients was performed and all patients underwent endomyocardial biopsy, echocardiography and coronary angiography to exclude myocarditis, ischemic cardiomyopathy and other forms of heart muscle disease.

Standard 12-Lead ECG

Standard 12-lead pre and post-operative ECGs were recorded at 25mm/sec, using a Hewlett Packard Equipment model 1700 with an interval of 45 days between both ECGs.

RESULTS

Pre-op findings: Most of the exams showed a sinus rhythm and the QRS duration averaged 0.133 sec. Left Atrial Enlargement (LAE) was shown in 13 cases (86.65%). Left Ventricle Hypertrophy (LVH) was found in 100% of cases. Left Bundle Branch Block (LBBB) was found in 8 cases (53.3%); one of these presented a -60° and the other seven had a normal axis. Left Anterior Superior Fascicular Block (LASFB) was seen in 4 cases (26.6%), one case presented a LASFB associated with a Right Bundle Branch Block (RBBB). Abnormal Q-waves simulating myocardial infarction were shown in 4 cases (26.6%), two of them in the inferior wall, one in the lateral wall and one in the inferior+anterior walls.

Post-op findings: Within the follow-up period we still found a sinus rhythm; the QRS duration showed practically no change. Both LAE and LVH were the same as before (86.6% and 100%). In what refers to LBBB, of the 8 cases previously found, 4 still showed the same axes; 3 cases showed a change in axes to -60°; the case in which the axis was -60° shifted to +180°. Considering LASFB: 1 case showed no change; a second shifted from -60° to +90°; the case where LASFB was associated to RBBB shifted from -90° to -150°. All 4 cases showing abnormal Q-waves simulating myocardial infarction (MI) showed an extension of them to the lateral wall (Q-waves in D1 and aVL). Their axes also showed a modification, 3 of them already mentioned above, and 1 shifting from -60° to 0°.Six cases where no abnormal Q-waves on the lateral wall were shown before surgery, had these presented in the post-op exams. Five of these cases also had their QRS axes modified: two from +60° to -60°; one from -30° to -150°, one from 0° to +30° and another from +30° to 0°.(Table I)

Table I

CASE	PRE BBB	OP MI	AXIS	q waves ECG	POST BBB	OP MI	AXIS	q waves ECG
01	LBBB	--	+ 60	--	LBBB	LAT	- 60	q D1, aVLTerSlow.
02	LBBB	--	0	--	LBBB	--	0	--
03	LASFB RBBB	Inf + Ant	- 90	D2,3,F V4,5,6	LASFB RBBB	Inf+Ant +LAT	-150	q-D1,2,3,F,L V,4,5,6
04	--	--	- 30	--	--	LAT	-150	q- D1,aVL
05	LBBB	--	0	--	LBBB	--	- 60	--
06	--	--	+ 60	--	--	--	+ 60	--
07	LBBB	--	0	--	LBBB	LAT	+ 30	q-D1 ,aVL
08	LASFB	Inf.	- 60	D2,3,F	--	Inf.+ LAT	0	q- D2,3,aVF D1,aVL
09	LBBB	--	+ 60	--	LBBB	LAT	- 60	q- D1,aVL
10	--	--	+ 30	--	--	LAT	0	q- D1,aVL
11	LBBB	Lat	- 60	D1aVL	LBBB	LAT	+180	QS- DI;aVL
12	--	--	0	--	--	--	+ 30	--
13	LBBB	--	+ 30	--	LBBB	--	+ 30	--
14	LASFB	Inf.	- 60	D2,3,F	LPIFB	Inf+LAT	+ 90	q-D2,3,F,Ter.Slow.
15	LASFB	--	- 60	--	LASFB	LAT	- 60	q- D1,aVL,V5,6

LBBB-Left Bundle Branch Block; LASFB - Left Anterior Superior Fascicular Block ;RBBB-Right Bundle Branch Block; LPIFB - Left Posterior Inferior Fascicular Block;MI -Myocardial Infarction;LAT - Lateral;TerSlow.- Terminal Slowing

DISCUSSION

The partial ventriculectomy, developed by the Brazilian surgeon Randas Batista, is being proposed as a very interesting option because it is a relatively simple surgery with no important contraindication. It is based on the Laplace law and consists in the resection of the left ventricle lateral wall to reduce its diameter. That author reports an improvement of the clinical conditions and ventricular output, with a short term mortality of 18% and medium term of 28%, and an actuarial survival of one year in 60% of cases[1]. In our group (15 patients) there were four deaths, one of arrhythmia in the immediate post-operative period and the others in the late postoperative period. Our purpose has been to investigate the effects of surgical remodelling in the heart's electrical activity brought by this new surgery technique, through electrocardiographic exams carried out in the pre and post-operative periods. The sinus rhythm found in both the pre and post-operative exams of most of the patients contrasts with the findings of ventricular tachycardia very difficult to control and of a high mortality rate. Ventriculectomy may have potential effects on complex interaction of factors involved in ventricular arrhythmia mechanisms through areas of fibroses and myocardial infarction, that were observed in our necropsy studies. Those regions of scar and infarction could modify the arrhythmogenic underlying process perhaps by new re-entrant ventricular mechanisms[2]. In the post-op period there was an intriguing evidence of decrease in the expression of electrical activation of the heart, shown in the decrease of left atrial enlargements and left ventricular hypertrophies as well as in left bundle branch blocks voltages, as compared to the pre-op voltages obtained (Brody's effect)[6-7]. The QRS axes modifications (80% of cases with abnormal Q-waves) evidenced the already mentioned alterations of the electrical activation of the heart in post-op and can reinforce the increased presence of BBB after surgery. Both alterations in QRS axes and increased BBB's could correlate to MI detected by increased levels of CKMB and in the necropsy of patients who died in the immediate post-op. The findings of MI can explain the presence of abnormal Q-waves in six cases of patients who developed such patterns after surgery, and also the extension of Q-waves to the left ventricle lateral wall in those four patients who showed these abnormal Q-waves in the pre-op exams.(fig.1 and fig.2)

Fig.1 - Ecg and Vcg (case 1 -Pre-op.) with BBB and LVH

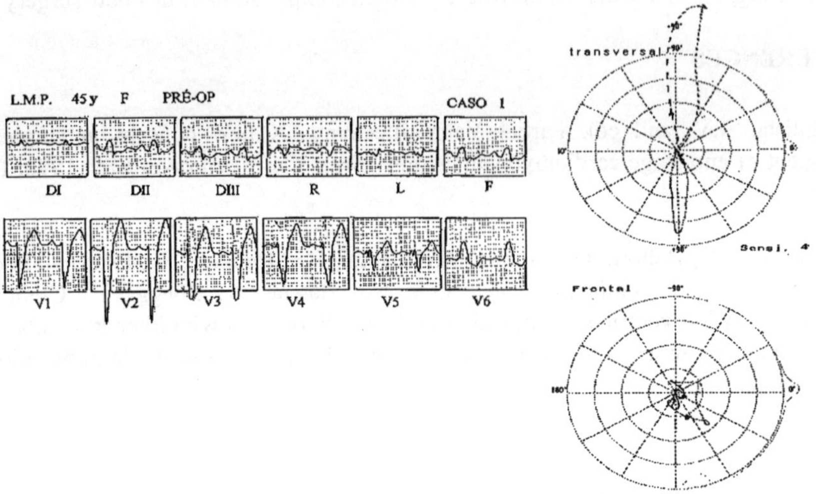

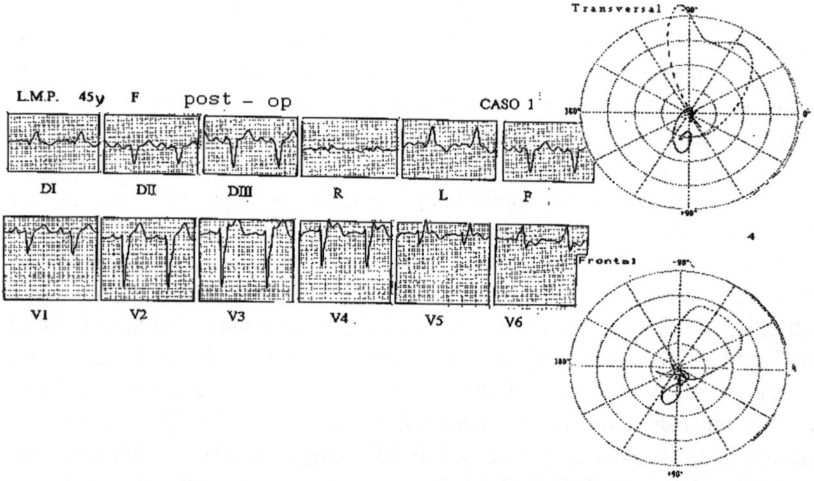

Fig.2 - Ecg and Vcg (case 1 - Post-op) - LBBB,LVH and presence of q waves (D1 and aVL) and terminal slowing.

CONCLUSIONS

Evidences of decreased voltages in the ventricular activation and the appearance of new Q-waves are frequently described after partial ventriculectomy. These findings suggest that acute MI may be a common complication of this new surgery.

REFERENCES

1- Batista, R.V. and col. Partial Ventriculectomy: A new concept in surgical treatment of end-stage cardiomyopathies. *Rev. Bras. Cir. Cardiovascular*. 1996; II: 1-6.

2- Bocchi, E.A.; Bellotti, G.; Moraes, A.P.; Bacal, F.; Moreira, L.F.; Esteves Filho, A.; Fukushima, T.; Guimarães, G.; Stolf, N.; Jatene, S.; Pileggi, F.. Clinical outcome after left ventricular surgical remodelling in patients with idiopathic dilated cardiomyopathy referred to heart transplantation. Short term results. In publication *(Circulation-97)*.

3- Bellotti, G.; Bocchi, E.A.; and col.. Partial Ventriculectomy outcome upon mechanical properties, shape and geometry of the left ventricle in patients with dilated cardiomyopathies. *Arq. Bras. Cardiologia.* 1996; 67: 395-400.

4- Chon,Jn. Structural basis for heart failure: ventricular remodelling and its pharmacologial inhibition. *Circulation* 1995; 91: 1504-7.

5- David A. Kass. Johs Ventriculectomy - A direct apllication of Laplace's law. Hopkins School of Medicine. *Arq. Bras. Cardiol.* 1996; 67: 401-402.

6- Pastore, C.A.; Moffa, P.J.; Moraes, A.; Tobias, N.; Kaiser, E.; Bacal, F.; Moreira, L.F.; Stolf, N.; Bocchi, E.; Bellotti, G.; Pileggi, F.. Pre and post-operative electrocardiographic aspects of patients submitted to the reductive ventriculectomy (Batista Operation). *XVIII Congress of the Cardiology Society of São Paulo. 1997; Abstract.*

7- Moffa, P.J.; Pastore, C.A.; Moraes, A.P.; Tobias, N.; Kaiser, E.; Bacal, F.; Moreira, L.F.; Stolf, N.; Bocchi, E.; Bellotti, G.; Pileggi, F. Analysis of pre and post-operative vectorcardiographic findings of patients submitted to the partial ventriculectomy (Batista Operation). *XVIII Congress of the Cardiology Society of São Paulo. 1997; Abstract.*

ANALYSIS OF PRE AND POST-OPERATIVE VECTORCARDIOGRAPHIC FINDINGS OF PATIENTS SUBMITTED TO THE REDUCTIVE VENTRICULECTOMY (BATISTA OPERATION)

Moffa, P.J.; Pastore, C.A.; Moraes, A.P.; Tobias, N.M.; Kaiser, E.; Bacal, F.; Moreira, L.F.; Bocchi, E.; Stolf, N.; Bellotti, G.; Pileggi, F.

Heart Institute of HC of FMUSP/UNIP- Al.Franca 797 - CEP 01422 - 000 - São Paulo - Brazil

ABSTRACT

With the purpose of studying vectorcardiographic aspects, 15 patients were evaluated, 13 male, between 38 and 68 years of age (average 49,7), who had been submitted to the reductive ventriculectomy surgery during the period January/95 to October/96, at the Heart Institute ,University of São Paulo,Medical School(Brazil). Each patient had a pre and a post-operative VCG carried out, follow up 45 days. Left atrial enlargement (86,6%) and left ventricular hypertrophy (100%) were the most constant finding pre and post operatively. Bundle branch and fascicular blocks were clearly evidenced in VCG's. Pre-op showed predominance of Left bundle branch blocks (53.3%), with an only case of a - 60° deviation. Left anterior fascicular blocks were seen in 4 cases (26.6%), 1 associated with right bundle branch block. Post-op showed 2 of those cases with left bundle branch blocks with a - 60° axis deviation, 1 case changed to normal axis, 1 case became a left posterior fascicular block. Evidences of myocardial infarction were seen in 4 cases pre-operatively, 2 with inferior, 1 with anterior and inferior and 1 with lateral infarctions. After surgery 6 more cases showed signs of myocardial infarction. All of these amount to 10 patients (66.6%) with signs of infarction after surgery ($p < 0,05$). 100% of cases showed lowered VCG loops voltage, decreasing aspects of left ventricular hypertrophy, myocardial infarction and bundle branch blocks. Important alterations in the vectorcardiogram were therefore observed in this study, deriving both from the surgical technique that has an effect similar to a myocardial infarction, as well as from the clinical consequences of the operation.

INTRODUCTION

Heart transplantation is an accepted therapy for end-stage heart failure in patients suffering from idiopathic dilated cardiomyopathy refractory to classic clinical methods. However this surgical procedure faces several important limitations, such as the donor shortage and the criteria selection. On the other hand, there are some other alternatives to minimize the difficulties of performing a heart transplantation[1]. The partial ventriculectomy, developed by the Brazilian surgeon Dr. Randas Batista , has been proposed as a very interesting option for treatment of refractory heart failure[2]. This new procedure can reverse some aspects of the cardiac remodelling like hypertrophy, dilation, change in left ventricular shape and augmented wall stress (Laplace law) and increased myocardial oxygen consumption[3-5]. The ventriculectomy is a relatively simple surgery and consists in the resection of a large wedge of wall muscle from the left ventricle lateral wall, beginning at the apex, extending between the papillary muscles, and ending proximal to the mitral annulus. The many alterations it brings about include modifications of electric cardiac activation. Classical methods as the Vectorcardiography, Electrocardiography and Body Surface Mapping can evaluate and quantify such alterations[6-7]. The purpose of this study was to analyse the repercussions of this surgery on the electrical activation of the heart employing the VCG.

METHODS AND MATERIAL

- The study population consisted of 15 patients, 13 male, from 38 to 68 (average 49.7) years of age. These patients were submitted to the Partial Ventriculectomy during the period ranging from January 1995 to October 1996. Each patient had a pre and post-operative VCG carried out, within a 45 days follow-up. A clinical evaluation of these patients was carried out and all underwent endomyocardial biopsy, echocardiography and coronary angiography to exclude myocarditis, ischemic cardiomyopathy and other forms of heart muscle disease.
- VCG was performed using a BSM system HPM 7000 unit (Fukuda Denshi Co.) in the pre-operative and in the post-operative, within a 45 days follow-up.
- The statiscal analysis was performed using a chi-square test and Fisher`s test exact test.

RESULTS

Pre-op findings: 13 cases (86.6%) showed Left Atrial Enlargement (LAE). 15 cases (100%) showed Left Ventricle Hypertrophy. The QRS loops evidencing Left Bundle Branch Block (LBBB) were seen in 8 cases (53.3%), one of them presenting a left axis deviation (-60°). 4 cases (26.6%) showed QRS loops with left and upward desviations characterizing Left Anterior Superior Fascicular Block (LASFB), one of them presenting LASFB associated with Right Bundle Branch Block (RBBB). In 4 cases (26.6%) QRS loops showed classic patterns simulating myocardial infarction(MI): two of them only in the inferior wall and associated with LASFB; one in the lateral wall associated to LBBB and a -60° axis; and one in the inferior + anterior wall associated with LASFB plus RBBB.

Post-op findings: LAE and LVH rates remained the same as in the pre-operative. LBBB pre-operatively seen in 8 cases suffered the following alterations: 4 cases (26.6%) maintained the same axes; 3 cases had axes shifted to -60°; the case with a -60° axis shifted to +180°. LASFB showed these alterations: 1 case from -60° to +90° (such change in the QRS loop suggests left posterior inferior fascicular block, LPIFB); 1 case had no modification; 1 case where LASFB was associated with RBBB preoperatively shifted from -90° to -150°. The 4 cases with pre-operative VCG patterns of MI showed an extension of these patterns to the lateral wall. QRS loops simulating MI on the lateral wall were found in six cases where no such patterns existed preoperatively. Of these, only one case showed no axis modification after loop patterns of MI appeared. The most frequent finding in the QRS loops suggesting lateral MI was a displacement to the right of the initial portion of the loop and the presence of a terminal slowing also located on the right.(Table I)

Table I

	PRE	OP			POST	OP		
n.	BBB	MI	AX	VCG	BBB	MI	AX	VCG
01	LBBB	–	+ 70	FP;ccw; inf TPccw;post	LBBB	LAT	- 60	FP cw;init.right; up TP cw;init.right;post
02	LBBB	–	0	nl	LBBB	–	0	nl
03	LASFB RBBB	Inf + Ant	- 90	FP ccw;up TP ,ccw;post	LASFB RBBB	Inf+ Ant +Lat	-150	FP ccw;up;right TP ccw;ant;right
04	–	–	- 30	FP ccw;up TP ccw;postt	–	LAT	-150	FP cw,up;right TP ccw;post;right
05	LBBB	–	0	FP ccw,up TP ccw,post	LBBB	–	- 60	FP ccw,up;left TP ccw,post;left
06	–	–	+ 60	nl	–	–	+ 60	nl
07	LBBB	–	0	FP ccw,eight TP cw,post	LBBB	LAT	+ 30	FP ccw,init.right;inf. TP cw,init.right;post.
08	LASFB	Inf.	- 60	FP ccw,up TP ccw,post	–	Inf.+ LAT	0	FP cw,init.right;up TP ccw,init.right,post.
09	LBBB	–	+ 60	FP ccw,inf TP cw,post	LBBB	LAT	- 60	FP ccw,init.right;up TP cw,init.right;post
10	–	–	+ 30	FP ccw,inf TP ccw,eight	–	LAT	0	FP cw,init.right;up TP ccw,init.right;
11	LBBB	Lat	- 60	FPcw,init.rig TPcw,init.rig	LBBB	LAT	+ 180	FP cw,init.right,inf. TP ccw,right,post
12	–	–	0	nl	–	–	+ 30	nl
13	LBBB	–	+ 30	nl	LBBB	–	+ 30	nl
14	LASFB	Inf.	- 60	FP ccw,up TP ccw,eight	LPIFB	Inf+ Lat	+ 90	FP cw,inf;left,TS TP ccw,post,left,TS
15	LASFB	–	- 60	FP ccw,up TP ccw,eight	LASFB	LAT	- 60	FP cw,init.right,up TP cw,init.right,post

LBBB- Left Bundle Branch Block; LASFB - Left Anterior Superior Fascicular Block; LPIFB- Left Posterior Inferior Fascicular Block;RBBB- Right Bundle Branch Block; MI- Myocardial Infarction; LAT-Lateral;CW- Clockwise;CCW-Counterclockwise;TS- terminal slowing; Init.right- initialy to the right

DISCUSSION

Short-term goals of medical therapy for heart failure are to relieve symptoms and improve quality of life. The long-term goal should be to prolong life by slowing, halting or actually reversing the progressive left ventricular dysfunction and dilation. In spite of favourable drug effects, progression of heart failure has been demonstrated in trials among patients receiving the best currently available therapy[4]. The complexity of heart failure syndrome contributes to the limited effectiveness of medical therapy in reaching these goals, stimulating the development of new drugs and surgical options.

One of the recent and very interesting options is the left ventricle partial ventriculectomy, developed three years ago by Dr. Randas Batista, an unconventional and relatively simple therapy for patients with idiopathic dilated cardiomyopathy with severe left ventricular dysfunction. However, despite the initial compelling results, data have inspired controversy in scientific areas and in the press[5]. In accordance with the above, the purpose of the present study was to investigate the effects of surgical remodelling following a partial ventriculectomy in the electrical activation of the heart, using the classic method of Vectorcardiography[6-7].

Same as in the ECG exams, a decrease in the QRS loops voltages was noticed in 100% of cases. The Brody's effect consists in increased voltages as the blood volume in the ventricular cavity increases. In this study the reductive ventriculectomy reduces the left ventricular cavity, hence decreases of voltages could be explained by the above described effect, although some authors question the validity of that explanation. In 11 out of the 15 cases there was a change in QRS loop axes (73.3%) ; 90% of this group also developed patterns of Myocardial Infarction in the post-operative. These could correlate with the ressection of the wall muscle from the left ventricle lateral wall, which results in alterations in the electrical acti vation of the heart. The effects of surgical remodelling on the heart's electrical activity can explain both the above alterations and the modifications of Bundle Branch Blocks patterns.

The QRS loop patterns in the VCG suggesting myocardial infarction were the above mentioned displacements to the right of the initial portion of the loops and also the terminal slowing on their right side. These patterns were seen in the exams of 6 patients who developed them after surgery and also in those 4 patients who had an extension to the left ventricle lateral wall of previously detected MI.(Fig.1 and 2)

Fig.1- Ecg and Vcg (Case 3 - pre-op) with RBBB + LASFB and patterns of MI (anterior + inferior)

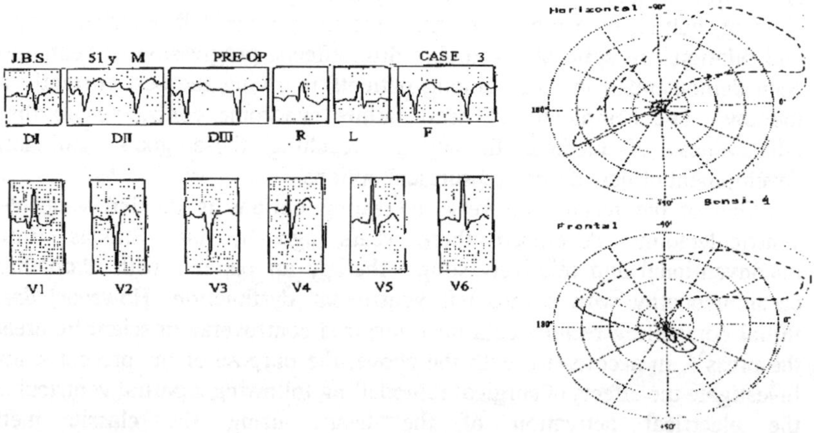

Fig.2- Ecg and Vcg (case 3 - post-op) with RBBB + LASFB and patterns of MI (anterior + inferior + lateral) . QRS loop changed to the right sugesting Lateral MI .

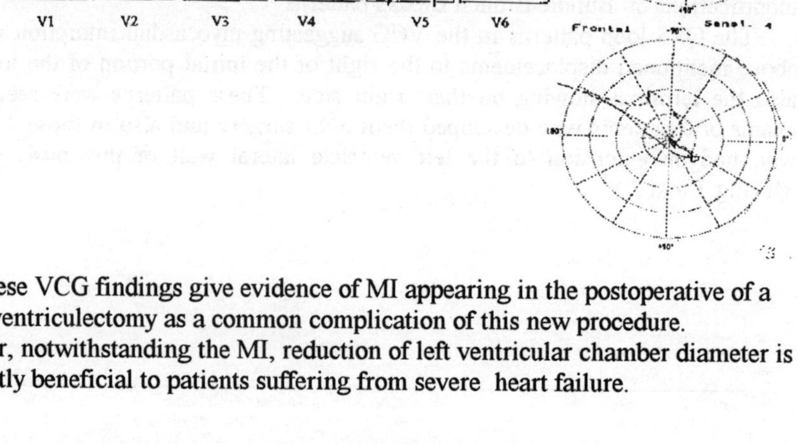

These VCG findings give evidence of MI appearing in the postoperative of a partial ventriculectomy as a common complication of this new procedure. However, notwithstanding the MI, reduction of left ventricular chamber diameter is apparently beneficial to patients suffering from severe heart failure.

CONCLUSION

The follow-up of this new surgery technique employing this classic method of examination has proven to be of great importance to understand the anatomic and electrical modifications that happen in the heart. The findings of this study suggest the occurrence of a myocardial infarction in 66.6% of the patients submitted to the partial ventriculectomy. Despite this evidence, an improvement in functional class was observed in all patients in the immediate postoperative. This fact demonstrates that the effect on geometry making the left ventricle less spherical results in a better physiological mechanism of contraction. An understanding of the modifications in the electrical activation shows that the findings suggesting myocardial infarction such as the ones described in this study are not definitely correlated with a poorer function of the heart. Indeed, this happens as part of a new surgical therapeutic procedure to partially reverse the anatomic remodelling process in heart failure.

REFERENCES

1 Boochi, E.A.; Bellotti, G.; Moraes, A.P.; Bacal, F.; Moreira, L.F.; Esteves Filho, A.; Fukushima, T.; Guimarães, G.; Stolf, N.; Jatene, S.; Pileggi, F..Clinical outcome after left ventricular surgical remodelling in patients with idiopathic dilated cardiomyopathy referred to heart transplantation. Short term results. *In publication (Circulation -97).*

2- Batista, R.V. and col. Partial Ventriculectomy: A new concept in surgical treatment of end-stage cardiomyppathies. *Rev. Bras. Cir. Cardiovascular*. 1996; II: 1-6.

3- Bellotti, G.; Bocchi, E.A.; and col. Partial Ventriculectomy outcome upon mechanical properties, shape and geometry of the left ventricle in patients with dilated cardiomyopathies. *Arq. Bras. Cardiologia*. 1996; 67: 395-400.

4- Chon Jn. Structural basis for heart failure: ventricular remodelling and its pharmacologial inhibition. *Circulation* 1995; 91: 1504-7.

5- David A. Kass. Ventriculectomy - A direct apllication of Laplace's law. Johs Hopkins School of Medicine. *Arq. Bras. Cardiol.* 1996; 67: 401-402.

6- Pastore, C.A.; Moffa, P.J.; Moraes, A.; Tobias, N.; Kaiser, E.; Bacal, F.; Moreira, L.F.; Stolf, N.; Bocchi, E.; Bellotti, G.; Pileggi, F. Pre and post-operative electrocardiographic aspects of patients submitted to the reductive ventriculectomy (Batista Operation). *XVIII Congress of the Cardiology Society of São Paulo. 1997; Abstract.*

7- Moffa, P.J.; Pastore, C.A.; Moraes, A.P.; Tobias, N.; Kaiser, E.; Bacal, F.; Moreira, L.F.; Stolf, N.; Bocchi, E.; Bellotti, G.; Pileggi, F. Analysis of pre and post-operative vectorcardiographic findings of patients submitted to the partial ventriculectomy (Batista Operation). *XVIII Congress of the Cardiology Society of São Paulo. 1997; Abstract.*

DECARTO TECHNIQUE IN RECOGNITION OF INFERIOR MYOCARDIAL INFARCTION AND LOCALIZED LVH INDISTINGUISHABLE BY STANDARD CRITERIA

T.A.SAKHNOVA, E.Sh.KOZHEMYAKINA
Cardiology Research Complex,
3rd Cherepkovskaya, 15a,
Moscow 121552, Russia

N.E.BARINOVA, V.G.TRUNOV, E.A.I.AIDU, L.I.TITOMIR
Institute for Problems of Information Transmission,
Russian Acad. Sci., B. Karetny 19,
Moscow 101447, Russia

This study demonstrates the capabilities of the DECARTO technique in distinguishing complicated cases of left hypertrophy with the standard electrocardiographic signs inherent in myocardial infarction and cases of true inferior myocardial infarction. The activation duration decartogram is found to be most informative for solving such a diagnostic task. In each of the three tested patients with localized interventricular septal hypertrophy which simulates the standard markers of infarction, the decartograms reveal the hypertrophied regions, thus facilitating the differential diagnosis.

1. Introduction

One of the difficult problems occuring in practical diagnostics is recognition of hypertrophied regions of the heart which are located at the superior or basal parts of the interventricular septum and which affect the propagation of the depolarization front in such a way that the standard electrocardiographic signs of old inferior myocardial infarction are imitated. In particular, the Qr or qS configurations may be observed in the standard leads II, III, aVF or orthogonal lead Y.

This investigation is intended for demonstrating possibilities to use the DECARTO technique (dipole electrocardiotopography) for distinguishing the aforementioned pathologic categories on the basis of visual and, in part, quantitative interpretation of the maps (decartograms) of activation duration, which are most sensitive to prolongation of the depolarization front propagation through the hypertrophied myocardium.

2. Subjects and Methods

The data were obtained from a male patient aged 41 years and two female patients aged 22 and 42 years with left ventricular hypertrophy localized mainly to the upper part of the interventricular septum (LLVH group) and ten males and females aged 34 to 62 years with old inferior myocardial infarction (IMI group). The diagnoses were verified by a complete clinical examination including roentgenography, echocardiography, scintigraphy, coronaroventriculography, and other tests. The 12-lead standard electrocardiogram and McFee–Parungao orthogonal electrocardiogram recorded in each patient revealed signs typical for the inferior myocardial infarction, particularly, during the ventricular depolarization (QRS complex). This posed great difficulties for differentiating the pathologic states under consideration. For this reason, the initial orthogonal electrocardiograms were processed by the DECARTO technique, which provides transformation of the orthogonal electrocardiographic signals into a mapping form on the basis of simple electrodynamical models (the method is described in detail elsewhere [1, 2]). In particular, during the depolarization phase (QRS) the cardioelectric generator is described by a uniform double layer with circular edge changing its size and position, and during the repolarization phase (ST-T) it is described by an impressed current uniformly distributed all over the ventricular wall and changing its density and orientation. These models allow us to construct a set of instantaneous maps (decartograms) depicting distributions of the heart wall states (resting state, activation state, i.e. presence of the depolarization front, and completely depolarized state), along with the heart surface landmarks, on the image sphere surrounding the heart. This sphere is cut along the right meridian and unrolled on a plane with retaining the elementary areas. As well, summary, or integral decartograms are constructed, including the isochrone maps representing the times of depolarization arrival and depolarization departure, the activation duration map representing the duration of activation state, and the ventricular gradient map representing the recovery delay. The isochrone maps are especially sensitive to the spatio-temporal dynamics of propagation of the depolarization front in the tangential direction with respect to the heart wall, and the activation duration map is especially sensitive to the wall thickness and velocity of the front in the radial direction with respect to the heart midpoint. Thus, the overloaded or hypertrophied regions of ventricles are characterized by increased values of the activation duration at the corresponding sites of the latter map [3]. The decartograms of all the patients were thoroughly analyzed by visual inspection and quantitative assessment of characteristic regions on the maps.

3. Results and Conclusion

It was found that in the IMI group the infarction scars of the inferior ventricular wall always manifested as inactive regions at the corresponding lower part of

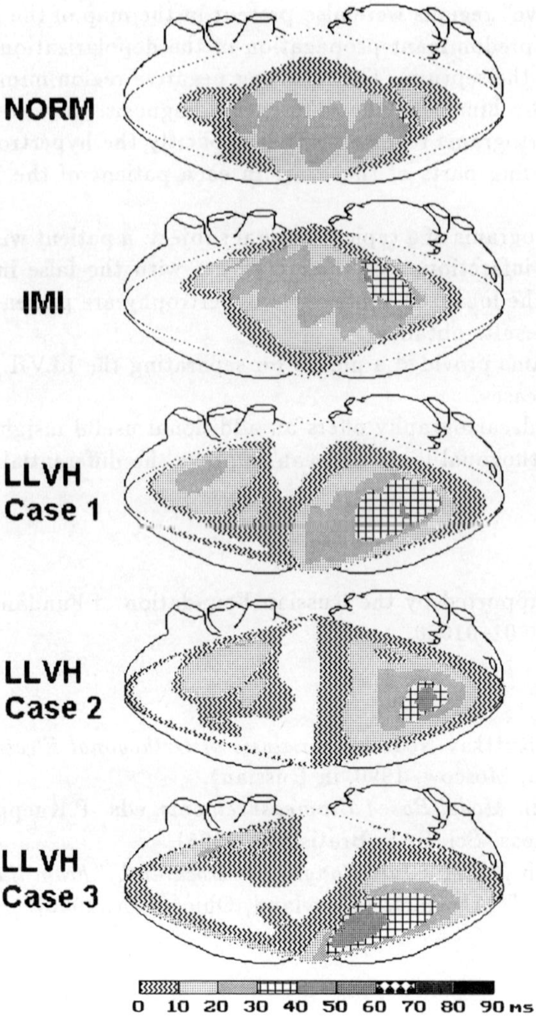

Figure: Orthogonal electrocardiograms (right) and activation duration decartograms of a normal subject (NORM) and patients with true inferior myocardial infarction (IMI) and localized left ventricular hypertrophy (LLVH). The presence of localized hypertrophy is manifested by the prolonged depolarization at superior basal part of the heart (left upper region of the map).

the map. Similar "inactive" regions were also present in the map of the LLVH group as a result of the predominant propagation of the depolarization front into the enlarged part of the septum. The resulting negative region mimics an inferior infarction, thereby hindering the differential diagnosis. However, the activation duration decartograms revealed rather explicitly the hypertrophied regions in the corresponding parts of the heart in each patient of the LLVH group.

The summary decartograms of a typical normal subject, a patient with the true inferior myocardial infarction, and three patients with the false inferior infarction simulated by the localized ventricular hypertrophy are presented in Figure to illustrate the results obtained.

Thus, the decartograms provided a means for separating the LLVH group from the true infarction cases.

It is concluded that decartography offers an additional useful insight into the data delivered by orthogonal leads and can improve the differential diagnosis.

Acknowledgements

This work was in part supported by the Russian Foundation of Fundamental Research, Project No. 96–01–01080.

References

1. L.I.Titomir and I.Ruttkay-Nedecky, *Analysis of Orthogonal Electrocardiogram* (Nauka, Moscow, 1990, in Russian).
2. L.I.Titomir et al, in *Model Based Biomeasurements*, eds. P.Kneppo, M.Tysler (Inst. Meas. Sci, SAS, Bratislava, 1995).
3. L.I.Titomir et al, in *XXIIIrd Int. Congr. Electrocardiol. "From the Cell to the Body Surface"*, Abstracts (Cleveland, Ohio, USA, 1996).

The QRS complex configuration in patients with acute myocardial infarction: its clinical significance and anatomical correlation

B. Ferreira, N. Lopes, P. Moffa, C. Pastore, N. Tobias, R. Kalil, C. Albuquerque, R. Santos, G. Bellotti, F. Pileggi. *Heart Institute University of São Paulo-SP-Brazil.*

ABSTRACT

The terminal portion of the QRS complex represents activation of the Purkinje fibers. Distortion of the terminal portion of the QRS (defined as emergence of the J point at a level above the lower half of the R wave or disappearance of the S wave in leads with RS configuration) occurs when ischemia is of great magnitude because these fibers are considerably more resistant to myocardial ischemia. The aim of this study was to investigate the correlation between distortion of the terminal portion of the QRS and in-hospital events: mortality, severe cardiac heart failure/shock ; left ventricular dysfunction, long term prognosis and the angiographic data. Patients with acute myocardial infarction submitted to thrombolysis were divided based on the initial ECG pattern in two groups: 42 with distortion of the terminal portion of the QRS (group A) and 78 without distortion of terminal portion of the QRS (group B) . There were no differences between groups in gender, age, incidence of anterior myocardial infarction (AMI), previous angina pectoris, previous AMI, hypertension, diabetes mellitus and smoking status. Results: The peak creatine kinase was similar in the two groups. The incidence of either death, severe congestive heart failure, or left ventricular ejection fraction<40%was higher in group A (45% vs 10%, $p < 0.0001$) and four year mortality tended to be higher in group A (7% vs 1%, $p = 0.237$). The single vessel disease was 60% in group A and 42% in group B (*p=0.108*) and the 90-minute TIMI flow 0,1 was similar in the two groups. In conclusion patients with the simple ECG pattern of distortion of the terminal portion of the QRS have worse in-hospital outcome and long term prognosis.

INTRODUCTION

Previous studies on the association between the admission electrocardiogram of patients with acute myocardial infarction and infarct size, high risk of ventricular arrhythmias, or in-hospital mortality have concentrated on the magnitude of ST segment elevation [1-4]. However, the major shortcoming of this method is that the magnitude of ST segment elevation is influenced not only by the extent and severity of ischemia, but also by variations in size and shape of the chest [5], location of the infarction [5], and geometry of the left ventricle [6]. Myocardial ischemia alters the QRS complex in a predictable manner in patients with variant angina and similar changes have been noted during transiet ischemia in dogs. This QRS changes consist of a modest increase of QRS duration and alteration in voltage of the terminal portion of the complex that can be represented by a vector directed towards the ischemic zone. Conduction velocity measurements in the animal preparation suggest that the QRS changes are due to conduction delay in the ischemic myocardium [7].

Previously , terminal distortion of the QRS on the acute myocardial infarction admission ECG was associated with increased in-hospital mortality [8-10], post-infarction left ventricular dysfunction [11],and worse long term prognosis [10]. The mechanism responsible for the association between terminal QRS distortion and adverse outcome is unknown. The aim of this study was to investigate the correlation between this ECG pattern and in-hospital events: mortality, severe heart failure/shock ; left ventricular dysfunction, long term prognosis and the angiographic data in patients with acute myocardial infarction given thrombolytic therapy.

METHODS

Study design: We studied 120 patients (21-70 years of age) who were admitted to the coronary care unit. All patients met these criteria: severe chest pain lasting at least 30 minutes, onset of chest pain less than 5 hours and ECG with ST segment of at least 0,2 mV measured 60 msec after J-point in at least two frontal plane leads or two precordial leads. All patients received thrombolytic therapy (actylise).
ECG analysis: The initial ECG was evaluated by 2 cardiologists, who had no knowledge of the clinical, angiographic and ecochardiografic data. Patients were allocated into the following 2 groups:
Group A) patients who had a distortion of the terminal portion of the QRS complex in $\geq$ 2 adjacent leads: defined as emergence of the J point at a level above the lower half R wave or disappearance of the S wave in leads with RS configuration (Figure IA).
Group B) patients who had no major changes in the morphology of the terminal portion of the QRS (Figure IB).
Clinical evaluation: The following data were recorded: age, sex, history of diabetes mellitus, hypertension, smoking status, previous AMI, previous angina, creatinine kinase levels, incidence of severe heart failure/cardiogenic shock and in-hospital mortality. The patients were followed for 4 years after the initial hospitalization for eventual mortality.
Left ventricular function: Echocardiography was done before hospital discharge.
Coronary angiographic analysis: Coronary stenosis of greater than 70 percent of the luminal vessels in any view was considered significant.
Statistical analysis: Mean values $\pm$ SD were calculated for continuous variables (age and serum creatine kinase levels). Chi-square tests was used to compare differences between discrete variables and Fisher exact test was performed in case of small numbers in each category. For continuous variables , differences between groups were analyzed by two tailed Student's *t* test. A p value < 0.05 was considered statistically significant.

Figure: IA) Admission electrocardiogram of a patient with anterior wall acute myocardial infarction with terminal QRS distortion. IB) Admission electrocardiogram of a patient with anterior wall acute myocardial infarction without terminal QRS distortion.

Figure IA

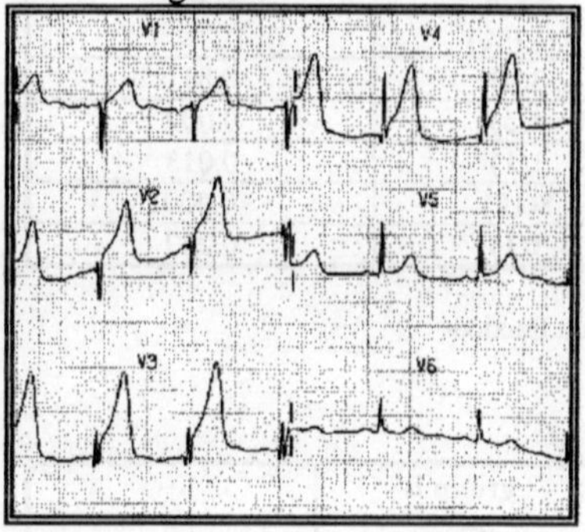

FigureIB

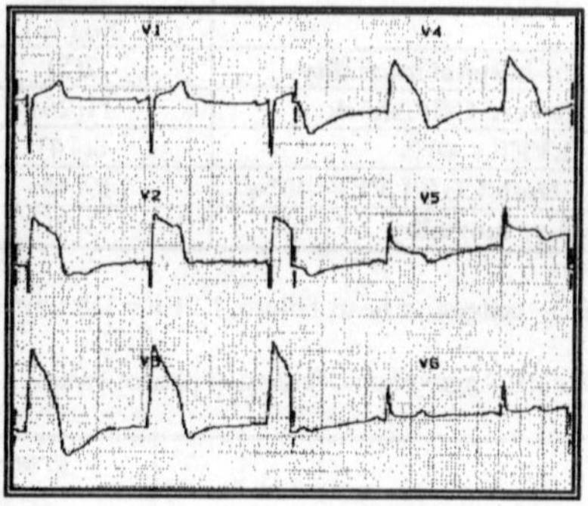

RESULTS

Clinical Characteristics: The study population included 120 patients: 42 patients in group A and 78 in group B (Table I). There were no differences in gender, age, incidence of anterior wall AMI, previous angina pectoris, previous AMI, prevalence of hypertension, diabetes mellitus and smoking status. Clinical outcome: The incidence of either death, severe congestive heart failure, or left ventricular ejection fraction < 40% was higher in group A and four years mortality tended to be higher in group A (Table II). No difference was found between the groups in the rates of 1 or multivessel disease. The rates of patients with 90-minute TIMI flow 0,1 (trombolysis without success) was similar in the two groups (table III). Peak serum creatine kinase was similar in group A 124.41$\pm$ 72.99 and in group B 120.99 $\pm$ 70.81 (p=0.083).

Table I: Clinical characteristics of patient groups.

	group A n=42 No.(%)	**group B n=78 No.(%)**	***P***
Men	35(83)	59(75)	0.457
Age	55.22±11.73	53.55±10.15	0.418
Previous angina	10(28)	22(28)	0.762
Hypertension	17(40)	41(52)	0.284
Diabetes mellitus	6(14)	12(15)	0.915
Current smoking	27(84)	45(57)	0.612
Previous infarction	2(5)	6(7)	0.818
Anterior AMI	21(50)	39(50)	0.848

AMI = acute myocardial infarction

Table II: Clinical outcome of patient groups

	group A n=42 No.(%)	group B n=78 No.(%)	*P*
In-hospital mortality	2(5)	3(4)	0.811
Severe CHF/shock	11(26)	4(5)	0.002
LVEF < 40%	6(14)	1(1)	0.013
Death/CHF/LVEF<40%	19(45)	8(10)	<0.0001
4-yr mortality	3(7)	1(1)	0.237

CHF = congestive heart failure; LVEF = left ventricular ejection fraction

Table III: Angiographic finding of patient groups

	group A n=42 No.(%)	group B n=78 No.(%)	*P*
single vessel disease	25(60)	33(42)	0.108
multivessel disease	17(40)	45(58)	0.108
TIMI flow 0 and 1 at 90 min	11(26)	31(39)	0.199

TIMI = Thrombolysis in myocardial flow grade

DISCUSSION

The terminal portion of the QRS complex represents activation of the Purkinje fibers [12]. Distortion of terminal portion of the QRS occurs when ischemia is of great magnitude because this fibers are considerably more resistant to myocardial ischemia as compared with contracting cardiac myocytes [13].

The surface electrocardiogram is a summation of the electrical vectors activating the left ventricle. During severe regional myocardial ischemia the electrical conduction in the ischemic Purkinje fibers is delayed. Thus, the electrical activation of the ischemic zone occurs relatively late [12,14] and the terminal vector of the QRS over the ischemic zone is less opposed by activation of the rest of the myocardium. This results in an increase in the R wave on leads in which the terminal vector is directed towards them (terminal R wave) and reduction in S wave amplitude in leads recording a complex with a terminal force directed away (terminal S wave).[12,14,15,16]

We found that patients with distortion of the QRS were associated with larger incidence of either death, severe congestive heart failure or left ventricular ejection < 40%. Despite the fact that in the group A there was no difference in 4-year mortality, there was a significant more prevalent left ventricular disfunction that is

considered the most important prognostic factor for long term mortality in post-acute myocardial patients. These observations support other studies where the electrocardiogram pattern was associated with worse prognosis [8,9,10]. Whereas terminal QRS distortion on admission may represent severe ischemia, the absence of such distortion despite prolonged ischemia may be related to differences in the collateral circulation and "preconditioning effects" due to preceding ischemic episodes. The presence of collateral circulation in smaller quantity in patients with distortion of the QRS could be related with prevalence of single vessel disease and less stimulus to the development of collateral circulation [17]. In this study patients in the group A tended to have a greater prevalence of single vessel disease than group B, however, the difference was no significant.

The history of previous angina serve as a "marker" for patients who may have experienced prior brief periods of ischemia (and therefore may have been preconditioned) before myocardial infarction. These preceding ischemic episodes confer a beneficial effect on in-hospital outcome after AMI [18], nevertheless no difference the groups was found regarding the incidence of previous angina.

We don't know yet the underlying mechanisms for the presence or absence of terminal QRS distortion on the admission ECG of patients with AMI, but we know that using this simple electrocardiographic sign it was possible the early identification of a high risk group, despite thrombolytic therapy, and more aggressive therapeutic approaches should be considered in order to improve prognosis.

REFERENCES

1. Nielsen BL. ST-segment elevation in acute myocardial infarction : prognostic importance. Circulation 1973; 48: 338-345.

2. Willems JL; Willems RJ, Willems GM, Arnold AER, Van de Werf F, Verstrate M. Significance of initial ST segment elevation and depression for the management of thrombolytic therapy in acute myocardial infarction. Circulation 1990; 82 : 1147-1158.

3. Bar FW, Vermeer F, de Zwaan C, Ramental M, Braat S, Simoons ML, Hermes WT, van der Laarse A, Verheugt FWA, Krauss XH, Wellens HJJ. Value of the admission electrocardiogram in predicting outcome of thrombolytic therapy in acute myocardial infarction: a randomized trial conducted by the Netherlands Interuniversity Cardiology Institute. Am J Cardiol 1987; 59: 6-13.

4. Birnbaum Y, Sclarovsky S, Ben-Ami R, Rechavia E, Straberg B, Kusniec J, Mager A, Sulkes J. Polymorphous ventricular tachycardia early after acute myocardial infarction. Am J Cardiol 1993; 71: 745-748.

5.Yusuf S, Lopez R, Maddison A, Maw P, Ray N, McMillan S, Sleight P. Value of electrocardiogram in predicting and estimating infarct size. Br Heart J 1979; 42: 286-293.

6. Lekven J, Chatterjee K, Tyberg JV, Parmley WW. Influence of left ventricular dimension on endocardial and epicardial QRS amplitude and ST segment elevation during myocardial ischemia. Circulation 1980; 61: 679-689.
7. Barnhill JE, Wikswo JP, Dawson AK, Gundersen S, Robertson RMS, Robertson D, Virmani R, Smith RF. The QRS complex during variant angina pectoris: studies in patients and in a canine preparation. Circulation 1985; 71: 901-11.
8.Birnbaum Y, Sclarovsky S, Blum A, Mager A, Gabbay U. Prognostic significance of the initial electrocardiographic pattern in a first acute anterior wall myocardial infarction. Chest 1993; 103: 1681-1687.
9. Birnbaum Y, Herz I, Sclarovsky S, Zlotikamien B, Chetrit A, Olmer L, Barbash GI. Prognostic significance of the admission electrocardiogram in acute myocardial infarction. J Am Coll Cardiol 1996; 27: 1128-1132.
10. Birnbaum Y, Kloner RA, Sclarovsky S, Cannon CP, McCabe CH, Davis VG, Zaret BL, Wackers FJT, Braunwald E. Distortion of the terminal portion of the QRS on the admission electrocardiogram in acute myocardial infarction and correlation with infarct size and long term prognosis (Thrombolysis in myocardial infarction 4 trial). Am J Cardiol 1996; 78: 396-403.
11. Hasdai D, Porter A, Birnbaum Y, Strahilevitz J, Sclarovsky S. Predicting postinfarction left ventricular dysfunction based on the configuration of the QRS complex and ST segment in the initial ECG of patients with a first anterior wall myocardial infarction. Cardiology 1996; 87: 125-128.
12. Holland RP, Brooks H: The QRS complex during myocardial ischemia: An experimental analysis in the porcine heart. J Clin Invest 1976; 57: 541-550.
13. DeHaan RL. Differentiation of the atrioventricular conducting system in the heart. Circulation 1961; 24: 458-470.
14. David D, Naito M, Michelson E, Watanabe Y, Chen CC, Morganroth J, Shaffenburg M, Blenko T. Intramyocardial conduction: a major determinant of R wave amplitude during acute myocardial ischemia. Circulation 1982; 65: 161-167.
15. Spekhorst H, SippensGroenewegen A, David GK, Janse MJ, Dunning AJ. Body surface mapping during percutaneous transluminal coronary angioplasty. QRS changes indicating regional myocardial conduction delay. Circulation 1990; 81: 840-849.
16. Barnhill JE, Tendera M, Cade H, Campbell WB, Smith RF. Depolarization changes early in the course of myocardial infarction: significance of changes in the terminal portion of the QRS complex. J Am Coll Cardiol 1989; 14: 143-149.
17. Reimer KA, Jennings RB. Myocardial ischemia, hypoxia, and infarction. In: Fozzard HA, ed. The heart and cardiovascular system. 2. ed. New York, Raven Press; 1992. p.1875-973.
18. Kloner RA, Shook T, Przyklenk K, Davis VG, Junio L, Matthews RV, Burstein S, Gibson M, Kenneth P, Cannon CP, McCabe CH, Braunwald E. Previous angina alters in-hospital outcome in TIMI 4. A clinical correlate to preconditioning ? Circulation 1995; 91:37-47.

STATISTICAL RECOGNITION OF RIGHT VENTRICULAR ENLARGEMENT ON THE BASIS OF DECARTOGRAMS

I.Ruttkay-Nedecky
Institute of Normal and Pathological Physiology, Slovak Acad. Sci., Sienkiewiczova 1, Bratislava 81371, Slovak Republic

V.G.Trunov, L.I.Titomir, M.G.Danilushkin
Institute for Problems of Information Transmission, Russian Acad. Sci., B.Karetny 19, Moscow 101447, Russia

G.A.Muromtseva, V.M.Shamarin
National Research Center for Preventive Medicine, Public Health Ministry of Russia, Petroverigsky 10, Moscow 101953, Russia

Statistical templates for distributions of the activation zones on instantaneous decartograms were constructed for three populations of children and youthes, including healthy subjects (norm), patients with congenital atrial septal defect (right ventricular dilatation), and patients with pulmonary stenosis (right ventricular hypertrophy). Diagnostical classifications were accomplished on the basis of a parameter characterizing the closeness of the particular patient's decartogram to the statistical template for the group considered and a few traditional ECG-parameters. The results confirmed the high informativity of the decartography.

1. Introduction

The instantaneous dipole electrocardiotopogram (decartogram) is a topographic representation of the orthogonal lead signals in the form of time evolution of the heart activation area, projected onto the unrolled quasiepicardium surface. Such a pictorial image facilitates the visual analysis, as well as computerized processing of electrocardiographic data [1, 2].

The aim of this study is to construct probability templates for the decartograms of ventricular depolarization for describing the states of right ventricular hypertrophy or dilatation and to use these templates for diagnosis.

2. Subjects and Methods

We retrospectively studied a population of children and youthes aged 1 to 24 years, investigated in the Institute of Normal and Pathological Physiology, Slovak Academy of Sciences (Bratislava).

Using Frank orthogonal electrocardiographic records and DECARTO technique (described in detail elsewhere [1, 2]), the instantaneous decartograms of ventricular depolarization were determined at the intervals of 10 ms over the QRS period of the heart cycle for the following groups: 48 healthy subjects (group I, norm); 55 patients with congenital atrial septal defect (group II, right ventricular dilatation), and 86 patients with pulmonary stenosis (group III, right ventricular hypertrophy). Then statistical templates (standards) for the distributions of the activation zones were constructed for group I, II, and III, as well as for total group II+III (Fig. 1).

The templates were obtained by accumulation of the decartograms of all patients in the studied group at each instantaneous depolarization map. On the resulting template map, the number of cases with the depolarization areas accumulated at each point defines the height of column at this point. The height of the column at a point on the map is the significance marker of this point. So, the templates represent the probability distributions for occurence of the depolarization area at a given map point and at a given time instant [3].

Diagnostical classifications of the subjects into group I and group II+III, or, alternatively, into group II and group III, were accomplished on the basis of a parameter characterizing the closeness of the particular patient's decartogram to the statistical template for the group considered. Quantitatively, the value of the closeness is determined as follows: the instantaneous decartogram of the tested patient at any time instant, for example, at 40 ms from the QRS onset (Fig. 1) is put on the template for the same instant, and the region of template under the depolarization area of the tested patient's decartogram is contoured. The sum of the significance markers of all template points in the contoured region represents the closeness of the patient's decartogram to the template for norm or any considered pathologic state at each depolarization instant.

The values of the closeness parameter for each time instant were subsequently used as diagnostical signs, along with the maximal magnitudes of the heart vector, in the statistical data processing by the voting method or the step-by-step voting method (Fig. 2).

3. Results

The following signs turned out to be most informative: for separation of group I and II+III, the closeness to the group II+III template at the instants 20,30, and 60 ms from the QRS complex onset; for separation of groups II and III, the closeness to the group III template at the instant 50 ms and closeness to the group II template at the instant 60 ms.

The sensitivity 85% with specificity 100% was provided in classification

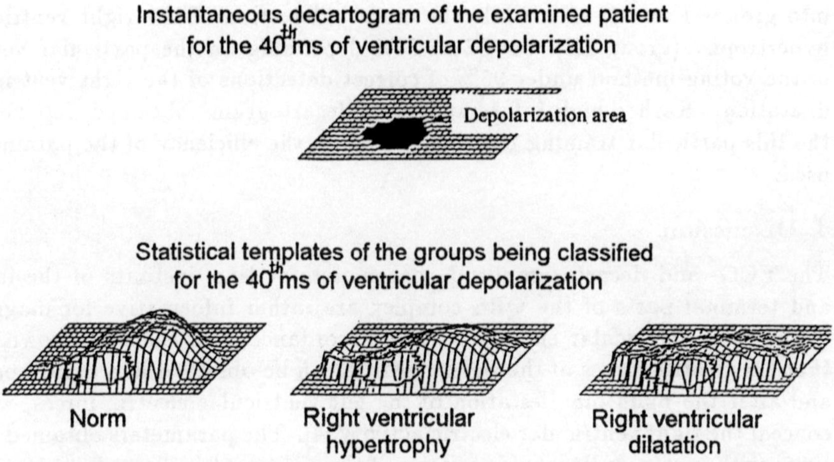

Figure 1: Instantaneous decartograms and statistical templates.

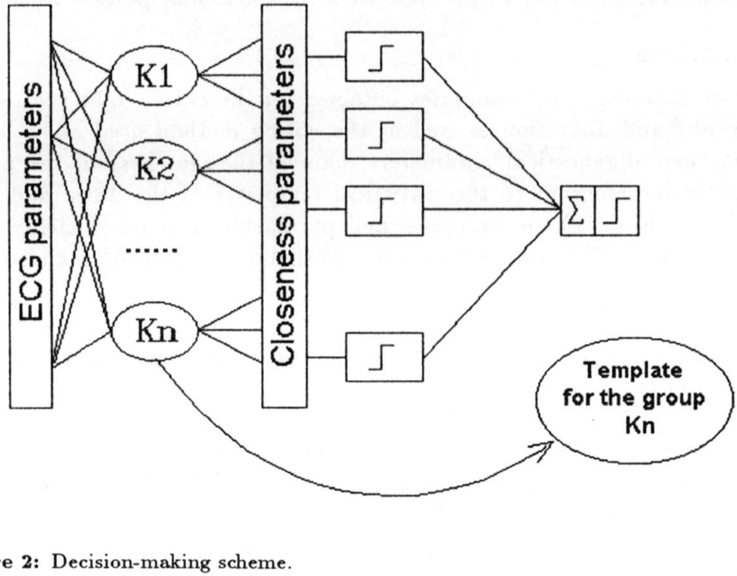

Figure 2: Decision-making scheme.

into groups I and II+III, while the correct detection of the right ventricular hypertrophy (group III) was 62 to 76% depending on the particular version of the voting method under 95% of correct detections of the right ventricular dilatation. Rather high informativity of decartograms obtained depends on the this particular training population and on the efficiency of the parameters used.

4. Discussion

The ECG- and decarto amplitude parameters at time instants of the initial and terminal parts of the QRS complex are rather informative for diagnosis of the right ventricular enlargement, in accordance with the well known idea that the electric forces of the right ventricle can be observed in a period before and after the main manifestation of the left ventricular electric forces, which conceal the right ventricular electric activity [4]. The parameters obtained here agree with vectorcardiographic criteria of the right ventricular enlargement [5].

The high informativity of decartograms demonstrated in this study depends upon the analysis of this particular training population of subjects. So, the results could be considered as an estimate of the limiting possible accuracy of recognition of the right ventricular hypertrophy and dilatation on the basis of decartograms. Further testing investigations will be carried out to reliably verify the informativity of the statistical classifications method used.

5. Conclusion

Statistical topographic templates obtained for the norm, right ventricular hypertrophy and dilatation as well as the voting method used allow us to formulate new diagnostical parameters, namely the closeness of the particular patient's decartogram to the statistical templates of the norm and different patologic cases. These templates and parameters can be efficienty used for computer processing of the cardioelectric signals in medical diagnostics.

References

1. L.I.Titomir, I.Ruttkay-Nedecky, Intern. J. Biomed. Comput. 20, 275 (1987)
2. L.I.Titomir et al., in Model Based Biomeasurements, eds. P.Kneppo, M.Tysler (Inst.Meas.Sci., SAS, Bratislava, 1995).
3. I.Ruttkay-Nedecky in Simulation of Systems in Biology and Medicine (Proc. Intern. Symp. Microfishes. Prague, E11–F01, 1988).
4. D.Durrer et al., Circulation 41, 899 (1970).
5. L.Bacharova, Atlas of Clinical Vectorcardiography (Kabel Publishers, Rockvill, 1993).

ASSESSMENT OF MYOCARDIAL VIABILITY WITH ELECTROCARDIOGRAPHIC ST-SEGMENT CHANGES INDUCED BY LOW-LEVEL EXERCISE

TAKUYA WATANABE, MD, YASUSHI AKUTSU, MD,
TAKASHI KATAGIRI, MD, TETUO MICHIHATA, MD*
*Third Department of Internal Medicine and *First Department of Surgery, Showa University School of Medicine, 1-5-8 Hatanodai, Shinagawa-ku, Tokyo 142, Japan*

OSAMU OKAZAKI, MD
Nora Eccles Harrison CVRTI, University of Utah, Salt Lake City, UT 84112, USA

KENICHI HARUMI, MD, FACC
Devision of Cardiology, Showa University Fujigaoka Hospital, 1-30 Fujigaoka, Midori-ku, Yokohama 227, Japan

We investigated whether the recovery of regional myocardial blood flow (RMBF) and left ventricular function after revascularization could be predicted preoperatively by low-level exercise-induced ST-segment changes. RMBF and cardiac output were measured with nitrogen-13 ammonia positron emission tomography at rest and during supine bicycle exercise (25 W for 6.5 min; 3 to 4 METS) in 28 of 72 consecutive patients with angiographically proven coronary artery disease before and after revascularization and in 9 healthy volunteers. Slowly upsloping, horizontal, or downsloping ST-segment depression of < 2 mm induced by low-level exercise may be a preoperative predictor of viable myocardium, whereas downsloping depression of ≧ 2 mm may be a predictor of severely impaired myocardium without visible collateral circulation.

INTRODUCTION

Identification of ischemic but viable myocardium is important in patients with coronary artery disease (CAD) who are candidates for revascularization. The aim of the present study was to evaluate whether low-level exercise-induced ST-segment depression can be used to predict preoperatively the recovery of myocardial ischemia and left ventricular (LV) dysfunction, as assessed by measurements of regional myocardial blood flow (RMBF) and cardiac output by simultaneous nitrogen-13 ammonia positron emission tomography (PET), after revascularization.

METHODS

Address for correspondence: Takuya Watanabe, MD, The Third Department of Internal Medicine, Showa University School of Medicine, 1-5-8 Hatanodai, Sinagawa-ku, Tokyo 142, Japan.

Subjects. Seventy-two consecutive patients with angiographically proven CAD (34 with angina pectoris and 38 with prior myocardial infarction) and without ST-segment abnormalities on resting ECG[a] underwent the PET study 1 week before revascularization. Of the 72 patients, 28 underwent the follow-up PET study 6 months after revascularization. Nine healthy volunteers underwent the control PET study. Informed consent was obtained from all patients and volunteers.

Coronary Angiography. Coronary angiography was performed whithin 1 week before the PET study. Coronary artery stenosis of ≧ 75% was defined as significant.[1] Collateral circulation was graded from 0 to 3 on the basis of collateral filling.[2]

ECG Exercise Testing in PET Study. A supine bicycle ergometer exercise at a fixed workload of 25 W continued for 6.5 minutes (total workload: 3 to 4 METS[b]) until severe chest pain, severe dyspnea, or serious arrhythmias developed.

ST-segment changes were evaluated in the 12-lead ECG with maximal ST-segment depression after 5 minutes of exercise. ST-segment depression was measured from the isoelectric PR-segment at 80 msec after the J-point.[3]

PET Study. The RMBF was measured by nitrogen-13 ammonia PET both at rest and after 5 minutes of supine bicycle exercise with previously described methods.[4] The LV wall was divided into 11 regions of interest and RMBF of each region was quantified from the radioactivity in heart tissue and arterial blood. Ischemic areas were defined in both patients with angina pectoris and patients with prior myocardial infarction as regions that showed an increase in RMBF of ≦ 10% (2 SD below the mean value [%] of healthy volunteers) with exercise in the territory of stenotic coronary arteries or as regions shown by abnormal Q waves on ECG to be infarcted.[4] Cardiac output was measured with the nitrogen-13 ammonia dilution method during the PET study.[4]

Statistical Analysis. Continuous variables are expressed as mean value ± SD and were compared by the Student's *t*-test between two groups and by the ANOVA among more than two groups. Categorical data were compared by the chi-square test. A p-value < 0.05 was considered statistically significant.

RESULTS

Patient Characteristics. In the PET study before revascularization, low-level exercise induced slowly upsloping ST-segment depression of 0.5 ≦ and < 1 mm in 45 patients (group A), horizontal or downsloping depression of 1 ≦ and < 2 mm in 19 patients (group B), and downsloping depression of ≧ 2 mm in 8 patients (group C) (Table 1). Age, the prevalence of prior myocardial infarction, and peak rate-pressure products during exercise did not differ significantly among the three groups. Multivessel disease was most frequent in group C and collateral circulation (grade 1

---

[a]ECG: electrocardiogram, electrocardiographic; [b]METS: metabolic equivalents.

Table 1: Baseline Characteristics of the Three Patient Groups.

	Group A (n = 45)	Group B (n = 19)	Group C (n = 8)
Demographic			
Age (yrs)	62.6 ± 7.3	64.4 ± 7.6	64.4 ± 6.7
Male	33 (73%)	14 (74%)	7 (88%)
Diagnosis			
Angina pectoris	24 (53%)	8 (42%)	3 (47%)
Prior myocardial infarction	21 (47%)	11 (58%)	5 (63%)
Coronary artery disease			
Multivessel disease	21 (47%)	11 (58%)	7 (88%)*
Collateral circulation	1 (2%)	10 (53%) †	1 (13%)
Low-level exercise			
Peak rate-pressure products (beats/min · mmHg)	14339 ± 3296	15274 ± 3182	15975 ± 2862

*$p < 0.05$ versus group A; † $p < 0.001$ versus group A.

to 3) was most frequent in group B.

The PET study after revascularization was performed in 11 of the 45 patients in group A, 12 of the 19 patients in group B, and 5 of the 8 patients in group C.

RMBF. Before revascularization, RMBF in ischemic areas at rest was similar in group C and groups A and B (46 vs. 49 and 50 mL, both p = NS) but was significantly lower in group C than in groups A and B (59 vs. 70 and 68 mL, both $p < 0.001$) during exercise. Figure 1 shows ischemic areas and changes in RMBF with low-level exercise. Ischemic areas were significantly larger in group C than in groups A and B. The RMBF increased with exercise in all regions (77 to 120 mL, 56%) in healthy volunteers. In group A, RMBF increased in both ischemic areas (31%) and surrounding areas (41%). In group B, RMBF increased insufficiently in ischemic areas (20%) and increased in surrounding areas (42%). In group C, RMBF increased still insufficiently in ischemic areas (17%) and increased in surrounding areas (41%).

After revascularization, RMBF in ischemic areas at rest improved significantly in groups A and B ($p < 0.05$, $p < 0.001$) but did not improve significantly in group C (Figure 2), and was significantly lower in group C than in groups A and B ($p < 0.05$, $p < 0.02$).

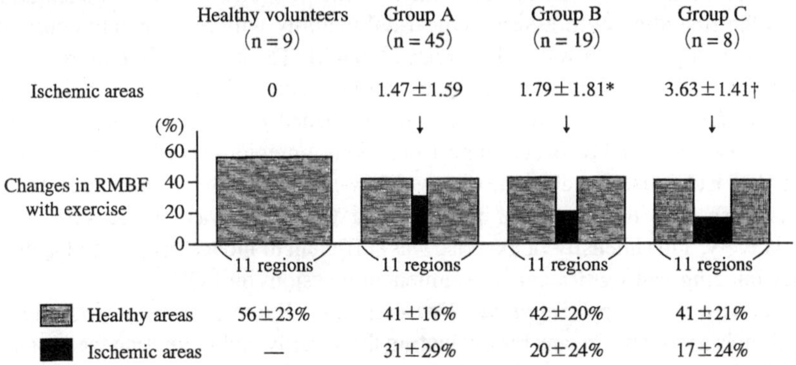

Figure 1: Ischemic areas and changes in RMBF with preoperative low-level exercise.
* $p < 0.05$ versus group A, † $p < 0.01$ versus group A.

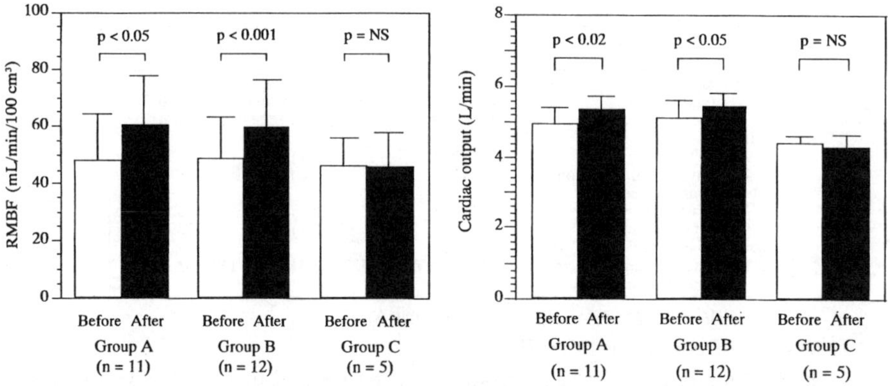

Figure 2: Recovery of RMBF in ischemic areas at rest and cardiac output at rest after revascularization.

LV Function. Before revascularization, cardiac output at rest was significantly lower in group C than in healthy volunteers (6.1 L/min) and groups A and B (each $p < 0.01$). After revascularization, cardiac output at rest improved significantly in groups A and B ($p < 0.02$, $p < 0.05$) but did not improve significantly in group C (Figure 2), and remained significantly lower in group C than in groups A and B (both $p < 0.05$).

DISCUSSION

Fluorine-18 fluorodeoxyglucose PET is an accepted standard with high diagnostic accuracy for identifying ischemic but viable myocardium.[5] As ECG exercise testing is now widely performed, its use in detecting myocardial viability has become attractive from both clinical and economic points of view. To our knowledge, this study is the first attempt to assess myocardial viability with ST-segment depression induced by preoperative low-level exercise (3 to 4 METS) by verifying improvements in RMBF and LV function as measured by simultaneous PET after revascularization.

Low-Level Exercise. According to recently published AHA/ACC guidelines,[1] low-level exercise (< 4 METS, Bruce stage 1 or less) is a precious standard for evaluating myocardial ischemia. In addition, we used low-level exercise in this study for two reasons. One was the safety of patients, and the other was to measure RMBF quantitatively. This intensity of exercise was sufficient to induce myocardial ischemia on PET imaging and significant ST-segment depressions on ECG.[4]

Significance of ST-Segment Depression. Exercise-induced ST-segment depression is a valuable means for evaluating the severity and predicting the prognosis of CAD. Goldschlager et al.[6] showed that the type of exercise-induced ST-segment depressions is related to the severity of CAD. Downsloping ST-segment depression suggests multivessel disease. Weiner et al.[7] reported that downsloping or ≧ 2 mm ST-segment depression indicates a higher frequency of adverse cardiac events and higher cardiac mortarity than do other types of ST-segment depression. In this study, exercise-induced slowly upsloping ST-segment depression of < 1 mm, horizontal or downsloping depression of 1 to 2 mm, and downsloping depression of ≧ 2 mm may indicate slight, moderate, and severe CAD and myocardial ischemia, respectively. Downsloping ST-segment depression of ≧ 2 mm was associated with severe ischemia in extensive myocardium in the territory of multivessel disease without visible collateral circulation.

Nonviable Myocardium. A lack of improvement in RMBF in ischemic areas after revascularization may be associated with less increase of RMBF in extensive ischemic areas with preoperative exercise. The RMBF in ischemic areas did not increase sufficiently with postoperative exercise only in group C, although sites of revascularization were proven to remain patent on follw-up angiography in all three groups. Possibly, myocardial oxygen consumption in ischemic areas did not increase with exercise despite the potential for supply of coronary flow with successful revascularization only in group C. Ischemic areas in group C patients may be irreversible myocardium that remains severely impaired after revascularization.

Conclusions. Our findings suggest that slowly upsloping ST-segment depression of < 1 mm and horizontal or downsloping depression of 1 to 2 mm induced by preoperative low-level exercise could predict the reversible myocardium of RMBF and LV dysfunction, whereas downsloping depression of ≧ 2 mm could predict the irreversible myocardium of RMBF and LV dysfunction after revascularization. Exercise-induced ST-segment changes are the hallmark in the assessment of myocardial viability in patients with severe CAD.

REFERENCES

1. Ryan TJ, et al. *Circulation* **88**, 2987 (1993).
2. Cohen M and Rentrop KP. *Circulation* **74**, 469 (1986).
3. Fletcher GF, et al. *Circulation* **91**, 580 (1995).
4. Watanabe T, et al. *Jpn Heart J* **38**, 207 (1997).
5. Baer FM, et al. *J Am Coll Cardiol* **28**, 60 (1996).
6. Goldschlager N, et al. *Ann Intern Med* **85**, 277 (1976).
7. Weiner DA, et al *Am Heart J* **105**, 749 (1983).

REVERSIBLE DECREASE OF DEPTH OF Q-WAVES FROM PREVIOUS INFARCTION DURING EXERCISE TESTING DUE TO MYOCARDIAL ISCHEMIA OF THE AREA OPPOSITE TO THE NECROSIS: A NEW DIAGNOSTIC INDEX OF ISCHEMIA

J.E. MADIAS, V. SINGH, C. TZIROS
Mount Sinai School of Medicine, New York, NY

An interaction of the scar from a previous myocardial infarction with transient myocardial ischemia of the contralateral to the necrosis heart territory can occur during exercise testing; this can lead to temporary reduction of the amplitude of Q-waves of the infarction. In 97 patients without ischemia of the contralateral to the infarct area the sum of Q-waves in mm were 21.7±12.3 and 22.4±12.5 at rest and peak exercise, respectively, (P=NS), while in 56 patients with such ischemia the sums of Q-waves were 27.3±15.5 at rest and 17.5±11.7 at peak exercise, respectively, (P<0.0005). Thus, exercise-induced ischemia in a cardiac region opposite a necrotic territory, reduces transiently the depth of infarctional Q-waves.

About 1 million patients survive an acute myocardial infarction (MI) each year in the USA. A sizeable proportion of this group is subjected to exercise testing (ET) to detect associated reversible ischemia, for risk stratification or preparation for revascularization. The low sensitivity of ET in patients with evidence of MI in the resting ECG is widely recognized. ST-segment changes, even when present, cannot be attributed with certainty to ischemia, since often they are due to dyskinesis, or they are reciprocal in nature. The sensitivity and specificity of ET is enhanced by the simultaneous implementation of thallium myocardial scintigraphy. However this modality is less available and more costly than the ET. Thus, the perpetual interest in devising additional ECG indices of ischemia, beyond the ones based on the traditional ST-segment displacement.

As a background to our hypothesis, the following points should be considered:

1) Wilson's "window theory" proposed that the Q-waves in the ECG of a patient with an MI are due to an altered balance of electrical potentials, which point opposite to the territory of partial or wall-to-wall necrosis, and are generated by the noninfarcted myocardium.[1,2] Consequently, transient ischemic compromise of this region could theoretically render it partially or totally, incapable in generating Q-waves.

2) The Q-waves of an old MI occasionally are reduced in amplitude, or disappear

when a new MI occurs in the myocardial region opposite the original necrosis.[3] This constitutes a scar-to-scar interaction leading to a "Q-wave counterpoise".

3) We have recently described a phenomenon dubbed "ischemic ST-segment counterpoise," which is characterized by the occurrence of a falsely negative exercise ECG in the presence of unequivocal myocardial ischemia involving heart territories opposite each other, as diagnosed by SPECT ^{201}Tl myocardial perfusion scintigraphy. The postulated mechanism in this occurrence was a cancellation of ischemic ST-segment vectors of equal magnitude and direction, but opposite sense, generated by the transiently ischemic regions facing each other.[4-6]

4) There is literature supporting the view that Q-waves are not only indicative of necrosis, but occasionally such changes occur transiently, and reflect ischemia in a myocardial territory, like for example in the course of attacks of unstable or Prinzmetal's angina.[7,8] Thus, transient ischemia can lead to temporary QRS alterations.

5) It has been previously shown that "new" Q-waves after aortocoronary bypass surgery are not always due to peri-operative MIs, but occasionally derive from unmasking of an old myocardial scar due to the improvement of myocardial blood flow, of the contralateral region to the old MI,[9] as a result of the revascularization procedure. We thought that the reverse could also be true, that is, disappearance of Q-waves due to contralateral to the MI transient ischemia.

6) Recently, we described another phenomenon, that , of the interaction of a scar from an old MI with transient ischemia in the contralateral to the MI myocardial region ("scar-ischemia counterpoise").[10] Accordingly, in a patient with MI and contralateral reversible ischemia, Q-waves disappeared transiently during ET ; in contrast, in a patient without ischemia in the opposite to the MI region, no such changes occured in the Q-waves of the ECG.

Based on the above experience, we postulated that stable Q-waves from a previous MI, either recent or old, might be modulated (decrease in amplitude, or even disappear) when transient myocardial ischemia of the contralateral heart territory occurs in the setting of ET.

To study this, 153 patients with history and ECG evidence of previous Q-wave MI, involving either the anterior or inferior walls of the heart, were subjected to exercise treadmill testing, in conjunction with ^{201}Tl myocardial perfusion scintigraphy.

SPECT analysis of the ^{201}Tl myocardial scintigrams was implemented to evaluate for the presence of fixed defects due to the myocardial scar, and regions of reversible myocardial ischemia; if the resting scintigram did not provide satisfactory differentiation between these two elements, radionuclide reinjection was employed. The patients were subgrouped to those with and without exercise-induced transient ischemia in the contralateral to the infarction myocardial territory.

Measurements of the infarcional Q-waves in mm were carried out using the ECGs, as derived from the conventional Mason-Likar electrode "hook-up;" the sums of the Q-waves from the resting, and peak exercise ECGs were calculated, and the percent change of these two measurements was derived.

Finally, the changes in the sums of Q-waves in the two subgroups of patients described above were compared.

Table 1

RESULTS

	N	ΣQR(in mm)	ΣQP(in mm)	%ΔΣQ
-OR	97	$21.7 \pm 12.3^{a,c}$	$22.4 \pm 12.5^{e,c}$	$+7.3 \pm 22.1^{b}$
+OR	56	$27.3 \pm 15.5^{a,d}$	$17.5 \pm 11.7^{e,d}$	-37.4 ± 18.7^{b}

a,c,e=P>0.05; b,d=P<0.0005

-OR=no ischemia in the contralateral to the infarction region; +OR= ischemia in the contralateral to the infarction region; ΣQR=sum of Q-waves at restΣQP=sum of Q-waves at peak exercise; %ΔΣQ=% change between ΣQR and ΣQP. "scar-ischemia counterpoise"

The results are shown on Table 1. Sums of Q-waves of patients without reversible ischemia in the contralateral to the MI territory remained stable between rest and peak exercise, while there was a reduction of this parameter by 37% at peak exercise in comparison with the measurements at rest in the patients with reversible ischemia in the opposite to the MI area.

It is of paramount importance to expand the ECG indices of ischemia, beyond the traditionally employed ST-segment deviations, in order to enhance the sensitivity and specificity of exercise ECG in the detection of myocardial ischemia. Analysis of exercise ECG in the presence of Q-waves due to previous MI is problematic, leading the investigator to avoid selecting such cases for his/her studies, and making the clinitian uneasy about the correctness of his/her interpretation; thus, implementation of the proposed ECG ischemic index for the large group of patients with prior MI undergoing exercise testing has enormous clinical implications.

We conclude that transient reduction in the depth of Q-waves during exercise treadmill testing constitutes a novel ECG indicator of reversible ischemia of the contralateral to the scar heart territory. It is postulated that the mechanism for this phenomenon is a form of "electrical stunning" of the ischemic region, which, by becoming partially incapacitated during exercise, cannot generate depolarization forces of the magnitude attained at rest.

References

1) Wilson Fa, Hill IG, Johnson FD: Am Heart J 10:903, 1935.
2) Wilson FN, Johnson FD, Hill IG: Am Heart J 10:1025, 1935.
3) Saikawa T, Abe M, Nakagawa M, et al: Jap Heart J 28:805, 1987.
4) Madias JE, Sheth K: Am J Noninvas Cardiol 8:194, 1994.
5) Madias JE, Mahjoub M, Valance J: J Electrocardiol 29:243, 1996.
6) Madias JE, Khan M, Manyam B: Clin Cardiol 20:489, 1997.
7) Haiat R, Chiche P: Chest 65:140, 1974.
8) Madias JE: Chest 82:279, 1982.
9) Basan MM, Oatfield R, Hoffman I, et al: N Eng J Med 290:349, 1974.
10) Madias JE, Manyam B, Khan M, Singh V, Tziros C: J Electrocardiol 30:97, 1997.

DIAGNOSTIC EFFICACY OF SEISMOCARDIOGRAPHY AND ELECTROCARDIOGRAPHY FOR THE DIAGNOSIS OF CORONARY ARTERY DISEASE DURING VELOERGOMETRIC TEST

L.GARGASAS, A.VAINORAS, G.JARUSEVICIUS
Institute of Cardiology, Kaunas Medical Academy,Sukileliu 17, Kaunas, Lithuania
E-mail: vytmi@kma.lt

The purpose of this study was to compare diagnostic accuracy of two methods-electrocardiography and seismocardiography for diagnosis of coronary artery disease. The results of study permit to conclude that seismocardiography is more sensitive method for coronary artery disease detection.

1.Introduction

Exercise electrocardiogram (ECG) is most available noninvasive test for coronary artery disease (CAD) detection but has a relatively low sensitivity (about 60%) especially for CAD in its early stages [1,2] Seismocardiography is noninvasive method for recording cardiac vibratory activity as a measure of cardiac contractile performance [3]. Seismocardiographic device detects and provides registration of low-frequency cardiac vibrations on the chest wall during ventricular contraction and during both early and late ventricular filling [4]. Seismocardiography is not a new method, was developed in the 1960s [5], but considerable technological advancements created conditions for development of modern seismocardiographic devices including improved ultrasensitive piezoelectric accelerometer, analogy-digital conversion, a microprocessor for digital signal-processing and automated wave analysis, neural network method is used for computerized interpretation [3,4]. Multicenter clinical trials revealed the seismocardiogram (SCG) being an informative and useful test for CAD detection, furthermore, SCG effectively complemented exercise ECG [1,3,4,6-9]. Therefore a modern seismocardiograph and software for computerized SCG analysis have been made in our institution [10]. The computerized ECG computer analysis system Kaunas have been developed ten years ago. The purpose of this study was to evaluate the accuracy of exercise SCG and compare it with accuracy of exercise ECG for early recognition of coronary artery disease.

ECGs and impedance cardiograms were obtained at rest in supine and upright position during veloergometric test at the moments of submaximal load, cessation of test and at three moments of the recovery period in supine position - immediately after load, two and six minutes after cessation of load. SCGs were obtained at resting in a supine position and at three above-mentioned moments of the recovery period. ECG was defined by program as abnormal when a horizontal or downsloping ST depression more than 0.1 mV has been detected in any lead. In the resting and postexercise SCG two criteria - systolic and diastolic have been estimated [6]: systolic criteria

$((AO\text{-}IM/IM\text{-}MC)_{Load} < (AO\text{-}IM/IM\text{-}MC)_{Rest})$ and $(AO\text{-}IM)_{Load} < (AO\text{-}IM)_{Rest}$;

diastolic criteria $(RF)_{Load} > (1{,}2RF)_{Rest}$

AO-IM and IM-MC are distance between points and RF is amplitude of RF wave (Figure 1.)

The developed system have been used for analysis of exercise ECG and postexercise SCG of 73 healthy persons and 46 patients with angiographycaly CAD but without myocardial infarction. Since this study have additional purpose to assess diagnostic accuracy of SCG for the diagnosis of preinfarctional stages of CAD, for all selected 46 patients coronary artery narrowing was less that 70%.

3.Results and discussion

Sensitivity, specificity and diagnostic efficacy of ECG and SCG criteria for CAD detection are listed in Table 1.

Table 1: Exercise electrocardiogram and seismocardiogram for detection of CAD

Criteria	Sensitivity %	Specificity %	Diagnostic efficacy %
ECG ST changes	48	89	73
SCG systolic parameter	59	89	76
SCG diastolic parameter	77	90	85
SCG systolic and diastolic parameters	87	89	88

In Figure 2 the sample of ECG and SCG changes of healthy person before exercise (a) immediately after exercise (b) and patient with CAD - c and d respectively. In this study cohort the sensitivity of ECG criterion was relatively low. It may be due inability to reach submaximal load and target heart rate in the

2.Methods and materials

The hardware of SCG computer analysis system is composed of a low-frequency accelerometer of piezoelectric type with linear response 0.5 - 600 Hz, sensitivity 0,9 V/g (g = 9,8 m/s^2), weight - 1 kg, an analog - digital converter (sample rate 500 samples/second). It is necessary to stress, that device for SCG registration and input into PC is not a separate equipment but part of the cardiosignals computer analysis system including 12 lead ECG, impedance cardiogram and, finally, SCG. It can be seen that such complex of the signals creates possibility to analyse the electric, hemodinamic and mechanical properties of the cardiac activity. Moreover, the synchronous registration of these signals enables more precise recognise the waves and characteristic points of signals by the way seismocardiogram (Figure 1).

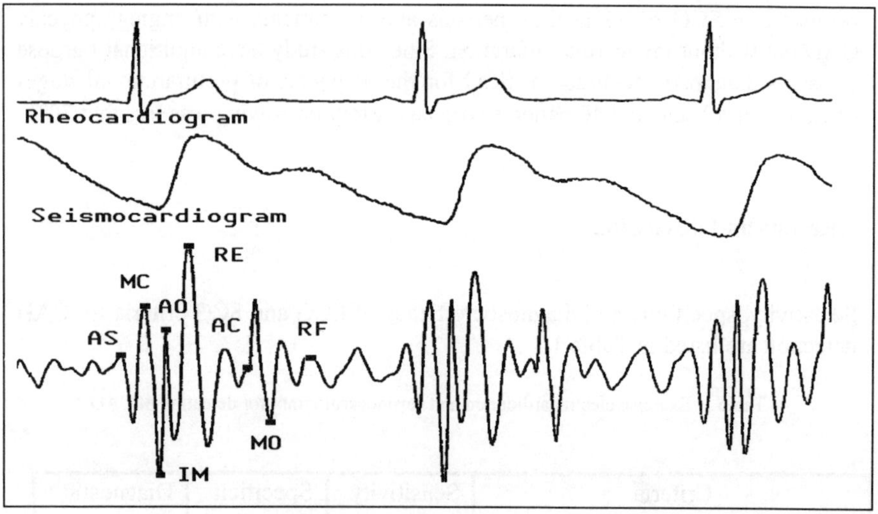

Figure 1: Simultaneous ECG, impedance cardiogram and SCG recordings and characteristic points of seismocardiogram (explanations in text).

According to methodology, proposed by D.M.Salerno and co-workers [4], the following waves and points are recognised and measured for SCG computerized interpretation: in the systolic interval - mitral valve closure (MC), aortic valve opening (AO), onset of rapid ejection in the left ventricular outflow tract (RE), peak velocity of flow in left ventricular outflow tract (PE), aortic valve closure (AC); in the diastolic interval - mitral valve opening (MO),peak velocity of transmitral flow in early diastole (RF), peak velocity of transmitral flow due to atrial systole (AS).

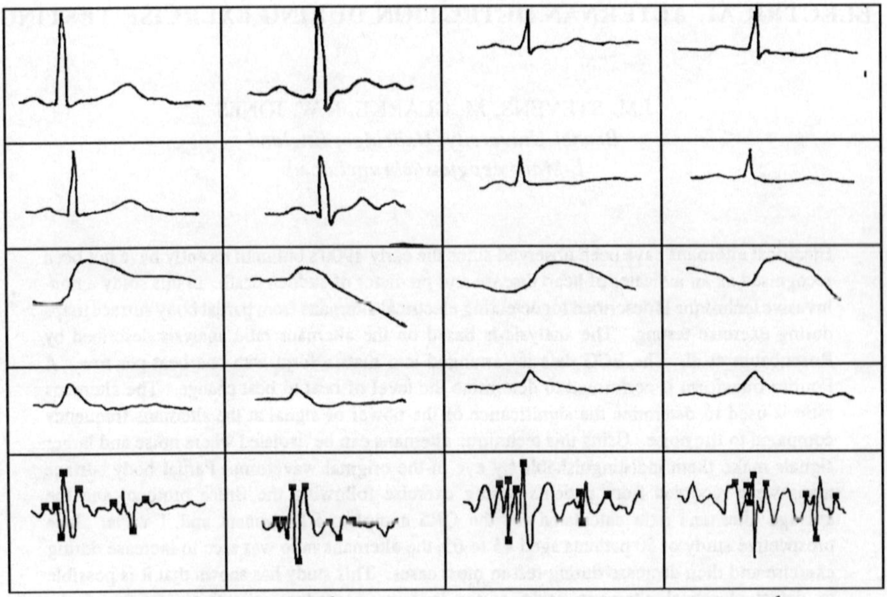

Figure 2. Veloergometric test results of healthy person J.G., 28 yrs, male (a,b) and patient S.A., 48 yrs, male with CAD (c,d).

one third part of patients with CAD. In addition as mentioned above all tested patients have moderate luminal diameter stenosis on angiography. Our results well coincide with results of investigation, performed by R.A.Wilson and coworkers [1].

In conclusion, the most sensitive criterion of CAD in this study was diastolic parameter of SCG which is based on the amplitude or area under the rapid diastolic filling wave. Increase of this amplitude in the postexercise SCG by 20% or more is a valuable indicator of myocardial ischemia and CAD.

References

1. R.A.Wilson et al, Am.J.Cardiol.D 71,536(1993)
2. R.Gianrossi et al, Circulation D80, 87(1989)
3. D.M.Salerno and J.Zanetti, J.Cardiovasc. Technol. D9,111(1990)
4. D.M.Salerno et al. Am.J.Cardiol. D68,201(1991)
5. R.M.Bayevsky et al, Cardiologia, D4, 87(1964)
6. D.M.Salerno et al, Am.J.Noninvaz.Cardiol.D6, 321(1992)
7. D.M.Salerno and J.Zanetti,Chest,D100,991(1991)
8. D.W.Crook et al, Cardiol. Elder., D2,401(1994)
9. R.S.Crow et al, Am.J.Noninvas.Cardiol., D8,39(1994)
10. L.Gargasas et al, Med.Biol.Engineer.Comput.,D34, Suppl.1, Part 1,401(1996)

ELECTRICAL ALTERNAN DETECTION DURING EXERCISE TESTING

J.M. STEVENS, M. CLARKE, R.W. JONES
Brunel University, Uxbridge, England
E-Mail: eepgjms@brunel.ac.uk

Electrical alternans have been observed since the early 1900's but until recently have not been recognised as an indicator of heart disease and predictor of sudden death. In this study a non-invasive technique is described for detecting electrical alternans from partial body surface maps during exercise testing. The analysis is based on the alternans ratio analysis described by Rosenbaum et al. The ECG data is arranged into matrix form with one beat per row. A Fourier transform is performed to determine the level of beat to beat change. The alternans ratio is used to determine the significance of the power of signal at the alternans frequency compared to the noise. Using this technique alternans can be isolated where noise and larger signals make them indistinguishable by eye in the original waveform. Partial body surface maps were recorded from patients during exercise following the Bruce protocol and the average alternans ratio calculated for the QRS-complex, ST segment and T-wave. In a prospective study of 50 patients aged 45 to 65, the alternans ratio was seen to increase during exercise and then decrease during rest in most cases. This study has shown that it is possible to detect electrical alternans using a non-invasive procedure, allowing a study of the phenomenon on the general population.

1 Introduction

The presence of electrical alternans was first noticed in the early 1900's but for a great many years they were seen as having no clinical significance. In more recent times, however, electrical alternans in electrocardiograms have been suggested as an indicator of ischaemia and a precursor to sudden cardiac death[1,2]. The lack of interest in electrical alternans could be due to the rarity of alternans that are large enough to be seen over noise and the normal ECG signal. Also, these visible alternans only manifest themselves after more obvious symptoms have come to light. However, modern signal processing techniques make it possible to detect electrical alternans of a much smaller magnitude, possibly before other symptoms are present[2,3].

1.1 Alternans Mechanism

The cause of electrical alternans is not fully understood, but it is suggested that poor perfusion of the cardiovascular system causes delayed repolarisation of the myocardium. This manifests itself as a 'weak' beat when the myocardium has not recovered sufficiently for a normal beat. This being the case we would expect to see an increase in alternans associated with an increase in the heart rate as the time for repolarisation is shorter and the heart is being worked harder.

1.2 Alternans Measurement

This beat to beat variation manifests itself as a variation in the amplitude of the electrocardiogram. The alternans are mostly small in magnitude, therefore signal processing is used to distinguish them from noise. The earliest measurements were made using the invasive technique of atrial pacing to elevate the heart rate to induce electrical alternans in patients deemed vulnerable to ventricular arrhythmias[2]. The work shows early detection of electrical alternans could be used to diagnose cardiac disease before other (potentially dangerous) arrhythmias occur. This study extends this work by showing that low-level electrical alternans can be detected with surface ECG measurement using exercise testing.

2 Methods

2.1 Data Source

Precordial body surface map data recorded from 50 patients aged 45-65 was used for the study. A full clinical history was available for each patient as all were involved in a long term prospective cardiological trial. Recordings were made at rest and then at increasing loads on a treadmill following the Bruce protocol. Further recordings were during the recovery period.

2.2 The Alternans Analysis technique

ECG data is arranged into matrix form with one beat per row and the power spectrum found of the beat to beat signal (the columns). The mean spectrum is found for the QRS, ST and T segments of the ECG. Since the alternans manifests itself as a beat to beat variation, we would expect a strong component at 0.5 cycles/beat (see for Figure 2 for a typical spectrum). The alternans ratio is used to enhance the measure, by determining by how much the alternans frequency power differs from the general noise. The alternans ratio is expressed as:

$$\textit{alternans ratio} = \frac{\textit{alternans peak} - \overline{\textit{noise}}}{\sigma_{noise} + 1} \qquad (1)$$

Where alternans peak is the value of the power spectrum at the alternans frequency and the noise is estimated over a pre-defined range of frequencies (noise window) well away from any expected signal components. To prevent the problem of very small σ_n, that may occur with small data sets, distorting the ratio unduly, we compensate by adding 1. The alternans ratio is calculated for the QRS-complex, ST-segment and T-wave.

3 Results

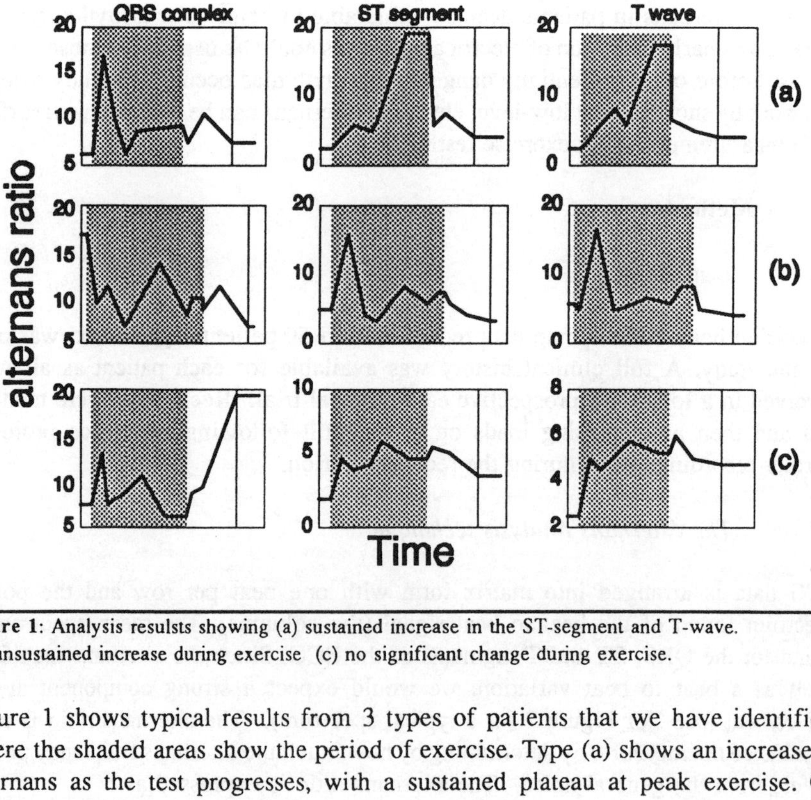

Figure 1: Analysis resulsts showing (a) sustained increase in the ST-segment and T-wave. (b) unsustained increase during exercise (c) no significant change during exercise.

Figure 1 shows typical results from 3 types of patients that we have identified, where the shaded areas show the period of exercise. Type (a) shows an increase in alternans as the test progresses, with a sustained plateau at peak exercise. On termination of exercise the alternans decreases towards its rest value. In this example the effect is most pronounced in the ST and T segments, though it has occasionally been seen in the QRS segment. We identify this as a positive test. Type (b) shows some variation in alternans ratio during exercise, but there is no sustained elevation. We identify this as an inconclusive test. Type (c) shows no significant change during exercise. We identify this as a negative test.

Of the 50 patients analysed, 40 were type a, 5 were type b and 4 were type c.

One patient was subsequently excluded with insufficient exercise to give a conclusive result. Unfortunately the clinical diagnoses were not available in time to allow sensitivity and specificity to be determined. These will be reported in a subsequent paper.

4 Discussion

The study has shown that a signal matching the expected characteristics of electrical alternans is detected during exercise using surface ECG measurements. The signal is not attributable to muscle noise as we would expect its value to fall more quickly at the end of exercise. Nor is the signal due to breathing, as this gives a prominent component at 0.2 cycles/beat, well below the alternans frequency.

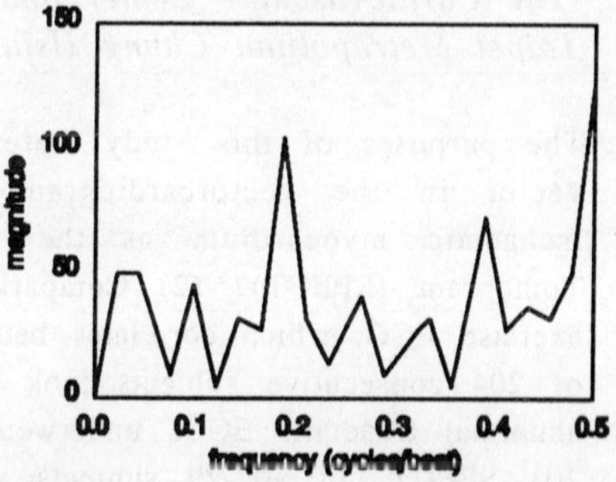

Figure 2: A sample power spectrum for the ST segment

5 Conclusion

This study shows electrical alternans can be detected by surface ECG measurement during exercise testing. This would allow measurements to be made on the general population permitting a wider study on the sensitivity and specificity of alternans as a predictor of cardiac events and giving promise as a clinical investigative tool.

Acknowledgements

The authors wish to thank EPSRC for the funding of this research.

References

1 E.A. Reader, et al. 'Notes upon alternation of the heart', *N Engl J Med*, Vol. 326, p271-2 (1992)

2 D.S. Rosenbaum, et al. 'Electrical alternans and vulnerability to ventricular arrhythmias', *N Engl J Med*, Vol. 330, p235-41 (1994)

3 W. Zareba, et al. 'Automatic Detection of Spatial and Dynamic Heterogeneity of Repolarization', *J Electrocardiol*, Vol. 27S, p66-72 (1994)

EXERCISE VECTORCARDIOGRAM OR TREADMILL EXERCISE ELECTROCARDIOGRAM VERSUS THALIUM-201 SINGLE-PHOTON EMISSION COMPUTED TOMOGRAM IN THE DIAGNOSIS OF MYOCARDIAL ISCHAEMIA.

W. CARSON, Y.K., CHEN*, C.Y. CHENG

The Cardiovascular Center and Nuclear Medicine Department, Taipei Metropolitan Chung Hsin Hospital, Taipei, Taiwan, R.O.C.*

The purposes of this study were: (1) Can the maximal spatial ST vector in the vectorcardiogram (VCG) indicate location of the ischaemic myocardium as the Single-Photon Emission Computed Tomogram (SPECT)? (2) Comparing the exercise VCG or treadmill exercise ECG, which correlates better with the SPECT results? A total of 204 consecutive subjects took a routine physical checkup, 42 had abnormal treadmill ECGs underwent exercise VCG and 180-degree Tl-201 SPECT. In all 29 subjects with the positive VCG and SPECT studies, the maximal spatial ST vector pointed to either the right-posterior-superior or the right-anterior-superior direction. However, all the positive SPECT images documented transmural myocardial ischaemia. VCG and treadmill ECG correlated with SPECT, the sensitivity was 97% and 93%, specificity was 67% and 25%, Kappa was 0.69 and 0.22, respectively. Therefore, the electrophysiological terminology of "subendocardium ischaemia" is misleading and suggested to be abandoned. Exercise VCG correlates better than a treadmill ECG with the SPECT results.

1 Introduction

There has been no report concerning exercise vectorcardiographic and single-photon emission computed tomographic study of myocardial ischaemia.

2 Methods

Two hundred and four consecutive subjects were admitted into two-and-half days physical checkup ward. Each subject performed a treadmill exercise test in a fasting state according to the standard Bruce protocol. Subjects with the abnormal treadmill exercise tests received further exercise VCG, and SPECT examinatios between four to six weeks later.

Each subjects received vectorcardiographic examinations as their baseline data.When they have reached target heart rate, fatigue, or chest pain during the treadmill exercise tests, Tl-201 isotope had been given. The second VCGs had been recorded. (A positive exercise vectorcardiographic examination had abnormal ST vector (0.1 mV in at least two planes in patients without ventricular enlargement. In patient with ventricular enlargement, additional changes in the morphology or in the direction of insciption of T loop in at lcast onc planc, was classified as a positive test.) Thereafter, the subjects had been transfered to the r-camera room. Single-photon emission computed tomographic perfusion pictures were recorded in five minutes after exercise, which was followed by reperfusion imaging four hours later. Tomograms obtained from reperfusion served as individual subjects` own control for determining ischaemic myocardium (photon-deficient area presented in perfusion images but which disappeared in the reperfusion images).

3 Results

Forty-two subjects had abnormal treadmill exercise ECGs received further VCG and SPECT examinations. They were 28 men and 14 women. Age ranged between 35 and 74 years (mean 55.02 (10.63). Duration of exercise time between treadmill ECG and exercise VCG was no significant difference. However, the peak heart rate of treadmill ECG was faster that exercise VCG and P = 0.0028. Further, the Fisher`s Exact test value was 0.491 revealed no gender difference of the SPECT results. VCG correlated with SPECT the sensitivity was (29/1+29) 97%, specificity was (8/4+8) 67%, Kappa value 0.69. Treadmill ECG correlated with SPECT the sensitivity was (28/28+2) 93%, specificity (3/3+9) 25%, and Kappa value 0.22. Three among the four had septal myocardial ischaemia on SPECT images. Nearly half of the subjects (12/25 = 48%) the maximal spatial ST vector revealed posterior component. The SPECT did have posterior myocardial ischaemia. However, all subjects the maximal spatial ST vector showed superior component, the SPECT did revealed inferior myocardial ischaemia except one. Further, all 29 subjects the maximal spatial ST vector had right component. The SPECT revealed myocardial ischaemia in the left ventricle. However, all the positive SPECT images documented transmural myocardial ischaemia whereas the maximal spatial ST vector in the exercise VCG suggested electrical "subendocardium" myocardial injury.

4 Discussion

The results are quite disappointing when comparing treadmill ECG with SPECT results. The better correlation between VCG with SPECT results could be due because both methods are 3-dimensional, VCG has LS plane, and changed morphology or inscription direction of the T loop under chamber enlargement can only be identified by the VCG. Among 29 subjects with both positive VCG and SPECT examinations, four had the maximal spatial ST vector pointing at right-anterior-superior octant. Three among the four subjects had SPECT documented septal ichemia. This is similar to 11 of 13 patients with thallium-201 scintigraphy documented anteroseptal ischaemia after treadmill test[1], or one type of the maximal spatial ST vector in patients with acute anteroseptal myocardial infarction in the Coronary Care Unit[2]. Twenty-five subjects had the maximal spatial ST vector pointing to the right-posterior-superior octant. All of them had right component of the maximal spatial ST vector that the SPECT showed left ventricular ischaemia. Almost all superior components of the maximal spatial ST vector had the SPECT revealed inferior ischemia except one. However, the posterior component of the maximal spatial ST vector had either anterior or posterior myocardial ischaemia documented on the SPECT. According to the present electrophysiological concept that the maximal spatial ST vector pointed to the right-posterior-superior octant the anterior or apical ischaemia in the SPECT must be subendocardial ischaemia, the posterior ischaemia in the SPECT must be transmural. However, to our surprise that all SPECT suggested "transmural" myocardial ischaemia.

One study[3] indicated that "Considered purely on a mathematical basis it is very doubtful whether epicardial S-T depression is always reciprocal to a subendocardial injury current". Based on our data, the ST segment depression on the treadmill ECG indicating "subendocardial" ischaemia shall be abandoned. We dare to predict that the terminology will follow the fate of Q waves wrongly indicating "transmural" myocardial infarction and step into the history.

Acknowledgments

This research has been supported by a grant from the Taipei Institute of Pathology. We are grateful for Schmidt Scientific Company Taiwan Limited for kindly allowed us to use their Mac-8 machine.

References

S. Abouantoun, S. Ahnve, M. Savvides, K. Witztum, D. Jensen, V. Froelicher, *Am Heart J* **108**, 933 (1984)

W. Carson, Y.Z. Tseng, *Int J Cardiol* **43**, 165 (1994)

A. Ekmekci, H. Toyoshima, J.K. Kwoczynski, T. Nagaya, T.M. Prinzmetal, *Am J Cardiol* **7**, 412 (1961)

THE CLINICAL SIGNIFICANCE OF THE ABNORMALITY OF ST-T SEGMENT IN THE AMBULATORY ECG RECORDINGS AT REST.......COMPARISON WITH THE RESULTS OF STRESS ECG, ECHOCARDIOGRAPHY AND CORONARY ARTERIOGRAPHY

M.MORITA
Soma General Municipal Hospital, 142 Tubogasako, Soma City 976, Japan

We investigated the significance of ST-T segment abnormality of rest ECG, by comparing with the results of stress ECG, echocardiography and coronary arteriography. The presence of ST depression and T wave inversion at rest ECG correlated with the presence of LVH in ECG and echocardiography. In those who have ST<-0.10mV and/or T<-0,.5mV, they have LVH in ECG and the extent of ST depression correlated with LVPWTd and LV mass. The presence of ST depression and/or T wave inversion is the additional methods for the extent of left ventricular hypertrophy.

Background and Purpose

ECG recordings at rest may be the most easily and repeatedly obtainable noninvasive method for the diagnosis of heart disease, but the interpretation of ECG findings are not necessarily clear. The changes of ST-T segment is most widely obtainable in ambulatory ECG recordings, and has been reported to be the suggestion of LVH since the study of Sokolow and Lyon, although the significance of ST segment depression and/or T wave incversion is not completely clear.

In order to make clear this problem, we investigated the significance of ST segment depression and/or T wave inversion, by comparing the rest ECG with treadmill test, echocardiography and coronary arteriography.

Subjects and Methods

One thousand and eight hundred subjects who has undertaken ECG recordings at rest were cotinuously enrolled in this study. The mean age was 64±15 years old. The sex ratio for male to female was 2:3. In ECG, the presences of ST segment depression and/or T wave inversion and the lead which has ST-T changes were investigated. The presences of LVH was investigated by Sokolow-Lyon's method and Romhilt-Estes score.

Treadmill teat was performed for 249 subjects in order to investigate the presence of symptomatic and asymptomatic coronary artery disease, and the HR-ST loop analysis was used. In HR-ST loop, peak ΔST, the slope of the line connecting the point of ischemic threshold and maximal ST depression (line 1) ($\Delta ST/\Delta HR$)

and the the angle between the line 1 and the line connecting the maximal ST depression and 30 seconds at recovery period (line 2).

Echocardiography was performed for 370 subjects , and IVSTd, LVPWTd, LVDd and LV mass (Devereux and Reichek, 1977). In echocardiography, IVSTd>12.8 mm and LVPWTd>11.5 mm were determined as LVH.

Coronary arteriography was performed for 67 subjects, and the presence of over 90% stenosis of coronary artery was regarded as coronary artery disease.

Results

Ki-square analysis between STdepression and/or T wave inversion and LVH and CAD was shown in Table 1. The presence of ST depression was correlarted with LVH in UCG and LVH in echocardiography, and loosely correlated with left venticular dilatation. No correlations were found between the ST-T changes and the parameters in treadmill teats. The correlations were found between the presence of coronary artery disease in coronary arteriography, although not so much subjects has underwent coronary arteriography.

Correlation between STdepression and/or T wave inversion and LVH and CAD was shown in Table 2. The correlations between ST depression and LVH in ECG and UCG was found though these were very loose. Those between T wave inversion and LVH in ECG and UCG were also found although the correlations were very looser than those of ST depression.

$\chi 2$ With ST<-0.05 mV in Rest ECG	Frequency/Total		$\chi 2$ With T<-0.20 mV
ST<-0.05 mV	**318/1547(25%)**		**110/1555 (7.1%)**
LVH (Sokolow-Lyon)	**449/1743(26%)**	**$\chi 2$=20.9 (p<0.0001)**	$\chi 2$=1.27 (p=0.26)
LVH (Romhilt-Estes Score>5)	**78/395(20%)**	**$\chi 2$=25.3 (p<0.0001)**	**$\chi 2$=6.99 (p=0.008)**
LVH in UCG (IVSTd>12.8 mm)	**33/309 (11%)**	**$\chi 2$=8.0 (p=0.0046)**	$\chi 2$=0.24 (p=0.62)
LVH in UCG (PWTd>11.5 mm)	**170/370 (46%)**	**$\chi 2$=4.4 (p=0.037)**	$\chi 2$=0 (P>0.9999)
Treadmill Positive	**39/249 (16%)**	$\chi 2$=2.3 (p=0.13)	$\chi 2$=1.44 (p=0.23)
CAG Positive	**14/67(21%)**	**$\chi 2$=8.2 (p=0.0042)**	**$\chi 2$=6.1 (p=0.01)**
Sinus/af		**$\chi 2$=6.8 (p=0.033)**	**$\chi 2$=20.8 (p=0<0.0001)**

Table 1.

The comparison of the correlation of ST depression, T wave inversion and left ventricular mass[1] between the subjects who has LVH in ECG or not were shown in Figure 1. In the subjects who has deeper ST depression and T wave inversion have the tendency of showing LVH in Romhilt-Estes score. In those who has LVH in Romhilt-Estes Score, The amplitude of ST depression and/or T wave inversion well correlated with left ventricular mass.

The presence of ST segment depression and/or T waveinversion were also found in higher age.

	Correlation With Rest ΔST	Correlation With Rest ΔT
Treadmill		
PeakΔST(mV)	r=-0.26 (p=0.14)	r=-0.22 (p=0.47)
ΔST/ΔHR(μV/bpm)	r=0.18 (p=0.30)	r=0.05 (p=0.87)
Recovery Index (Degree)	r=-0.32 (p=0.15)	r=-0.64 (p=0.09)
ECG		
SV1+RV5 (mV)	**r=-0.35 (p<0.0001)**	**r=-0.18 (p<0.03)**
Romhilt-Estes Score	**r=-0.41 (p<0.0001)**	**r=-0.34(p<0.0001)**
UCG		
IVSTd (mm)	**r=-0.35 (p<0.0001)**	r=-0.04 (p=0.69)
PWTd (mm)	**r=-0.33 (p<0.0001)**	**r=-0.34(p=0.0004)**
LVDd (mm)	r=-0.02 (p=0.79)	r=-0.03 (p=0.74)
LV Mass(Gram)	**r=-0.33 (p<0.0001)**	r=-0.19 (p=0.08)
Age	**r=-0.24 (p<0.0001)**	r=-0.12 (p=0.27)
Heart Rate	r=-0.04 (p=0.55)	r=-0.03 (p=0.96)

Table 2.

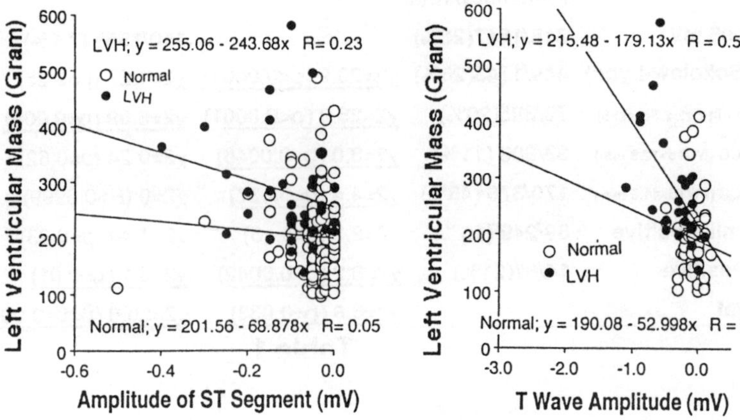

Figure 1.

Discussion

The presence of repolarization abnormality has been reported to be correlated with age and the severity of left ventricular hypertrophy, the ST segment depression and T wave inversion being deeper when they are advanced age and left ventricular hypertrophy[2]. The result of this study supports this result, although very few study have resulted about the amplitude of ST segment depression and the extent of LVH, the results of this study is useful because in especially younger population who has left ventricular hypertrophy, the amplitude of ST segment depression reflect the left ventricular hypertrphy.

On the contrary, the slight depression opf ST segment in who does not show left ventricular hypertrophy has been reported to be non-specific ST changes. The subjects who has slight ST-T changes have lower tendency of showing left ventricular hypertrophy and did not correlate with left ventricular mass. Nonetheless, the diagnosis of " nonspecific ST-T changes" should be made when correlated with echocardiography.

Conclusion

The presence of ST-T changes suggested that, the extent of ST-T changes reflect the extent of left ventricular hypertrophy. Presence of ST-T changes were not affected well with the presence of coronary artery disease in the clinical settings of screening.

In ST-T changes, the higher the extent of left ventricular hypertrophy in electrocardiography and echocardiography and the amplitude of ST-T changes reflected well with the left ventricular mass.

The slight ST-T changes did not correlate well with left ventricular hypertrophy, although the presence of heart disease should be persued not only by interpreting the findings of electrocardiography, but also the clinical and family history of disease and risk factors of cardiac disease was considered for diagnosing heart disease.

Although ST-T changes are not sufficient for the diagnosis of heart disease except in who has left ventricular hypertrophy, the presence of heart disease should be made with taking the family history, the risk factors for heart disease, and the clinical course into consideration.

References

1. R. Devereux and N. Reichek, *Circulation,* D55, 613 (1977).
2. A. Bayes de Luna in *Clinical Electrocardiography*, ed. A. Bayes de Luna (Futura, Publishing Company, Inc., Mount Kisco, New York, USA, 1993).

LOCALIZATION OF CORONARY ARTERY NARROWINGS BY EXERCISE-INDUCED CHANGE OF ELECTRICAL AXIS AND ST DEPRESSION WITH R-WAVE AMPLITUDE CORRECTION IN SINGLE-VESSEL CORONARY ARTERY DISEASE

S.SHIMIZU,MD, F.MATSUBARA,MD, M.YANASE,MD, T.HIDAKA,MD, M.WATARAI,MD, Y.SHIGA,MD, F,TAKATSU,MD,
Division of Cardiology,Department of Internal Medicine,
Anjo Kosei Hospital,Anjo,Aichi,Japan

This study investigated whether culprit coronary artery can be localized by the change of frontal plane electrical axis and the site of maximal ST depression with R-wave amplitude correction during exercise stress test in standard 12 leads electrocardiogram. Rightward axis changes were seen in 83% of RCA narrowings and 71% RCA narrowing could be localized by the site of ST depression in the leads of Ⅱ, Ⅲ,aVf. LAD narrowing could be localized by the site of ST depression in the leads of V3,4,5,6. While LCX narrowing could not be localized by these methods.

1 Background

Exercise testing is a useful non-invasive test to detect the presence of coronary artery disease.Many cardiologists have tried to evaluate the presence of ischemia and also to predict the location of coronary artery narrowings using exercise testing.Several reports have discussed correlation between the the leads of ST depression and location of narrowings[1,2,3] . But,significant correlation has not been found[1,2,3]. It has been reported that the magnitude of ST depression was influenced by the R-wave amplitude[4,5]. And we have found that the electrical axis change was observed during transient ischemia such as coronary angioplasty (PTCA) or exercise testing.

2 Methods

2.1 Study population

We studied 89 patients of stable angina pectoris with single-vessel coronary narrowing (≧75% luminal diameter stenosis, LAD:49, RCA:24, LCX:16) and ≧ 0.1mV ischemic ST-segment depression during exercise stress test. None of 89 had bundle branch block , abnormal Q wave , atrial fibrillation or flutter. Their mean age was 63(range 41 to 81).

2.2 *Exercise testing*

Master's two step test was performed. Length of exercise was decided according to the severity of angina or physical condition. All drugs were withdrawn at least 48 hours before the exercise test.

2.3 *Axis change*

Angles of axes were measured before(θ 1) and after(θ 2) exercise. Averaged data of axes of 5 consecutive beats were obtained to exclude the effect of breathing. Difference of angles(θ 2- θ 1) was defined as a change of axis. In analysis we divided into 3 groups, rightward change(≧5° rightward change), leftward change (≧5° leftward change) and no change(5° > change). The relationship between the location of narrowing and the axis change was evaluated.

2.4 *ST depression with R-wave amplitude correction*

ST depression was measured at 60 ms after J point and R-wave amplitude was also measured from the baseline to the peak of the R wave. Averaged data of ST depression and R-wave amplitude of 5 consecutive beats were obtained at supine rest and after exercise. ST depression with R-wave amplitude correction was defined as the exercise-induced ST depression(ΔST) divided by the R-wave amplitude of the same lead. In this way the lead of maximal ST depression was determined. In analysis the leads were divided into 3 groups , inferior leads(II , III ,aVf), anterior leads(V3-V6) and lateral leads(I ,aVl).

2.5 *Cardiac catheterization*

Cardiac catheterization was performed within I day after the exercise test. Coronary arteriography and left ventriculography were performed by the Judkins or Sones technique. Coronary arteriograms were analyzed by 2 or more angiographers without knowledge of the clinical and exercise test findings. The degree of percent luminal diameter stenosis was classified according to the

American Heart Association reporting system.

2.6 Statistical analysis

The difference of axis change and the site of maximal ST depression with R-wave amplitude correction among 3 vessels was analyzed by Fisher's test. The change of mean axis in each vessel was analyzed by paired t-test. The ability to localize coronary artery narrowings in each vessel was evaluated in sensitivity ,specificity and accuracy. A p value of <0.05 was considered as significant.

3 Result

3.1 Axis change

Mean axis altered from 25.8 ± 21.5 to $37.0\pm27.0°$ in 24 patients of RCA narrowing(axis change was $+11.2\pm12.8°$:$p<0.01$), from 39.7 ± 30.3 to $39.1\pm33.3°$ in 49 LAD patients(axis change was $-0.5\pm10.3°$:NS), from 40.4 ± 24.6 to $41.5\pm35.3°$ in 16 LCX patients(axis change was $+1.1\pm15.4°$:NS).

Of the 24 patients of RCA narrowing, 20 patients showed rightward axis change(83.3%:$p<0.01$), and 4 patients did leftward change. Of the 49 LAD patients,15 patients showed rightward change, 16 patients did no change and 4 patients did leftward change(NS). Of the 16 patients of LCX narrowing, 7 patients showed rightward change , 3 patients did no change and 6 patients did leftward change(NS).

3.2 The lead of maximal ST depression

In RCA patients,17 patients showed maximal ST depression in inferior leads(70.8%:$p<0.01$) , 6 patients did in anterior leads and 1 patient did in lateral leads. In LAD patients,43 patients showed maximal ST depression in anterior leads(87.8%:$p<0.01$) , 6 patients did in inferior leads. In LCX patients,11 patients showed in anterior leads(68.7%:NS) ,4 patients did in inferior leads(25.0%:NS) and 1 patient did in lateral leads(6.3%:NS).

4 Discussion

This study investigated whether culprit coronary artery could be localized by change of frontal plane electrical axis and the site of maximal ST depression with R-wave amplitude correction during exercise stress test in standard 12 leads electrocardiogram.

In the present study , patients with RCA narrowing had a tendency to show rightward frontal plane electrical axis change during exercise stress test. But no tendency of axis change was obtained in LAD or LCX narrowing. RCA narrowing could be localized by clinically distinguishable ≧5° rightward change of electrical axis (sensitivity 83.3%,specificity 66.2%,accuracy 70.8%). Although the precise explanation for this difference in axis change is unclear at present, but it may be assumed that altered ventricular conduction induced by RCA ischemia lead to the change of frontal axis. And it may be also assumed that the ischemia of posterior fascicle of left bundle branch mainly fed by only RCA, caused the tendency of right axis deviation.

Both RCA and LAD narrowing could be localized by the site of maximal ST depression with R-wave amplitude correction (RCA:sensitivity 70.8%,specificity 84.6%,accuracy 80.9%, LAD:sensitivity 87.8%,specificity 57.5%,accuracy 74.2%) LCX narrowing could not be localized by the methods we tried in this study.

These findings were thought to become useful parameters for the prediction of culprit coronary artery.

References

1. Dunn RF *et al*, Am J Cardiol 1981;48:837-843
2. Abouantoun S *et al*, Am Heart J 1984;108:933-941
3. Kubota I *et al*, Am Heart J 1985;110:949-955
4. Hollenberg M *et al*, Am J cardiol 1985; 56:13-17
5. Hakki A *et al*, JACC 1984;3:1155-1160

COMPARISON OF THE VARIABILITY OF SPECIFIC POTENTIAL AND LEFT VENTRICULAR MASS IN CONGENITAL AORTIC STENOSIS

L. BACHÁROVÁ
Institute for Heart Research SAS, Dúbravská cesta 9
842 33 Bratislava, Slovak Republic

E. VANŽUROVÁ, K. KANÁLIKOVÁ
Slovak Institute for Heart Diseases, Pod Krásnou Hôrkou 1
833 48 Bratislava, Slovak Republic

J. BACHÁR
Economic University, Dolnozemská cesta 1
851 01 Bratislava, Slovak Republic

The aim of the study was to analyze the specific potential of myocardium (SP), calculated as a ratio of maximum spatial QRS vector magnitude (QRS_{max}) and left ventricular cross-sectional area (LVAA), in left ventricular hypertrophy due to pressure overload in a group of 78 patients aged from 3 to 24 years with congenital aortic stenosis diagnosed as coarctation of aorta, subvalvular stenosis, and valvular stenosis, respectively. No significant correlation was observed between age and QRS_{max}. Significant correlation was found between age and LVAA or LVM, respectively ($r = 0.4519$, $p < 0.01$, $r = 0.5203$, $p < 0.001$). SP values correlated inversely with age ($r = -0.3760$, $p < 0.05$). QRS_{max} values were associated positively with LVAA ($r = 0.4171$, $p < 0.0001$) and LVM ($r = 0.5004$, $p < 0.001$). The variability of LVM, expressed as a value of minimum-maximum range, was the highest in the age group 11 to 15 years. The variability of QRS values was the highest in the youngest age group (< 10 years), they decreased in older age groups. As well, the range of SP values was highest in the age group < 10 years, and they decreased considerably with increasing age. No significant differences of QRS_{max} were observed between diagnostic subgroups. The highest values of left ventricular mass (LVM) and LVAA were found in the subgroup of subvalvular stenosis, however the differences between the subgroups were not significant. Significant difference of SP was found between the subgroups of coarctation of aorta and of subvalvular stenosis. Values of QRS_{max} correlated positively with LVM and LVAA in coarctation of aorta and valvular stenosis. No correlation between QRS_{max} and LVM or LVAA was found in the subgroup of subvalvular stenosis. These findings suggest that the different trends of the variability of LVM, QRS_{max}, and their ratio SP in the youngest age groups could reflect anatomical and structural changes related to the growth and development of LVH, which are not followed proportionally by the increase of the QRS amplitude. The decrease of SP and the lack of significant correlation between QRS_{max} and LVM and LVAA in the subgroup of subvalvular stenosis could be interpreted as different passive electric properties of the myocardium in subvalvular type of stenosis as compared to valvular stenosis and coarctation, respectively, possibly reflecting structural differences of myocardial tissue.

1 Introduction

Congenital aortic stenosis is a natural clinical model to study the relationship between increase of left ventricular mass and behavior of QRS voltage in left ventricular hypertrophy due to pressure overload. Increase of left ventricular mass during the period of childhood and adolescence is modified by the pathological growth of left ventricle and depends on the severity and duration of stenosis. Additional pathological factors which could modify the QRS voltage, as ischemic heart disease, can be practically excluded.

The aim of this study was to study the relationship between left ventricular mass and maximum QRS vector magnitude, and to analyze the specific potential calculated as a ratio of maximum spatial QRS vector magnitude and left ventricular cross-sectional area, in various types of aortic stenosis.

2 Material and Methods

The study group consisted of 78 subjects (22 females, 56 males) aged from 3 to 24 years (average age 11.99 years) with left ventricular overload due to congenital aortic stenosis and echocardiographic signs of LVH. 18 cases were diagnosed as coarctation of the aorta, 12 as subvalvular aortic stenosis, and 52 as valvular aortic stenosis, respectively. Patients with QRS conduction abnormalities or cardiac decompensation were not included into this study.

McFee-Parungao physically corrected orthogonal electrocardiograms were recorded using a Hewlett-Packard 1520A Vectorcardiograph system. The X, Y, Z components of instantaneous QRS vectors at 10 ms intervals from the onset of QRS were measured manually from the vectorcardiographic loops projected onto horizontal and left sagittal planes. The spatial instantaneous QRS vectors magnitudes were calculated as $\sqrt{(X^2+Y^2+Z^2)}$. The maximum spatial QRS vector magnitude (QRS_{max}) was used for further analysis.

M-mode echocardiograms were recorded using a Toshiba 160 echocardiograph. Values of IVS, EDD and LVPW were used for calculation of left ventricular activation area (LVAA)[1]:

$$LVAA = [IVS^2 + LVPW^2 + EDD(LVPW + IVS)] * \pi/2$$

SP was calculated as a ratio of QRS_{max} and LVAA[1]:

$$SP = QRS_{max} / LVAA$$

Left ventricular mass was calculated at end-diastole using the formula[2]:

$$LVM = 1.04\,([EDD + LVPW + IVS]^3 - EDD^3) - 13.6\ g$$

The Kolmogorov-Smirnov test was used for testing the fitting of data to normal distribution. Differences between subgroups were tested using analysis of variance and t-test for continuous variables and by χ^2 test for categorical variables. Relations between variables were assessed using simple regression, and by multiple regression. Probability $P < 0.05$ was considered to be statistically significant. Data are presented as mean $\pm$ S.D.

3 Results and Discussion

The basic descriptive statistics for the whole study group is given in Table 1. The QRS_{max} values exceed the upper normal limits in 52.56 % of cases (95 percentile for age groups according to Liebman[3] were used as upper normal limits). No significant correlation was observed between age and QRS_{max}. As expected, significant correlation was found between age and LVAA or LVM, respectively ($r = 0.4519$, $p < 0.01$, $r = 0.5203$, $p < 0.001$). SP values correlated inversely with age ($r = -0.3760$, $p < 0.05$). QRS_{max} values were associated positively with LVAA ($r = 0.4171$, $p < 0.0001$) and LVM ($r = 0.5004$, $p < 0.001$).

TABLE 1: Results of basic descriptive statistics for the whole study group.

	$\bar{x}$	**S.D.**	**min. -max.**
IVS	10.45	2.50	6 - 18
EDD	41.45	7.26	25 - 60
LVPW	10.5	2.32	6 - 18
LVAA	17.27	5.09	7,16 - 28.31
LVM	172.53	76.49	40.91 - 356.46
QRS_{max}	3.08	0.93	1.23 - 5.38
SP	187.64	61.60	61.28 - 380.86

IVS: interventricular septum thickness in diastole (mm), EDD: end-diastolic internal diameter of left ventricle (mm), LVPW: left ventricular posterior wall thickness in diastole (mm), LVAA: left ventricular activation area (mm^2), LVM: left ventricular mass (g), QRS_{max}: maximum spatial QRS vector magnitude (mV), SP: specific potential of myocardium (mV/mm^2).

The variability of LVM, QRSmax. and SP values, resp., expressed as a value of minimum-maximum range, is presented in Table 2. The variability of QRS_{max} and LVM showed different trends with increasing age. The variability of QRS values was the highest in the youngest age group (< 10 years), they decreased in older age groups. On the contrary, the range of LVM values was the highest in the age group 11 to 15 years. Similarly to the variability of QRS_{max}, the range of SP values was highest in the age group < 10 years, and they decreased considerably with increasing age to about 30% of the values in the youngest age group (< 10 years). In the diagnostic subgroups the average values of QRS_{max} were lowest in the subgroup of coarctation of aorta and highest in the subgroup of other types of stenosis, but the differences were not statistically significant. The highest values of LVM and LVAA were found in the subgroup of subvalvular stenosis, however the differences between the subgroups were not significant.

Significant difference of SP was found between the subgroups of coarctation of aorta and of subvalvular stenosis.

TABLE 2: Variability of LVM, QRSmax and SP in age groups.

age		LVM	QRSmax	SP
< 10	range	238,01	3,97	319,58
	x	117,22	2,79	210,63
11 - 15	range	269,48	3,45	209,20
	x	202,05	3,42	182,19
16 - 20	range	245,95	2,70	148,29
	x	221,43	2,88	150,82
> 20	range	154,23	2,06	81,65
	x	224,79	3,26	160,00

LVM: left ventricular mass (g), QRS_{max}: maximum spatial QRS vector magnitude (mV), SP: specific potential of myocardium (mV/mm^2, range: value of minimum maximum difference

Values of QRS_{max} correlated significantly with LVM and LVAA in diagnostic subgroups of coarctation of aorta and valvular stenosis. No significant correlation between QRS_{max} and LVM or LVAA was found in the subgroup of subvalvular stenosis.

These findings suggest that the different trends of the variability of LVM, QRS_{max}, and their ratio SP in the youngest age groups could reflect anatomical and structural changes related to the growth and development of LVH, which are not followed proportionally by the increase of the QRS amplitude. The decrease of SP and the lack of significant correlation between QRS_{max} and LVM and LVVA in the subgroup of subvalvular stenosis could be interpreted as different passive electric properties of the myocardium in subvalvular type of stenosis as compared to valvular stenosis and coarctation, respectively, possibly reflecting structural differences of myocardial tissue.

Acknowledgment

Supported in part by grant 2/4046/97 from the VEGA, Slovak Republic

References

1. L Bachárová: in: *Comparative approaches to medical reasoning*, ed. ME Cohen, DL Hudson (World Scientific, Singapore 1995)
2. RB Devereux, N Reicheck, *Circulation* **55**, 613 (1977)
3. J Liebman, at al. in: *Vectorcardiohraphy 2,* ed. I Hoffman, et al. (North-Holland Publishing Company, Amsterdam - London 1971)

VII. Electrocardiologic Monitoring of Myocardial Rejection

INFLUENCE OF CIRCADIAN RHYTHM ON INTRAMYOCARDIAL ELECTROGRAMS FOR NON-INVASIVE REJECTION MONITORING AFTER HTX

B.GRASSER, F.IBERER, G.SCHREIER*, S.SCHAFFELLNER, G.PRENNER, T.ALLMAYER, A.WASLER, B.PETUTSCHNIGG, H.MÜLLER, P.KASTNER*, M.SCHALDACH+, H.HUTTEN* UND K.H.TSCHELIESSNIGG

Karl - Franzens University of Graz, Austria
Division of Surgery, Department of Transplantation
Chirurgische Klinik Graz, LKH, Fach 37
A-8036 Graz, Austria
Phone +43 316 385 4444, Fax +43 316 385 4446

+ Zentralinstitut für biomedizinische Technik, Erlangen, Germany

* Technical University Graz, Austria

CHARM („computerized heart acute rejection monitoring“) is a new, non-invasive method for graft surveillance after heart transplantation. Intramyocardial electrograms are recorded via a telemetric pacemaker system with fractally coated electrodes. Rejection sensitive markers have been defined, which correlate to the results of the endomyocardial biopsy. Biopsy-proven rejection grade 2 or higher safely can be detected. The circadian rhythm influences the rejection sensitive parameter (8.00 a.m. versus 4.00 p.m.) and systolic blood pressure. Moreover, the rejection sensitive parameter is affected by the pacing frequency. Successful monitoring of steroid rejection therapy and the early detection of steroid refractory rejection episodes has been reported. The future perspective of non-invasive graft monitoring is the reduction of the number of endomyocardial biopsies and tailored immunosuppressive therapy.

1 Introduction

Progress in immunosuppression after heart transplantation (HTX) can be achieved either by more specific immunosuppressive drugs or by the improvement of therapy control, which reduces side effects related to immunosuppressive therapy. The endomyocardial biopsy (EMB), the current golden standard of rejection surveillance, cannot be repeated daily. CHARM („computerized heart acute rejection monitoring“) is a new, non-invasive method for graft surveillance after HTX. Intramyocardial electrograms are recorded via a telemetric pacemaker system with fractally coated electrodes. Major advantage of non-invasive cardiac rejection monitoring is the unrestricted access to intramyocardial electrograms at any time of the day. Non-invasive rejection monitoring is a tool for daily rejection diagnosis.

2 Materials and Methods

2.1 Transplant procedure, pacemaker implantation and patient management

The transplant procedure is performed according to the technique described by Shumway and Lower (1). During HTX, two unipolar, epimyocardial, fractally-coated, screw-in electrodes are implanted. Electrodes with fractal surface allow the detection of the ventricular evoked response at the pacing electrode. The first electrode is screwed-in to the right ventricular outflow tract, about 4 centimeters from the pulmonary valve, as near as possible to the ventricular septum, - site of first epicardial breakthrough of the ventricular depolarisation, more comparable spontaneous recordings, improved ventricular contraction pattern after stimulation (2,3). The other electrode is implanted preferable to the lateral wall of the left ventricle which presumably enables differentiation of left or right ventricular dilatation. Both electrodes are connected to a Biotronik Physios CTM pacemaker (Biotronik, Berlin/Germany) which is implanted subcutaneously in the left upper abdominal wall.

Between measurements, the pacemaker is programmed in AAI or VVI mode, other parameters (hysteresis, pacing rate) are programmed according to the patient´s spontaneous heart rhythm. Induction therapy (polyclonal antibodies) and triple drug maintenance immunosuppression are given. Regular sheduled EMB's are performed - according to the guidelines of the International Society for Heart and Lung Transplantation (4) - in order to compare the results to the analysis of intramyocardial electrograms. The immunosuppressive regimen is guided by the results of the EMB.

2.2 CHARM data aquisition, rejection and infection sensitive parameters

On biopsy days, one minute sequences of the paced intramyocardial electrogram of both electrodes are recorded at each electrode (pacing frequency preferable 100 beats/minute). Additionally recordings on non-biopsy-days are performed at each outpatient visite or during adverse events (rejection, infection, major changes of therapy, heart failure). Recordings of the ventricular evoked response are done with a notebook-based system and under standardized conditions: i.e. patients are resting in supine position for at least 5 minutes before data aquisition. Sampled data are sent via internet to a central workstation at the Technical University. Rigorous signal morphology checking and averaging is done to avoid beat-to-beat variations, ectopic beats and artefacts resulting from electromagnetic fields. Within a few minutes, patient reports return via internet which contain trend curves of the parameters extracted from intramyocardial electrograms.

The Rejection Sensitive Parameter (RSP) is defined as the decrease or increase of the descending side of the t-wave (t-slew rate) of the ventricular evoked response. We described the Infection Sensitive Parameter (ISP) as the time between the calibration pulse and the cross-over of the 0-line with the descending side of the t-wave.

3 RESULTS

3.1 System configuration

Currently, we use a a unipolar, bifocal pacemaker system with both electrodes on the ventricles. Variations extracted from recordings of intramyocardial electrograms are influenced by myocardial rejection and are used to detect rejection. For that purpose, each patient is used as its own reference and consecutively, the accuracy of rejection diagnosis by endomyocardial electrograms depends on the reproducibility of the myocardial depolarisation pattern. Unipolar right ventricular evoked responses reflect changes of the electrical activity of the heart significantly less dependent from the position of the electrode than intramyocardial electrograms during spontaneous beating (5). With respect to beat-to-beat variations and to the long term reproducibility of the intramyocardial electrogram, the signal morphology of the ventricular evoked response was significantly more comparable to that of spontaneous heart beats (6). We assume, that paced sequences are more comparable as they originate from the electrode implantation site as the unique point of initial myocardial depolarisation. Pacing via the observation electrode achieves reproducible ventricular depolarisation. No signal disturbances are caused by the polarisation artifact of the pacing electrode because of the fractal electrode surface.

3.2 Clinical studies

In a single-center study, a favourable correlation between results of endomyocardial biopsies and the results of the analysis of intramyocardial electrograms using Mikros Biogard pacemakers (Biotronik, Berlin/Germany) has been reported (negative predictive value for rejection grade 2 or higher 99%, positive predictive value 17%), (7). The introduction of the currently used bifocal pacemaker Biotronik Physios CTM offers the recording of two independent signals and enables more accurate data aquisition.

Successful monitoring of steroid rejection therapy and the early detection of steroid refractory rejection episodes has been published (8). From 1992 to 1996, 89 biopsy-proven rejection episodes (grade 1b or higher, ISHLT classification) have been detected in 29 patients. Rejection therapy consisted of daily 1000 mg Methyprednisolone for 3 days, the control biopsy was performed on day 4-6. VERA (ventricular evoked response amplitude) was recorded at the day of the biopsy which indicated rejection therapy (1,27±0,43 mV), during therapy (1,55±0,54, p<0,0001) and at the day of the control biopsy (1,51±0,54, p<0,0001). The increase of VERA correlated to the improvement of the biopsy result. Patients without improvement of the biopsy result presented with significantly lower increase of VERA (6±20 % versus 25±23 %). Non-invasive rejection monitoring enables the estimation of the effects of rejection therapy during application and indicates steroid refractory rejections before biopsy results are available.

Biopsy-proven rejection grade 2 or higher safely can be detected. Nevertheless, infection influences the rejection sensitive parameters in the same manner as rejection does (negative predictive value for rejection grade 2 or higher 99%, positive p.v. 17%). Differentiation between rejection and infection would increase the value of this method. We found, that a decrease of the RSP during severe infection was associated to a longer duration of the signal (infection sensitive parameter): 360 (350-370) versus 430 (380-490) ms. During rejection, no prolongation of the signal could be found. Patients with severe infections had significantly higher ISP. A decrease of RSP and increase of ISP was observed during rejection and simultaneous clinical infection, a decrease of RSP and no changes of ISP was observed during rejection.

3.3 Influence of circadian rhythm and pacing frequency on the rejection sensitive parameters

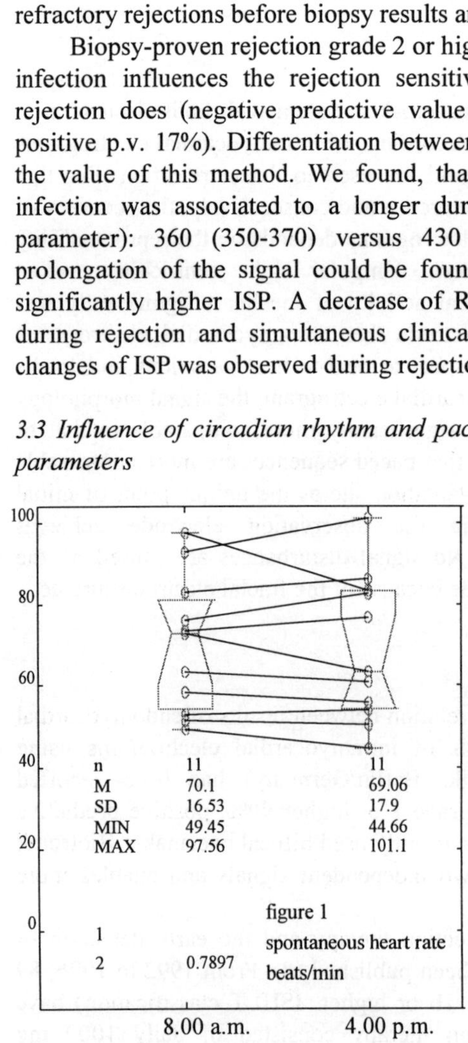

Data on the influence of the circadian rhythm on intramyocardial electrograms of denervated hearts after HTX are not published yet. The influence of the time of the day on spontaneous heart frequency, blood pressure and the rejection sensitive parameter has been investigated in 12 patients (10 men, 17 to 68 years, mean age 52±12), data were obtained at 8:00 a.m. and 4:00 p.m.. Data are presented as mean and standard deviation, statistical analysis between the morning and afternoon measurements were performed by the two-tailed, unpaired Wilcoxon test. Spontaneous heart frequency did not differ between 8.00 a.m. and 4.00 p.m. (figure 1).

During spontaneous beating and during pacing with a pacing rate of 100 beats/minute, systolic blood pressure was significantly higher in the morning (figure 2, 3).

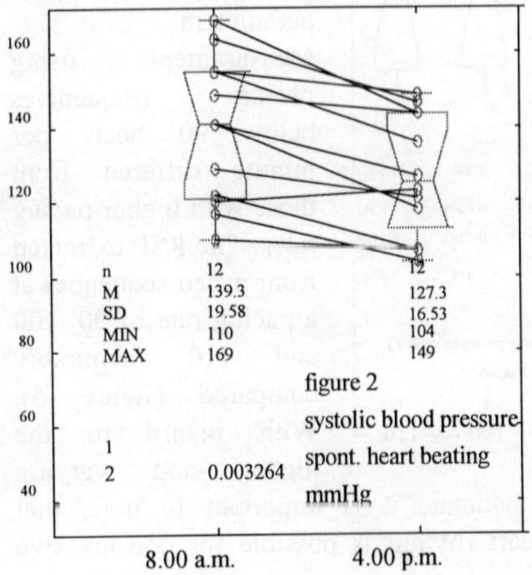

figure 2
systolic blood pressure
spont. heart beating
mmHg

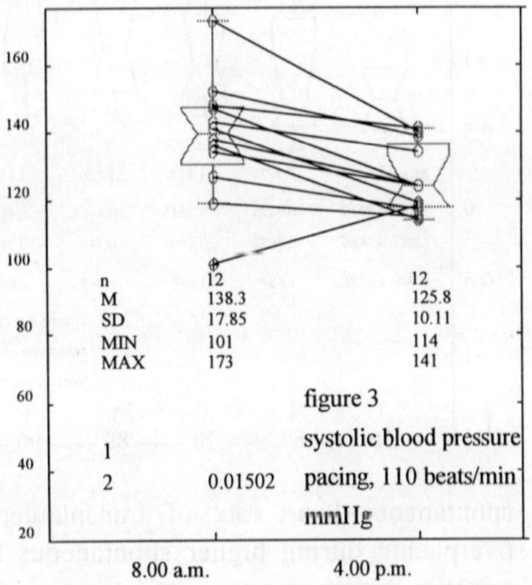

figure 3
systolic blood pressure
pacing, 110 beats/min
mmHg

We assume, that the application of antihypertensive drugs, which takes place at 8.00 a.m., immediately after the measurements, influenced this results.

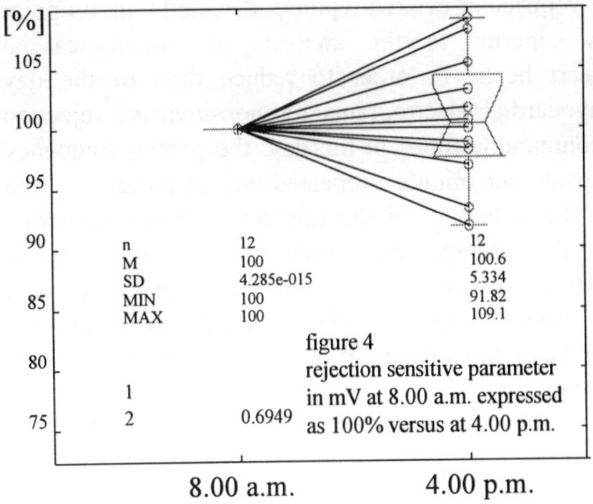

figure 4
rejection sensitive parameter in mV at 8.00 a.m. expressed as 100% versus at 4.00 p.m.

With regard to the rejection sensitive parameter, no statistical significance could be found between the measurements obtained in the morning, or in the afternoon, but intraindividual differences (up to 7 % of the morning value, at the same heart rate) were noted (figure 4). In order to reduce influences of the time of the day, routine measurements should be sheduled at the same time of the day.

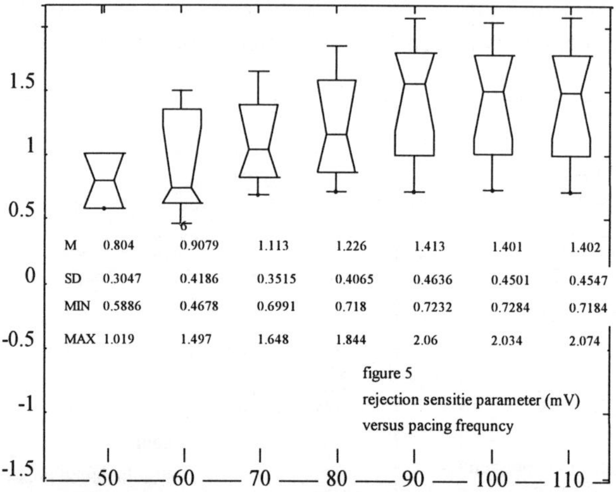

figure 5
rejection sensitie parameter (mV)
versus pacing frequncy

The pacing frequency influenced rejection sensitive parameters. Measurements using pacing frequencies below 90 beats per minute differed from those with higher pacing rates. The RSP extracted from paced sequences at a pacing rate of 90, 100 and 110 favourably compared (figure 5). With regard to the higher and varying spontaneous heart rate of transplanted patients, it is important to note, that overpacing during higher spontaneous heart rhythm is possible for non-invasive rejection monitoring.

4 Discussion and Conclusion

In conclusion, the analysis of the ventricular evoked reponse, detected with unipolar fractally coated electrodes, is superior to the analysis of intramyocardial electrograms of spontaneous heart beats. In order to reduce time of the day variations, recordings of intramyocardial electrograms for non-invasive rejection monitoring should be taken at comparable times of the day, the pacing frequency should be between 90 and 110 beats per minute. Repeated non-invasive rejection monitoring might be a tool for the reduction of the number of endomyocardial biopsies. This would reduce fluoroscopy exposition time, avoid surgical complications such as ventricular perforation, tricuspid valve insufficiency and pneumothorax. Consecutively, CHARM might enable the guidance of tailored immunosuppressive therapy after heart transplantation because of the unrestricted access to intramyocardial electrograms.

References

1. Lower RR, Stofer RC, Shumway NE. J.ThoracCardiovasc Surg;41:196-204(1961)
2. Wyndham C, Meeran M, Smith T, et al. Circulation 59, 1: 161-8 (1979)
3. Iberer F. Acta Chirurgica Austriaca 22; Supplement 85, 1-14 (1990)
4. Billingham ME, Cary N, Hammond E, et al. J Heart Lung Transplant 9:587-93 (1990)
5. Schreier G, Kastner P, Hutten H, et al. Conference Proceedings 18th Annual International Conference of the IEEE Engineering in Medicine and Biology Society, Amsterdam, Soetekouw, Nijmegen, The Netherlands (1996)
6. Schreier G, Hutten H, et al. Proceedings of the 17th Annual International Conference IEEE-EMBS, pp 33-34, Montreal (1995)
7. Auer T, Schreier G, Hutten H, et al. J Heart Lung Transplant 15:993-8 (1996)
8. Grasser B, Schreier G, Iberer F, et al. Transplantation Proceedings, Vol 28, 6:3276-7 (1996)

THE POSSIBILITIES OF USING THE WIGNER'S TRANSFORMATION OF HR ECG FOR NON-INVASIVE DETECTION OF ACUTE GRAFT REJECTION AFTER HEART TRANSPLANTATION

M. BERNADIC, I. SULKOVA, P. HUBKA, B. MLADOSIEVICOVA, H. PETRASOVA, I. HULIN

Institut of Pathophysiology, Faculty of Medicine, Comenius University, Sasinkova 4, 811 08 Bratislava, Slovakia
E-mail: bernadic@fmed.uniba.sk

I. SLUGEN

Institut of pathology IVZ, Limbova 5, 833 05 Bratislava, Slovakia

R. HATALA, Z. SCHREINEROVA, E. SCHRAMEKOVA, J. FABIAN

Slovak Heart Institut, Pod Krasnou horkou 1, 833 48 Bratislava, Slovakia

For the judgement of the state of the myocardium in patients with transplanted heart it is not possible to use the etalon of "SA ECG standards" produced from the sets of healthy subjects. Rejection can be detected only by an intraindividual comparison. There is no absolute spectral parameter which indicates rejection. Therefore, the main advantages of HR ECG: it is non-invasive method, it can be performed quickly, and it is specific to the whole heart.

1. Introduction

Heart transplantation (HTx) is a therapeutical method for patients with severe heart failure, the status of which defies other available procedures (1,4). The aim of HTx is to prolong life and to improve its quality. It is obvious, that patients after HTx need continuous specific intensive care which determines their further life (1,3). It especially involves the threat of acute graft rejection and complications of the primary disease.

Currently in Slovakia, 38 patients have been subdued to HTx. The patients are regularly subdued to EMB with a three-month frequency. The endomyocardial biopsy (EMB) is the only method on the basis of which it is possible to evaluate the status of transplanted heart in relation to graft rejection.

The limitations of this invasive method represent some reasons why, new methods and procedures are being sought. The main problem of our study is to define the possibilities of HR ECG, espetially its frequency domain analysis, to detect of acute heart rejection in long-term non-invasive monitoring after HTx.

2. The set of patients and methods

From July 1995 to the present date we have repeatedly been recording the SA ECG in 38 patients, who were subdued to HTx within the period from 1987 to 1996. In some cases the registration of SA ECG was performed as many as 10 times.

2.1. ECG, HR ECG signal recording
We used the ART 1200 EPX device to record simultaneous orthogonal X,Y and Z leads and standard ECG. The recording of ECG signal was performed in patients in supine position 24 h before EMB and 3 h after EMB.

2.2. Time domain analysis
The data were filtered using a bidirectional digital filter (25 to 250 Hz, 40 to 250 Hz and 80 to 250 Hz). The 3 leads were combined in a root-mean-square vector.

2.3. Gliding window fast Fourier transform analysis
By GW FFTA we ascertained the area ratio (7). We used a 40 ms window which was moving through the entire ventricular complex. The values of area ratio were used in the construction of curves for each lead and for composite lead. The peak expresses the ratio of the selected frequencies in favour of higher frequencies, or the decrease in lower frequencies.

2.4. Time and frequency domain analysis
Spectro-temporal mapping is a combination of bouth time and frequency domain analysis in the form of spectro-temporal maps.

2.5. Wiegner`s transformation
Wiegner`s distribution describes the spectrum of the given signal taking into consideration its unstationary character. The method results in spectro-temporal mapping. We can acquire a review of the dynamics of changes in the proportion of individual frequencies during ventricular activation.

3. Results

The typical ECG of Htx patients is sinus rhythm and RBBB. In the period of positive EMB non-significant decrease of QRS amplitude and T wave abnormalities we can find. In spectro-temporal mapping we analysed composite leads. The normality factor was uncalculated for QRS compex, for ST-T segment was in EMB positive period lower 10 % of EMB negative one. The changes are not significant.

During the 3 month period (6 investigations of the same patient) the changes of energy in the QRS frequency spectrum in the area 70-110 Hz were significant. Within the QRS complex there are no significant changes of the frequency spectrum between two analysed situations. The picture of a complete spectrum of frequencies was gained by Wiegner`s transformation. It is apparent, that inside the ventricular complex the bulkiness of the spectrum is the largest, as well as the high frequencies are clearly visible.

4. Conclusions

The results of our study imply that for the judgement of the state of the myocardium in patients with transplanted heart it is not possible to use the etalon of "SA ECG standards" produced from the sets of healthy subjects. Rejection can be detected only by an intraindividual comparison. There is no absolute spectral parameter which indicates rejection. The comparison especially in the area of QRS 70-110 Hz frequency analysis can represent a marker of the approximating rejection episode, vice versa, the return to the values of negative EMB is a sign of compensatory state. Intraindividual comparison of the HR ECG requires reproducible electrode locations, the same technical equipment and most important is an experienced person to registrate and evaluate results. Therefore, the main advantages of HR ECG: it is non-invasive method, it can be performed quickly, and it is specific to the whole heart.

References

1. ACC expert consensus document. JACC, 27, 1996, 1, 238-249.
2. M.G. Dear et al.: Cardiovasc Res 1973, 7:687-695.
3. J. Fabián et al.: Bratisl lek Listy 1997, 5:243-248.
4. R. Haberl et al.: Circulation 1987, 1:101-108.
5. I. Hulin et al.: Can J Cardiol 1993, 9:789-796.
6. M. Weber et al.: Transplant Proc 1990, 4:1460-1461.

HIGH-RESOLUTION ECG AS A PART OF COMPLEX CARE FOR PATIENTS AFTER ORTHOTOPIC HEART TRANSPLANTATION A CASE REPORT

I SULKOVA , M BERNADIC , P HUBKA , B MLADOSIEVICOVA , H PETRASOVA , I HULIN
Institute of Pathophysiology , School of Medicine , Commenius University , Sasinkova 4 811 08 Bratislava, Slovakia

R HATALA , Z SCHREINEROVA , E SCHRAMEKOVA , J FABIAN
Institute of Cardiovascular Diseases,Bratislava,Slovakia

I SLUGEN
Institute of Pathology , IVZ ,Bratislava,Slovakia

In the postoperative period after orthotopic heart transplantation is the early detection of allograft rejection one of the most important factors in management of these patients. The standard current method is endomyocardial biopsy, however because of its invasive character and the inability to provide information about the global cardiac status , reliable noninvasive diagnostic methods are still needed. The purpose of our study is to evaluate the possibilities of noninvasive electrophysiologic approaches in early detection of heart rejection. Signal-averaged ECG { SA ECG} recordings were obtained repeatedly 6-8 times in 38 patients with heart transplantation as a part of regular controls at the Institute of Cardiovascular Diseases in Bratislava. Preliminary results are documented in case report of 46-year old man after heart transplantation for dilated cardiomyopathy {1994}. The recordings were obtained 24 hours before and 3 hours after biopsy . SA ECG recordings were analyzed in the time domain after high-pass filtering at 25 and 40 Hz . Three parameters were studied - filtered QRS duration , duration of potentials below 40 μV and root-mean-square voltage of last 40 ms of QRS. There were no correlations between positivity of endomyocardial biopsy and positivity of SA ECG at 25 Hz high-pass filtering. At 40 Hz high-pass filtering there is a positive correlation between the findings of EMB and SA ECG. We suppose that SA ECG will become a component of complex long-term monitoring of heart transplant recipients in detection of allograft rejection.

1 INTRODUCTION

In the postoperative period after orthotopic heart transplantation is the early detection of allograft rejection one of the most important factors in management of these patients. The standard current method is endomyocardial biopsy, however because of its invasive character and the inability to provide information about the global cardiac status, reliable noninvasive diagnostic methods are still needed.
With the use of cyclosporine previously useful noninvasive diagnostic means,as decrease in electrocardiographic voltage, have become insensitive in detecting

rejection episodes. High-resolution ECG represents a new and promising approach in recognition of acute rejection in patients receiving cyclosporine. Several investigators eveluated the utility of signal-averaged ECG in the early phase after heart transplantation, only few of them in chronic phase . The results of these investigations are rather difficult to interpret. The recordings are analyzed in time domain and frequency domain analysis. Some investigators advocate time domain analysis in detecting rejection{Lacroix et al. 1992} ,others consider frequency domain being more appropriate {Haberl et al. 1990}. In frequency domain analysis an appropriate analytic algorithm is needed. Recently the use of FFT of SA ECG predominates but no conclusive results have been obtained till now using this method. Frequency analysis is a rapidly evolving field and also other analytic algorithms such as Wigner's distribution , wavelet transform have to be investigated.

2 CASE REPORT

A 46-year old man underwent orthotopic heart transplantation for dilative cardiomyopathy in 1994. He is regularly controled at the Institute of Cardiovascular Diseases in Bratislava. Clinical characteristic:NYHA I,arterial hypertension WHOII, hyperlipoproteinaemia, weight- 100 kg, height - 186 cm

SA ECG recordings were obtained using ART 1200 EPX at every control , 24 hours before endomyocardial biopsy and 3 hours after the procedure. The recordings were analyzed using time-domain analysis after high-pass filtering at 25 and 40 Hz, fast Fourier transform and Wigner' s distribution.Simson's criteria for detection of late potentials were used . The results were correlated with the biopsy findings. As positive biopsy findings were considered the stages mild-2 and moderate-3 of acute rejection.

3 RESULTS

In the time-domain analysis in frequency range 25 - 250 Hz there is no correlation between positivity of late potentials and positivity of biopsy. In the frequency range 40 - 250 Hz there is a correlation between two positive biopsy findings and positivity of late potentials. One biopsy finding was negative for acute rejection ,but the late potentials {LP} were present.

Table 1 : Time-domain analysis results
0/no rejection 1/nonsignificant rejection 2/mild 3/moderate Positivity of LP-according to Simson's criteria two of the three measured parameters have to be positive

25-250 Hz			40-250 Hz			EMB
f QRS /ms/	LAS/ms/	RMS 40 /μV/	f QRS /ms/	LAS /ms/	RMS 40 /μV/	
122	40	21.8	120	42	11.5	
124	29	25	124	43	13.7	2,3
119	42	21.1	118	45	10.2	
122	27	27.4	121	44	14.9	0,1
119	29	22.3	117	46	13.2	
123	28	26.9	123	37	15.9	2,3

4 DISCUSSION

The results of time-domain analysis in this patient show that the value of late potentials in detection of allograft rejection after heart transplantation is low. In the frequency range 40 - 250 Hz there is a positive correlation between two acute rejection episodes and presence of late potentials,however the late potentials are positive also without acute rejection . Also because high percentage of the patients has right bundle branch block , late ventricular potentials are inappropriate for noninvasive evaluation of acute rejection.

Frequency domain-analysis seems to be a more promising method , but the interpretation is at present time rather difficult . Comparing FFT and Wigner's distribution we think,that the second one has a greater potential to become succsessfull .

5 CONCLUSION

This case report showed that the late potentials have low value in prediction of acute rejection and that in future frequency - domain methods need to be investigated more properly in order to find noninvasive markers of acute rejection after orthotopic heart transplantation. Wigner's distribution seems to be a promising method but further investigation have to be done to detect its value in this field.

6 REFERENCES

1. Weber M, Haberl R, et al : Fourier Analysis of the Surface Electrocardiogram: A new noninvasive method to detect acute rejection after orthotopic heart transplantation in humans.Transpl Proc 22,No4,1990
2.Haberl R, et al :Frequency analysis of the surface electrocardiogram for recognition of acute rejection after orthotopic transplantation in man. Circulation 76,No. 1 ,1987
3.Lacroix D, et al:Signal-averaged electrocardiography and detection of heart transplant rejection:Comparison of Time and Frequency domain analyses JACC 19, No. 3, 1992
4.KerenA,et al: Heart transplant rejection monitored by signal-averaged electrocardiography in patients receiving cyclosporine. Circulation 70 suppl I,I-124,1984

VIII. Standards for Core ECG Laboratories

ECG CORE LABS

G. S. WAGNER
Duke University Medical Center, Durham, NC 27710, USA

ECG core labs for clinical trials have been developed during the past 20 years and now function independent from each other without standard methods, without certification as core labs, without certification for technicians, without archiving their records and without a stable future unless there is more formal development and scientific documentation of their value.

Clinical research has the potential to be a thriving business - the strange union of science and economics, but art is necessary to create this union, not creative art - like that required to put a painting on a canvas, but cooperative art. Art that cooperates with and facilitates nature.

New potentially therapeutic compounds will be developed that must be tested in randomized multicenter, often global clinical trials with names like GISSI, ISIS, BARI, GUSTO, PURSUIT, TRIM. These have either potential for solving or causing cardiovascular problems (or both), with effects measurable by the ECG. There are often strict ECG criteria for either inclusion or exclusion of experimental subjects and often study end points definable by ECG. But, we as a scholarly society of ECGers are not prepared well for this challenge.

We have a century old method that has been used qualitatively not quantitatively. Every physician believes that he is an expert at ECG interpretation and know all there is to know. Our trainees do not really learn how to read ECG's but sign off on computerized readings, based on automated analysis programs that none of us believe are scientifically optimal and certainly not quantitatively accurate. The Selvester QRS scoring system for estimating MI size, the Minnesota Code for describing serial ischemic changes, and other quantitative methods have been validated for 20 years, but do not appear routinely in any commercially available ECG system.

We use a 12-lead acquisition system with common misplacement of chest electrodes, and after years of body surface mapping, not a single new body surface site routinely added for improved diagnostic capability.

Recording of higher frequencies have been possible for decades, but have not been introduced into serious clinical use.

We do not have standard criteria for acute or re-infarction even in the absence of confounding factors such as bundle branch block or ventricular hypertrophy.

So, we have a large task. In the context of scholarly societies such as ICE, ISCE, AHA, ESC, ACC, NASPE and CIC, we must form a scholarly subsociety, a new kind of University without walls of our own laboratories or our own Universities. A university of ECG core labs for clinical trials with a constitution, a written document forged by task forces from our scholarly societies with a faculty of us from the various global laboratories with the interest, ability and stature to set the standards, govern their implementation, mentor future scholars and establish our archives, with manuscripts that test our hypotheses by statistically rigorous methods.

These are the challenges of this workshop and the workshops that should follow each time we gather in our scholarly societies, to evaluate the science of clinical electrocardiography, electrophysiology to a position in the business or clinical trials as a professional society of core laboratories.

We have a name, "Core Lab Orators", an official color, purple, a newsletter, unofficial seminars and now today, thanks to Drs. Bacharova and Rautaharju our 1st official workshop.

CODING OF SERIAL ECG CHANGES USING AN ADAPTION OF THE NOVACODE FOR Q-WAVE MYOCARDIAL INFARCTION IN A LARGE MULTICENTER CLINICAL TRIAL: THE BYPASS ANGIOPLASTY REVASCULARIZATION INVESTIGATION EXPERIENCE

BERNARD R. CHAITMAN, M.D.
SOPHIA H. ZHOU, PH.D.
KAREN STOCKE, BS, MBA
IGOR GUSSAK, M.D., PH.D.
MARK MILLER
St. Louis University ECG Core Laboratory, 1034 South Brentwood, St. Louis, Missouri 63105
PENTTI M. RAUTAHARJU, M.D., PH.D[+]
[+]EPICARE Center, Bowman Gray School of Medicine, Medical Center Blvd., Winston-Salem, NC 27157
Correspondence Address: Bernard R. Chaitman, M.D., St. Louis University Health Sciences Center, 3635 Vista Avenue, St. Louis, Missouri 63110, chaitman@slu.edu

Abstract

The Bypass Angioplasty Revascularization Investigation (BARI) of patients with multivessel coronary disease randomized 1829 patients to PTCA or CABG and the remainder into a Registry. Patients were followed for a minimum of 5 years with ECGs acquired at baseline, scheduled follow-up intervals, and for admissions associated with a suspect ischemic event. All ECGs were classified using Minnesota code criteria. A serial ECG classification program adapted from the Novacode was used to adjust for intrinsic weakness and instability at decision boundaries in the Minnesota code. Of 4,244 patients, a 2 grade Minnesota code Q wave worsening was noted in 568 patients (13.4%) using Minnesota code criteria alone compared to 367 (8.6%) after the adapted Novacode was applied. The incidence of grade 1 Minnesota Code Q wave worsening was decreased from 16.4% to 6.1% after the adapted Novacode was applied. In conclusion, the use of the standard Minnesota code in this multicenter clinical trial in patients with multivessel coronary disease indicates that additional coding rules are necessary to adjust for intrinsic weaknesses in the Minnesota code resulting from a biologic variability and coding variation.

Introduction

All rest and exercise ECGs associated with BARI were interpreted and classified at the St. Louis University Core ECG Laboratory. The aim of this report is to examine a limited set of serial coding rules that facilitate the classification of Q wave myocardial infarction using the Minnesota Code (MC).

Serial Comparison Program

The BARI protocol required ECGs at baseline, pre- and postprocedure, at the 6-week follow-up evaluation, annually during the follow-up period, and if the patient was admitted for a suspected cardiac event(1). The standard MC is generated automatically from ECG measurements by using a customized computer program for three anatomic lead groups.

The serial comparison program used in the BARI trial identifies the most recent ECG tracing and proceeds to generate consecutive paired ECG comparisons using the MC. A hierarchical system of classification based on the NOVACODE is used to generate comparisons between Q waves, ST-segment changes and T waves (2). Those ECGs with factors rendering the noncodable (eg, ECGs with missing leads) are identified and passed over, so that the paired comparison can be made with the next available suitable codable tracing. Grade 1 and 2 Q, ST, and T wave changes are programmed into the serial comparison computer software system. The St. Louis University serial comparison program uses 0 to indicate no change, +1 or +2 to indicate a grade 1 or 2 progression to a higher or more severe MC level, and –1 or –2 to indicate a grade 1 or 2 regression to a lower or less severe MC level. The program is flexible and prints a new serial comparison result for analysis when previous missing tracings or an edited ECG is inserted at any point during the process. The coding rules adjust for minimal change in R amplitude, Q amplitude or duration, ratio of Q/R amplitudes, and minimal changes that result from placement of a single precordial chest lead (Table 1). The program permits editing based on the serial comparison coding rules while maintaining the original measurement and code matrices.

Results

Of 36,781 protocol ECGs expected at the Core ECG Laboratory as of March 1995, 31,034 (84%) were received and 30,870 were analyzed. Of 31,034 ECGs available for coding, 10,373 (33%) were transmitted electronically to the Core

Laboratory, 12,935 (42%) were original paper tracings, and 7,726 (25%) were photocopied documents. Of 14 sites, 11 transmitted at least 20% of their tracings electronically; 6 transmitted 20-40% of their tracings electronically, and 5 transmitted more than 40% but less than 60% of their tracings electronically.

Frequency of Override Rules

Of 4,244 patients analyzed, 568 and 697 patients had a grade 2 or grade 1 MC Q wave progression, respectively, as of March 1995. Application of St. Louis University coding rules resulted in 201 and 438 overrides of a patient's file for grade 2 and grade 1 MC Q wave progressions, respectively (Table 2).
Thus, of 4,244 patients, the incident rate of major serial Q wave progression was 13.4% if no override rules were applied as compared with 8.6% when the coding rules were applied. As expected, application of coding rules were more frequent for grade 1 Q wave changes, and the incident rate of minor serial Q wave progression codes was reduced from 16.4 to 6.1% after application of St. Louis University coding rules.

Discussion

The new set of coding rules described here supports previous reports indicating the need to adjust for serial changes in the MC that result from minor biologic and technical variation and instability at the decision boundaries(2-4).

The notable differences in serial comparison output between the standard MC and the St. Louis University program indicate that the uncorrected MC overestimates the frequency of grade 1 and grade 2 Q wave progression and regression owing to trivial biologic variation(4,5). A major problem of individual ECG coding without serial waveform comparison is that Q, ST, and T wave changes may occur as a result of biologic variation, and minimal changes in Q wave duration or amplitude or Q/R ratio may result in a progression or regression leading to an increased false positive rate of myocardial infarction(4-6). The St. Louis University serial ECG comparison program addresses the need to identify myocardial infarction by rapidly generating and identifying any major or minor changes in the serial comparison of Q, ST, and T codes in consecutive ECGs of a patient. Verification rules address the parameters and in addition, allow for the possibility of erroneously located chest leads.

Table 1. Serial Comparison Rules Used in St. Louis University Program That Indicate Which Recorded Changes are Significant

1. Change in Q wave duration ≥ 20 ms
2. Change in R amplitude ≥2 mm, including initial R waves in the inferior and anterior lead groups
3. Change in Q amplitude ≥2 mm (particularly for MC1.2.6 for the inferior site)
4. Change in ratio of Q/R amplitude ≥75% for chest leads; 50% for change for limb leads
5. At least two precordial leads display changes sufficient to change a code (eg, MC1.3.2->MC1.2.7 does not indicate significant change)
6. Initial R wave in V1 is ignored for the purpose of all MC1.3.2, 1.2.7, 1.1.7 or 1.1.6
7. MC1.1.2 (Q=40 ms in any chest lead) reserved for coding anterior infarcts in the presence of right bundle branch block

Table 2. Summary of Changes in ECG Serial Comparison by the Using Minnesota Code and St. Louis Program University in the BARI Study by Number of Patients

	MC		SLUP	
Change	n	%	n	%
Grade 2 serial Q progression*	568	13.4	367	8.6
Grade 1 serial Q progression*	697	16.4	259	6.1
Grade 2 serial Q regression	139	3.3	121	2.9
Grade 1 serial Q regression	314	7.7	223	5.3
Presence of any serial Q change	1,718	40.5	970	22.9
Total patients	4,244		4,244	

*Definition of grade 2 and grade 1 Q progression and regression are shown in Appendix 2. MC, Minnesota code; SLUP, St. Louis University Program; BARI, Bypass Angioplasty Revascularization Investigation

References

1. BARI Investigators, *Circulation* 84(suppl V), V-1 (1991).
2. Rautaharju PM et al, *J Electrocardiol* 24,179 (1992).
3. P Rautaharju et al, Controlled *Clin Trials* 7,47S (1986).
4. B Chaitman et al, *J Electrocardiol* 29,265 (1996).
5. Blackburn H et al, *Circulation*. 21, 1160 (1960).
6. P Rautaharju in *Electrocardiography in epidemiology and clinical trials*, ed. P Macfarlane, T Lawrie (Elmsfort, New York, 1989).

EXPERIENCE WITH A CORE ECG/VCG LABORATORY IN SLOVAKIA

L. BACHÁROVÁ

Institute for Heart Research SAS, Dúbravská cesta 9

842 33 Bratislava, Slovak Republic

A brief review of the experience with the performance of a ECG/VCG laboratory in Slovakia (former Czechoslovakia) is given. The computer analysis in Slovakia started in the seventies, when the 12-lead ECG 5600 C interpretative system and the orthogonal 3-lead system 1530 B AVA interpretative system were tested. The AVA system was selected for utilization in preventive cardiologic programs and gradually implemented to home produced electrocardiographs and computer. On the basis of AVA Program a software package "KardioSys was developed for the computerized analysis of orthogonal electrocardiogram and vectrocardiogram. The ECG/VCG Laboratory processed, analyzed and archived electrocardiograms for research purposes, epidemiological and clinical trials, as well as for cardiological preventive and clinical practice. Since the activity of the laboratory was finished in 1994, a new project is prepared with the aim to create and manage an independent not-for-profit center, which will provide focused services for electrocardiological research, preventive and clinical cardiological practice, and will serve as a Core ECG Laboratory.

The beginning of the computer analysis of electrocardiograms in Slovakia is dated in the early seventies. The Research Institute of Medical Bionics (RIMB) was founded in Bratislava with the main task to introduce and utilize the computer technique in health care system in Slovakia (former Czechoslovakia) and the computerized electrocardiography was one of the subtasks.

As the first step the available software was tested, the 12-lead ECG 5600 C interpretative system[1] and the orthogonal 3-lead system 1530 B AVA interpretative system[2]. At that time, the AVA system was selected for utilization in preventive cardiologic programs since it was found that computer processing of physically corrected orthogonal ECG leads was more rational and more apt for further development..

The RIMB obtained the original version of the AVA Program from Prof. Pipberger in 1975 running at the HP 2100 minicomputer and later on in 1977 a later version of this program running on a CDC 3200 minicomputer. The AVA software was gradually implemented into home produced computers and electrocardiographs. The local technical background for the computerized electrocardiography in seventies in Slovakia consisted of:

- electrocardiographs CHIRAKARD 601 TK, produced by a Slovak firm CHIRANA. It was a 6 channel electrocardiograph, allowing to register also X,Y,Z Frank electrocardiograms and its advantage was an analogue output of the ECG signal. After a small adaptation CHIRAKARD 601 TK could be used as an input signal for computer analysis. Based on this experience with the ECG signal processing the advanced series of electrocardiographs CHIRASTAR was later developed by CHIRANA.

- computer technique: the development and production of the Slovak minicomputer was initiated in the seventies. The first Slovak minicomputer used for ECG signal processing was a 16 bits minicomputer RPP 16, later on SM 3/20 and SM 4/20, comparable with PDP 11 minicomputers. Parallelly the a/d converters and modulator/demodulators were developed, tested and produced. In the eighties the PC computers were introduced.

The Pipberger's AVA Program for Frank ECG data processing and analysis was further developed in RIMB and the developed software package "KardioSys" provided the following possibilities and outputs:

- conclusions of the original AVA Program including the identification of a patient, a table of basic time and amplitude parameters of P-wave and QRS-T of X, Y, Z Frank electrocardiograms. The diagnostic conclusion provided heart rate and rhythm evaluation and diagnostic conclusion of P and QRS-T presented as a diagnostic probability,
- detailed table of parameters: X, Y, Z coordinates of the spatial vectors in 10 ms intervals from the onset of QRS complex, and in eighths of the QRS duration, respectively. As well values of spatial magnitude, elevation and azimuth of the instantaneous QRS spatial vectors in the sane intervals, parameters of the maximum spatial QRS and T vectors and other characteristics of the orthogonal electrocardiogram and vectorcardiogram,
- vectorcardiograms: planar projections of spatial QRS and T loops projected on the horizontal, left sagittal and frontal planes, together with the scalar X, Y, Z electrocardiograms and time function of the spatial magnitude of QRS-T vector for selected heart beat,
- detailed vectorcardiographic diagnostics of the localization of myocardial infarction[3],
- decartograms: topographic presentation of orthogonal electrocardiogram using the biomathematical model according to Titomir[4] presented as integral and instantaneous maps of activation,
- 12-lead electrocardiogram derived from Frank electrocardiogram, using Dower transformation equations,
- ECG database for cardiovascular screening and epidemiology.

The RIMB participated as well in the development of the computerized 12-lead ECG analysis and automated Minnesota coding.

The diagnostic efficiency of the AVA program was repeatedly reevaluated, brief summary is given in Table 1. Results obtained with AVA program implemented into Slovak measurement and computer technique were comparable with published data.

The ECG/VCG Laboratory of the RIMB served as a research laboratory, as well it provided diagnostic vectrocardiographic and electrocardiographic services and consultations for cardiological practice.

Table 1: Summary of diagnostic accuracy of AVA program evaluated in Slovakia.

Authors	used computer	reference method	false positivity %	false negativity %
Ruttkay-Nedecký,I.[5]	HP 2100	12-lead ECG	33.1	7.7
Renker, B. et al.[6]	RPP 16	12-lead ECG	34.7	2.9
Bachárová,L. et al.[7]	SM 4/20	VCG	10.1	4.5

Main research topics:

- physiological variability and normal values of orthogonal electrocardiogram, vectrocardiogram and decartogram,
- cardiovascular screening and epidemiology, in adults, adolescents and school children,
- evaluation of the effect of antihypertensive drugs in clinical trials,
- assessment of left ventricular hypertrophy,
- developmental changes in healthy school children and adolescents.

The ECG/VCG Laboratory served as well as a diagnostic and consultancy laboratory for the clinical needs of cardiologists in Bratislava and in Slovakia.

A database of about 4 000 vectorcardiograms was created. The archive obtained records from screening and epidemiological surveys, as well as of cardiac patients indicated to the ECG/VCG Laboratory.

The Research Institute of Medical Bionics was transformed to the National Center for Health Promotion in 1993, and the ECG/VCG Laboratory finished its performance in 1995/1996.

With respect to cardiovascular morbidity and mortality and their negative trends in Slovakia, the need for re-establishing a core ECG laboratory in Slovakia is substantial. Our aim is to create and manage an independent not-for-profit center, which will provide focused services for electrocardiological research, preventive and clinical cardiological practice, and will serve as a Core ECG Laboratory.

Acknowledgment

Supported in part by grant 2/4046/97 from the VEGA, Slovak Republic.

References

1. R.A. Balda in *Trends in Computer-Processed Electrocardiograms*, ed. J.H. van Bemmel, J.L. Willems (North Holland, Amsterdam, 1977)

2. H.V. Pipberger *Automated ECG Analysis System* (Research Center for Cardiovascular Data Processing VAH, Washington 1975)
3. I.Ruttkay-Nedecky et al., *Vectorcardiogram of focal ischemic myocardial lesions* (Final Report SPZV VII-4-2, Bratislava 1974)
4. L.I.Titomir and I. Ruttkay-Nedecký *Int. J. Biomed. Comput.* **20**, 275 (1987)
5. I. Ruttkay-Nedecký *Evaluation of Hewlett-Packard Interpretative System for 12-lead ECG 5600 C* (RIMB, Bratislava, 1983), in Slovak
6. B. Renker et al., *Vnitř. lék.* **28**, 241 (1982), in Slovak
7. L. Bachárová et al., *Bratisl. lek. Listy* **86**, 603 (1988), in Slovak

ECG ANALYSIS BEYOND CORE LAB DUTY
EXPERIENCE FROM THREE SCANDINAVIAN TRIALS

PETER CLEMMENSEN, MD, PhD, LENE HOLMVANG, MD, FREDE LYCK, MD, PHILIP HASBAK, MD, GALEN S. WAGNER, MD, PEER GRANDE, MD, PhD.

The Heart Center, Rigshospitalet, Copenhagen University Hospital, Denmark, and Divison of Cardiology, Duke University Medical Center, Durham, NC, USA.

Abstract

Introduction. Core labs have well defined tasks but these are often defined by a scientific body where the experts from various core labs are not necessarily represented. The present report briefly describes the results of electrocardiographic (ECG) substudies beyond core lab duty in 3 clinical trials.

Methods. Single core lab analysis with blinded evaluation of standard ECG´s. The substudies were designed by the core lab investigators and subsequently approved by the different steering committees.

Results. In the ISIS 2 trial (Second International Study of Infarct Survival) intravenous streptokinase was compared to placebo with or without aspirin in a large factorial design mortality study. Previous studies had shown hat final AMI size could be predicted from the acute ST-segment changes in the absence of thrombolytic therapy. An ECG substudy was conducted (n=73) to study the relationship between acute ST segment changes and final QRS score estimated acute myocardial infarct (AMI) size. Patients who received streptokinase were considered as one group and patients who did not receive streptokinase as a control group. Final AMI size, which was estimated from the QRS score, was predicted from the admission standard ECG by previously developed formulas based on ST elevation. In the 40 control patients there was no change from ST-predicted to final QRS-estimated AMI size (median 18% vs 18%). In the 33 patients in the streptokinase group there was a significant decrease from predicted to final AMI size (median 22% vs 16%; p< .0002). This decrease was found for both anterior (24% vs 19%; p< .03) and inferior (22% vs 12%; p=0.001) AMI locations. Thus, intravenous streptokinase significantly changes the relation between predicted and final AMI size, demonstrating the potential of the standard ECG for non-invasive evaluation of myocardial salvage after thrombolytic therapy. This method has subsequently been used as a surrogate endpoint in later clinical studies.

In the TRIM study (Thrombin Inhibition in Myocardial Ischemia) patients with acute ischemic syndromes were randomized to a specific thrombin inhibitor (Inogastran, intravenously) or placebo. The purpose of the ECG substudy (n=472) was to determine the prognostic value of the presenting ECG in this patient population. Furthermore, the agreement between core lab analysis and local investigator interpretation of acute ischemic ECG changes was studied by kappa statistics. All standard admission ECG´s were analyzed and divided into four subgroups: ST segment elevation with or without Twave inversion (n=75; 16%), ST segment depression with or without T wave inversion (n=59; 13%), isolated inverted T-waves (n=199; 42%), and no ST-T change (n=139; 29%). Patients were followed for 30 days for the following endpoints: death, myocardial infarction, refractory angina, and recurrent angina. At the end of follow-up the event rate was 52%. Serious adverse events, defined as death, AMI or refractory angina leading to revascularization, occurred in 51 patients (11%). The majority (70%) of events occurred early within the first 3 days in hospital. Patients with ST-segment depression on admission had the worst outcome with a 24% risk of a serious cardiac event compared to only 11% in the remaining population (log-rank survival analysis, p=.0003). Isolated inverted T-waves and ST-segment elevation was not associated with an increased risk. In a comparative study between local investigator ECG interpretation and blinded analysis by core lab experts it was found that the agreement was very satisfactory for ECG changes where pattern recognition was involved (i.e., bundle branch block; kappa = 0.84) . However, when subtle quantitative ECG changes were necessary to determine if specific criteria were met the agreement was rather poor (i.e., ST-segment depression; kappa = 0.38 and ST-segment elevation: kappa = 0.06). Thus, standard ECG ST-segment depression in patients who present with acute ischemic syndromes is an ominous sign. Also, this study demonstrates the discrepancies between investigators and core labs even for routine variables normally considered relatively simple.

In the DANAMI trial (n=1008) patients admitted with first AMI received thrombolytic treatment and those with predischarge inducible ischemia were randomized to either conservative or invasive treatment. The patients were followed for 12 months. The purpose of the ECG substudy was to compare the evolution of the Selvester QRS score during follow-up in patients treated conservatively or by revascularization. A total of 817 patients had evaluable ECG´s from randomization,

3, 6 and 12 months. In the entire population, the median ECG estimated AMI size was 15% of the left ventricle at randomization decreasing to 12% at 12 months follow-up ($p<0.00001$). There was no difference in the reduction from baseline to 12 month ECG estimated AMI size when the patients were grouped according to randomization. When grouped according to actual treatment (PTCA, CABG or no invasive treatment) the QRS score normalization was not significantly different among the three subgroups. When comparing the overall resolution rate of QRS abnormalities in this population with the findings from 3 other studies conducted in the pre-thrombolytic era, an improvement in terms of additional QRS resolution could not be demonstrated in revascularized patients. However, the size of the infarcts, estimated by QRS score, were smaller at baseline in the DANAMI study than in studies from the pre-thrombolytic era. Thus, invasive treatment following thrombolysis after first AMI does not seem to influence the previously demonstrated normalization of QRS abnormalities over time.

Discussion. The design of a given clinical trial often stimulates researchers to generate substudies from core lab data. These studies have the potential to provide important knowledge about normal and disease states, extending beyond the primary objectives of a clinical trial. The optimal use of these resources requires the early involvement of core labs when planning a trial. This will also serve to stimulate the collaboration between core labs and their sponsor. Furthermore, the dialogue between sponsor and various core labs should be increased to overcome the inherent "conflict of interest" between the sponsor whose main interest could be safety or a balanced randomization and the core lab investigators who based on their scientific insight might propose more in depth analysis of the data to provide new knowledge about pathophysiological mechanisms.

The grave discrepancy between investigator and core lab interpretations of relatively simple ECG abnormalities in patients with acute ischemic syndromes underlines the importance of core lab involvement to ensure high quality unbiased analysis of clinical data, and further data on this issue should be published to stimulate the development of uniform requirements for all core lab activities.

IMPROVED IDENTIFICATION OF ACUTE MYOCARDIAL INFARCTION WITH 16-LEAD ECG

J. AHMAD, M.D., R.H.S. SELVESTER, M.D., Q.M. JALEEL, M.D., M.H. ELLESTAD, M.D.
Memorial Heart Institute of Long Beach, 2516 Atlantic Avenue
Long Beach, CA 90804, USA

In large randomized thrombolytic trials for acute myocardial infarction (MI) 75-80% of patients were not considered candidates, having not met the 12-lead ECG criteria of ST elevation in 2 contigous leads. In this study we evaluated 4 added leads, V4R, V7, V8, & V8R in 165 sequential patients who had this 16-lead ECG on admission and a sign out diagnosis of acute MI. ST elevation was presaent in 2 or more contiguous leads in 69 (41%); 8 (12%) more did not meet these ST criteria in their initial 12-lead ECG but did so in extra back leads indicating acute posterior MI; 35 (51%) of the 69 had inferior MI and 14 of these had 100uv or more ST elevation in V4R diagnostic of acute right ventricular (RV) MI; 11 of this high risk subset (rr=7) were not suspected clinically. Thus the 4 extra leads generated criteria not seen in the 12-lead ECG, that increased the number of acute MI candidates for urgent revascularization interventions by 19 (28%).

1. Introduction

In the large randomized multicenter trials [1-3] for evaluation of thrombolytic therapy of acute myocardial infarction (MI) a large number (75-80%) of those with a final diagnosis of acute MI failed to meet the 12-lead ECG entry criteria for the study. A major portion of acute MI patients were therefore not considered candidates for revascularization. One in 10 meeting entry criteria also met exclusion criteria. The remainder failed to show acute ST elevation in 2 contiguous leads of their admission 12-lead ECG even though having signs, symptoms, and laboratory findings leading to a final diagnosis of acute MI. Kornrnreich et al.[4,5] in large multigroup comparisons utilizing body surface ECG maps have shown that the best discrimination of anterior, inferior and posterior infarcts from each other, from left ventricular hypertrophy and from normals required 4-6 leads outside the standard 12 leads. Lux, et al.[6] recently reported that 96-99% of the discriminant power was found in 4 extra leads in addition to the standard 12.

Saetre, et al.[7] demonstrated that 16-lead ECGs provided excellent separation of acute anterior, posterior and inferior ischemia in patients undergoing balloon occlusion of left anterior descending, circumflex and right coronary arteries during angioplasty. In an earlier blinded study Madrid, et al.[8] had shown that 4 extra ECG leads on the back and right anterior chest (Cube vectorcardiograms) were 95% sensitive, 95% specific for posterior MI from left circumflex occlusion compared to 65%, 95% for the 12-lead ECG. Recent reports [9,10] of the 16-lead

ECG found a significant increase in acute posterior and rignt ventricular (RV) MI patients as potential candidates for urgent revascularization. The purpose of this study is to evaluate the 16-lead ECG of 4 extra leads, V4R, V7, V8, and V8R proposed by one of us (RHSS [11]) in patients who had a discharge diagnosis of acute MI.

2. Methods

The 16 simultaneous lead ECG was recorded at 500 samples/sec on a commercially available ECG digital cart (HP Pagewriter XL). The 500sps data was transferred via diskettes to a PC for off-line analysis and plotting of the data. Plotting routines developed by us were used to display Hi-gain ECG and 3D phase plots ie, Cube and derived Frank vectorcardiograms using the simultaneous 16-lead data. The 16-leads were visually assessed as a quality control of the computerized measurements of ST used as entry criteria of the study. The criteria of ST elevation for the ECG diagnosis of acute MI were: 1). $\geq$ 1 mm in 2 or more contiguous limb leads, 2), $\geq$ 1 mm in V4R (with inferior ST changes), and 3) $\geq$ 2 mm in 2 or more contiguous leads V1-V5, $\geq$1 mm in V6. $\geq$ 0.75 mm in V7, V8, V8R.

Table 1. Distribution of infarcts by location and with 16-lead ECG on admission

410. codes	Infarct Location	2 yr Totals	Adm 16lead
.0, .1	Anterior	160 (22.1%)	36 (22%)
.2, .4	Inferior	152 (21.0%)	39 (24%)
.3	Inferior-posterior	23 (3.2%)	12 (7%)
.5, .6	Posterolateral	28 (3.9%)	10 (6%)
.9	Non specified	125 (17.3%)	23 (14%)
.7	Subendocardial	234 (32.4%)	45 (27%)
	Totals	723	165

During the 2 year period ending Mar. 31, 1995, 7520 patients were admited to the Chest Pain Center of the Memorial Medical Center. A final diagnosis of MI was made in 723 (10.3%). The distribution of infarcts by location is shown in Table 1. A 16-lead ECG was recorded on admission in 177 (24.5%). Twelve patients with Left Bundle Branch Block or ventricular pacing were not included in this study. The remaining 165 were the final study group made up of 108 males (26–94yrs, median 61) and 57 females (35–91 yrs, median 69). The racial mix was 70% white, 11% black, 10% oriental, 7% hispanic, and 2% other.

3. Results

Excluding the patients with ventricular pacing or LBBB, 165 patients had a final discharge diagnosis of acute MI. The criteria of ST elevation in two or more contiguous leads used in thrombolytic trials was met in 69 (41%). In addition to the 69, 8 (12%) did not have 2 contiguous leads of ST elevation on their

Figure 1. Acute posterior MI: No 2 leads with ST criteria in 12-lead ECG but present in 16-lead.

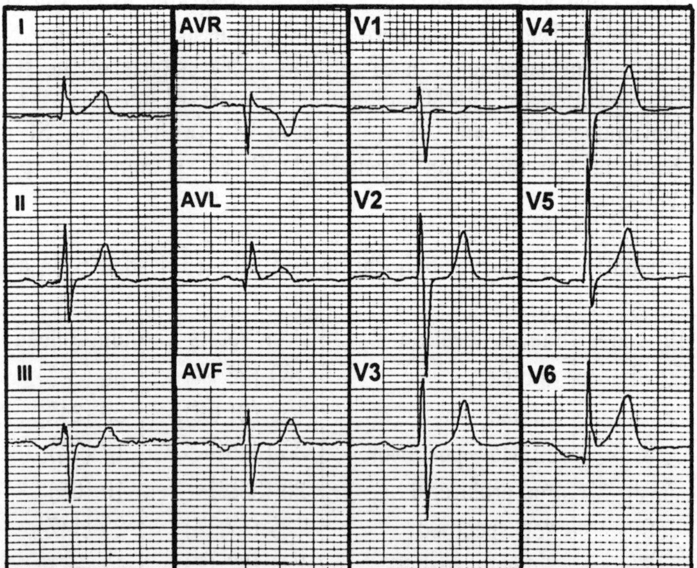

initial 12-lead ECG as used in the trials, but this criterion was met with extra back leads indicating acute posterior MI (see Fig. 1.). Acute ST elevation in 2 or more contiguous inferior leads was present in 35 patients, 14 of these had ST criteria in initial lead V4R, diagnostic of acute RV MI, 11 were not clinically suspected. Thus the 4 extra leads generated criteria not seen in the standard 12-lead ECG that increased the number of acute MI candidates for consideration of urgent revascularization interventions by 19 (28%).

4. Discussion

There are two groups of patients with 16-lead ECGs positive for STT change of acute MI not recognized on the 12-lead ECG: 1). Inferior MIs with a diagnosis of RV MI by extra lead V4R that were not otherwise suspected clinically. This group is reported to have a relative risk of 7 for acute mortalty and are prime candidates for early thrombolysis with a 4-fold reduction in risk (9). 2). Circumflex occlusions and acute posterior MIs who did not meet the criteria of ST elevation in 2 or more contigous leads of the 12-lead ECG but did so with extra back leads. An important capability of the 16 simultaneous lead ECG is the Hi-gain Hi-Fi (500sps) ECGs and 3D (XYZ) phase plots. The predischarge ECG/VCG plotted this way has been shown to be 97% reliable at predicting new MI in follow up tracings whether suspected or "silent," clinically and/or by 12-lead ECG criteria.[11] In the next phase of this ongoing study we will test these findings in this acute community hospital setting.

Acknowledgments

Study supported in part by grants from Genentech Inc, S.San Francisco, CA and the Memorial Medical Center Foundation, Long Beach, CA, USA.

References

1. ISIS-2 Collaborative group, Lancet. V2, 349 (1988).
2. GISSI-2, Lancet. V336, 65 (1990)
3. The GUSTO investigators, The New England J of Med. V 329, 673 (1993).
4. Kornreich F. et. el. J Electrocardiol. 22 Suppl, 169 (1989)
5. Kornreich F. Montague TJ. and Rautaharju PM. Circ. 87(3), 773 (1993).
6. Lux, Kornreich , et al. J Electrocardiol. 28 Suppl, (1995)
7. Saetre HA et al., J. of Electrocardiol. 24 Suppl, 153 (1992).
8. Madrid WL et al., Proceedings of the Emgineering Foundation Conference, Computer Interpretation of the Electrocardiogram XI.
9. Zehander, Kasper et al. N Eng J Med 328(14): 981 (1993).
10. Zalenski, Cooke et al., Ann Emerg Med 22(5): 786 (1993).
11. Selvester RHS. J Electrocardiol. 28 Suppl, 216 (1995)

RECOMMENDATIONS FOR CONSISTENT PLACEMENT OF THE CHEST ELECTRODES IN CLINICAL TRIALS AND EPIDEMIOLOGICAL STUDIES

P. M. RAUTAHARJU, F. S. RAUTAHARJU, L. P. PARK

The Epidemiological Cardiology Research Center (EPICARE), Department of Public Health Sciences, Bowman Gray School of Medicine, Winston-Salem, North Carolina, USA

E-mail: pentti@beowulf.phs.bgsm.edu

The primary purpose of the recommendations introduced here is to reduce systematic bias in ECG electrode placement and thus to enhance procedural comparability between clinical trials and epidemiological studies. Key recommendations call for precise identification of critical anatomical landmarks such as the left midclavicular and midaxillary lines. Formulation of well defined procedures is recommended for centralized training of ECG technicians at the onset of clinical trials. The overall goal is to maintain the systematic bias in chest electrode placement in clinical trials and epidemiological studies within 2 cm of the correct locations defined by a standardized procedure.

1 Background

Both systematic and random variations in electrode placement are large,[1,2] resulting in ECG amplitude and waveform variations[3] which may deteriorate the stability of ECG classification. Electrode locating errors are largely due to inconsistent definitions of critical anatomical landmarks such as the left midclavicular line, and poorly standardized procedures and technical difficulties in finding correct chest electrode positions particularly in women and in obese persons.

The primary purpose of the recommendations introduced here for consideration by the Working Group on Standardization of Criteria and Procedures for Core ECG Laboratories is to enhance the procedural comparability between various clinical trials and epidemiological studies.

2 Training of ECG technicians

A detailed step-by-step procedure for electrode placement needs to be specified and rigorously observed in training of ECG technicians at the onset of the study. A major emphasis of the training session should focus on the learning of proper palpating techniques for locating critical anatomical landmarks.

The use of a non-toxic marking pen after careful identification the correct position of each electrode improves electrode placement accuracy.

3 Placement of Limb Electrodes

The placement of limb electrodes on shoulders or the torso should be avoided. It should be noted that ECGs recorded with modified electrode locations as a reference ECG for exercise (Mason-Likar system) are distorted[4] and they cannot be corrected computationally with adequate accuracy.[5]

4. Placement of Chest Electrodes

4.1 Electrodes V1 and V2.

Step 1. Stand on the left side of the study participant. Locate the sternal angle between the index and middle finger of your right hand. With fingers wide apart and palpating with a fairly firm pressure, move them up and down until confident that the sternal angle is between your middle and index fingers.
Step 2. Palpate the second rib where it joins the sternal angle, and the second intercostal space below the second rib.
Step 3. Repeat the procedure twice to palpate the third rib, third intercostal space, the fourth rib and the fourth intercostal space.
Step 4. A the level of the fourth intercostal space, mark a small cross in the midsternal line as the correct reference level for V1 and V2.
Step 5. Palpate and mark the locations of V1 and V2 at the right and left sternal borders. It is important to place these electrodes so that the conduction part of the electrode is exactly at the sternal border and not too far laterally or on the sternal bone itself.

4.2 The level of V4, V5 and V6

Step 1. From V2, palpate the fourth intercostal space with the middle finger of the right hand, move the finger laterally about 2-3 cm in the fourth intercostal space.
Step 2. Place your index finger below the fifth rib. With the fingers wide apart and moving them up and down with as firm a pressure as possible without undue discomfort to the study participant, keep palpating the fifth rib while moving your fingers laterally at a slight angle downwards until you are approximately 5 cm (2 inches) from V2. The intercostal spaces there run more horizontally.
Step 3. Palpate the fifth intercostal space under your index finger. At this level make a small cross at the midsternal line below the V1-V2 reference mark. This is

the correct horizontal level for electrodes V4, V5 and V6.

4.3 Left midaxillary line and the location of V6

Step 1. Move the left elbow of the patient laterally without deviating anteriorly or posteriorly. Identify the midpoint of the left axilla between the anterior and posterior folds as the starting point of the left midaxillary line.
Step 2. Trace the midaxillary line from the axilla in the central plane of the thorax down until the exact horizontal level of the reference mark at the lower sternum for V4-V6 level without deviating from the central plane anteriorly or posteriorly. At this level mark the exact location of V6.

4.4 Locations of V4, V3 and V5.

Step 1. Use the Heartsquare ruler[6] to locate V4 at 45° angle between the midsternal and the left midaxillary lines.
Step 2. Mark V3 position at halfpoint in a straight line between V2 and V4.
Step 3. Mark V5 position at halfpoint in a straight line between V4 and V6.

3.5 Locations of V4, V3 and V5. Alternative method

Step 1. Using a flexible measuring tape with a metric scale, measure the curvilinear distance to the nearest 0.5 cm from V6 to the mark at the midsternal line at the lower sternum.
Step 2. Mark V4 position at halfpoint between V6 and midsternal line.
Step 3. Mark V3 position at halfpoint in a straight line between V2 and V4.
Step 4. Mark V5 position at halfpoint in a straight line between V4 and V6.

Discussion

The procedures recommended here differ in certain aspects from the traditional procedure followed in chest electrode placement. The left midclavicular line is identified as a meridional line running at a 45° angle between the midsternal and left midaxillary lines, or approximated for V4 location at the halfway point between V6 and the midsternal line. It can be assumed that the midsternal line can be located with a relatively small error, and subsequently the locations of V3, V4 and V5 are predetermined with reasonable precision, provided that proper care is taken in marking the location of the left midaxillary line.

The EPICARE procedure recommends the placement of all chest electrodes in women on the breast rather than under the breast as often done in clinical ECG laboratories. While it is true that V4 and V5 amplitudes are occasionally attenuated in women with an abundant amount of breast tissue, the overall effect of breast size is not significant in comparison with the dominant effect of the thorax size and shape. (Rautaharju et al, unpublished data). Locating the electrodes under the breast causes uncontrollable variability in electrode placement which can be a problem in serial comparison. A compromise can be offered here regarding the placement of V4 and V5 in women with large pendulous breasts. The horizontal level of the insertion point of the breast to the chest wall can be used as to guide the placement of these electrodes. If this level is more than 2 cm below the correct reference level for V4 and V6, all chest electrodes should be placed on the breast as defined. If this level is within 2 cm from the exact horizontal level of V4, V4 and V5 may be placed under the breast. V3 should always be placed on it's exact location on the breast, to retain the consistency of left ventricular hypertrophy criteria (Cornell voltage).

The EPICARE Center experience indicates that with well planned quality control procedures, it is an attainable goal to control systematic bias in chest electrode placement within 2 cm from the correct positions defined by the ECG protocol. A considerably more difficult task is to reduce random variations in electrode placement in successive recording sessions. To alleviate this problem in future clinical trials, documentation of the following three measurements of chest electrode positions at the baseline examination is suggested, to be used to determine electrode locations in subsequent follow-up recordings:1) linear distance from sternal notch to V1-V2 level; 2) linear distance from V1-V2 level to the reference mark for V4-V6 level at the lower sternum; and 3) curvilinear distance from midsternal line to V6.

References

1. M.J. Zema et al, J. Electrocardiol.**13**, 135 (1980).

2.W. Wenger et al, J Electrocardiol **29**, 179 (1996).

3. M.V. Herman et al, Clin. Cardiol. 14, 469 (1991).

4. P.M. Rautaharju et al, J. Electroacardiol. **13**, 109 (1980).

5. H.K. Wolf et al, in Advances in Cardiology, Electrocardiology, ed. H. Abel (Karegel Publishing Co., Basel, 1976)

6. P. M. Rautaharju et al, J. Electrocardiol. **9**, 35 (1975)

CODING EXPERIENCE AT THE GLASGOW CORE ECG LABORATORY.

PETER W. MACFARLANE.

University Department of Medical Cardiology, Royal Infirmary, Glasgow, Scotland.

JULIE KENNEDY.

University Department of Medical Cardiology, Royal Infirmary, Glasgow, Scotland.

SHAHID LATIF.

University Department of Medical Cardiology, Royal Infirmary, Glasgow, Scotland.

ABSTRACT.

The ECG Computing Laboratory at the University of Glasgow currently acts as the Core Laboratory for eight clinical/epidemiological studies. In effect, digital ECGs are transmitted by telephone from within the United Kingdom and other European countries for interpretation and coding using Minnesota code rules. In addition, serial comparison is also undertaken centrally. This paper reviews recent experiences.

1. INTRODUCTION.

An interest in the use of computers for ECG analysis developed in the University of Glasgow Department of Medical Cardiology in 1964. Since then, the process of development of software has continued to the point where the routines for basic 12-lead ECG interpretation have been distributed world-wide commercially. The software used was described in 1990(1). Criteria for the paediatric ECG have also been developed and an outline of the approach to interpretation of the paediatric ECG has also been reported(2).

In 1984, there was an interest in using the Minnesota Code for a population study and so routines were developed for coding the ECG according to the published rules(3). Later, with the location of the West of Scotland Coronary Prevention Study (WOSCOPS) in the University of Glasgow, there was a need to develop methods for serial comparison of ECGs according to Minnesota Code rules(3,4). Methods for serial comparison had already been developed in Glasgow a number of years previously both for the three orthogonal lead ECG(5) and for the 12-lead ECG(6).

The approach used is summarised briefly.

2. METHODS.

Within the Glasgow Program, an average beat is calculated from an 8 or 10 second recording. From this, measurements of all relevant wave amplitudes and durations together with selected intervals are obtained. It was therefore decided to use these averaged measurements for Minnesota coding rather than use the Minnesota Code rules for the presence or absence of waves in a majority of beats.

The software was initially written in Fortran for the PDP11 series computers and then slightly adapted for use on the Micro VAX II series of machines. However, when

WOSCOPS commenced, ECG management was based on the MINGOCARE system marketed by Siemens-Elema. With this facility, ECGs were interpreted in SICARD 440 machines in different locations and the measurement matrix, together with the interpretation and waveforms, transmitted to the management system.

With the co-operation of Siemens-Elema, the routines for coding according to Minnesota Rules were incorporated into the management system. The codes themselves were mapped onto 128 numbers (0-127) so that when an ECG was received in the management system by telephone, it was immediately coded with the results being stored in the database in the minimum of space and the output produced at the earliest opportunity with waveforms, a basic interpretation according to the Glasgow criteria and Minnesota Codes (Figure 1).

In order to undertake serial comparison, it was necessary to extract the measurement matrices from the ECGs being compared and input them to a separate PDP11 computer for analysis. During the WOSCOPS Study, this was generally done overnight to spread the load on the computing system with results being printed at that time.

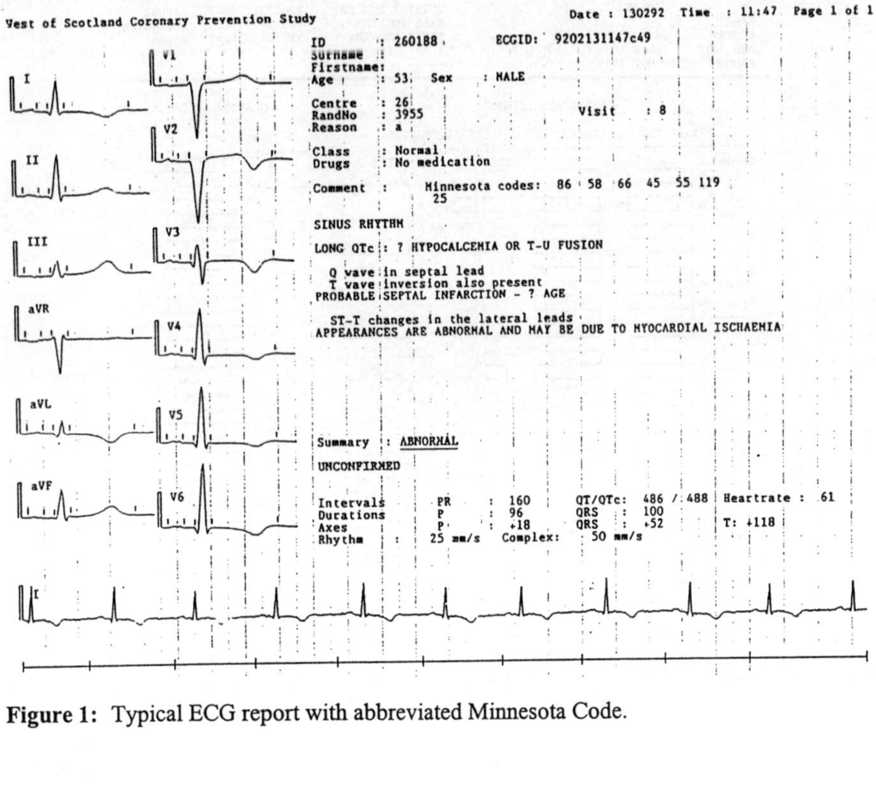

Figure 1: Typical ECG report with abbreviated Minnesota Code.

An example of the output format of the serial comparison is shown in Figure 2. Essentially, the baseline interpretation is printed together with the codes from the most recent ECG and if a serial change is detected, then a tick mark is printed in the relevant box.

Two types of serial comparison are allowed by Minnesota Coding. One relates to a straightforward comparison of codes whereas the second allows measurements to be compared. Both forms of serial comparison were utilised with results printed on the output form.

The ECG management facility allows over-reading to be undertaken. All study ECGs are reviewed by an experienced individual who decides whether the quality of the ECG is sufficiently accurate to allow the coding to be accepted. If not, a form of manual over-read has to be utilised and the codes reinserted into the ECG by an experienced technician using the management system over-reading facility. When this is done, a further serial comparison can then be undertaken and an updated printout produced.

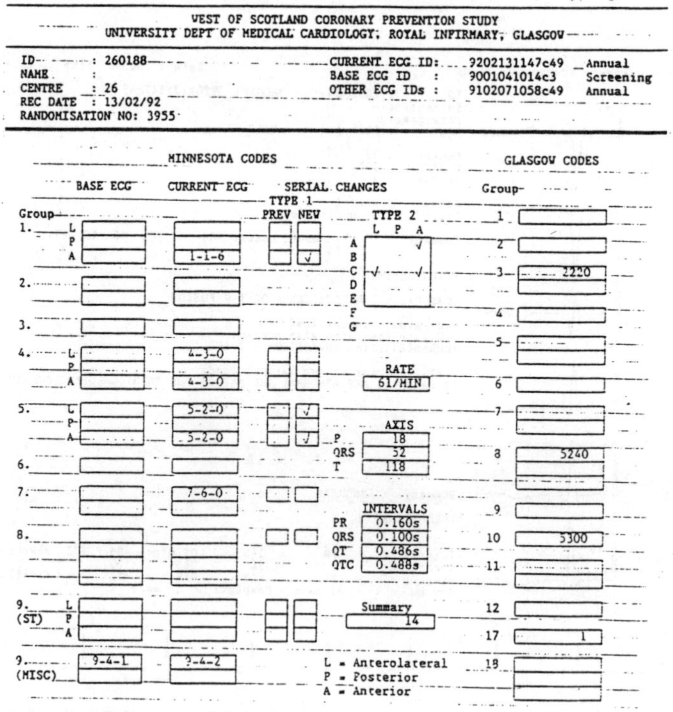
WEST OF SCOTLAND CORONARY PREVENTION STUDY
UNIVERSITY DEPT OF MEDICAL CARDIOLOGY, ROYAL INFIRMARY, GLASGOW

ID : 260188
NAME :
CENTRE : 26
REC DATE : 13/02/92
RANDOMISATION NO: 3955

CURRENT ECG ID : 9202131147c49 Annual
BASE ECG ID : 9001041014c3 Screening
OTHER ECG IDs : 9102071058c49 Annual

MINNESOTA CODES

Group		BASE ECG	CURRENT ECG	SERIAL CHANGES TYPE 1 PREV	NEW
1.	L				
	P				
	A		1-1-6		√
2.					
3.					
4.	L		4-3-0		
	P				
	A		4-3-0		
5.	L		5-2-0		√
	P				
	A		5-2-0		√
6.					
7.			7-6-0		
8.					
9. (ST)	L				
	P				
	A				
9. (MISC)		9-4-1	9-4-2		

TYPE 2

	L	P	A
A			√
B			
C	√		√
D			
E			
F			
G			

RATE
61/MIN

AXIS
P 18
QRS 52
T 118

INTERVALS
PR 0.160s
QRS 0.100s
QT 0.486s
QTC 0.488s

Summary
14

L = Anterolateral
P = Posterior
A = Anterior

GLASGOW CODES

Group	
1	
2	
3	2220
4	
5	
6	
7	
8	5240
9	
10	5300
11	
12	
17	1
18	

Figure 2: Minnesota Coding report form with serial changes output corresponding to Figure 1.

3. COLLABORATIVE STUDIES.

The Glasgow Lab has acted as the ECG Core Laboratory for the following studies in recent years. The Study Centres are also indicated.

1. West of Scotland Coronary Prevention Study. (Glasgow).
2. British Regional Heart Study. (London).
3. Whitehall II Study. (London).
4. Wandsworth Heart and Stroke Study. (London).
5. Early Diabetes Intervention Trial. (Oxford).
6. Fasting Hyperglycaemia Study. (Oxford).
7. British Genetics of Hypertension Study. (London/Glasgow).
8. The MRC Clinical Research Initiative in Heart Failure. (Glasgow).

Studies 1, 2, 3 each had over 6,000 subjects enrolled initially. In addition, another major multi-centre international trial is presently being designed and the ECG Core Laboratory will be in Glasgow, while a further small collaborative study with a Dutch research team is currently being piloted.

4. CODING PROBLEMS.

Without doubt, the single biggest problem in coding for such trials is the quality of the ECG recording. For each trial, the nursing staff involved have either visited Glasgow to be given training or else one of the Glasgow team has visited the Trial Centres to give a course to the staff involved in ECG recording.

As part of this talk, every type of fault seen in early studies is clearly explained with a warning that without fail, a similar problem will be encountered in the new study for which training is being given! Todate, the warnings have always proved correct! The Glasgow Program was modified to report faulty limb lead electrode connections as decribed by Haisty et al(7).

It appears to be inevitable that nursing staff who perhaps have not been accustomed to recording electrocardiograms daily for several years, will make common errors such as wrongly connecting limb leads. In addition, however, problems related to noise are among those which give the most difficulty. Inevitably, they lead to measurement error and faulty coding. However, as described elsewhere, reviewer over-reading is feasible with the management system in use.

Another problem encountered has been failure to find a recording despite the fact that nursing staff insist that it was made. In all probability, this means that staff failed to save the ECG in memory so that it could be transmitted to the Core Lab at a later stage.

5. DISCUSSION.

The facility described has proved relatively resilient in facilitating ECG coding for large clinical trials. Indeed, the methodology outlined above was used in WOSCOPS where it has been shown(8) that minor ECG abnormalities, such as Codes 4-2, 4-3, 5-2, 5-3, carry significant prognostic value in middle-aged men with hyperchoesterolaemia. In fact, in the 55-64 year age group, these minor ECG abnormalities on a univariate analysis carry the highest risk ratio of all variables studied including smoking, history of hypertension etc. It is probably worth noting that another significant point is that the Minnesota Code appears to be deficient in dealing with anteroseptal myocardial infarction where there are low R waves in the anteroseptal leads V2 to V4. Indeed, unless there is reversed R wave progression, there is no code for low R waves. Given an ECG with low R in V2 - V4 and the presence of almost pathognomic ST-T changes, it was found necessary to supplement Minnesota Coding by utilising the interpretation from the Glasgow ECG Analysis Program in order to reach a diagnosis of anterior myocardial infarction.

In conclusion, the system has shown itself to be of value in facilitating ECG analysis in major trials of considerable clinical importance. While the Minnesota Code is by no means perfect, it still remains the most commonly used coding scheme by which trials of varying types may be compared.

6. RECOMMENDATIONS.

In terms of recommendations for Core Laboratories, perhaps the principal concern has to be the standard of recording and it may be that all nursing/cardiological staff involved in clinical trials should be issued with a certificate of competence in ECG recording. As regards running a Core Laboratory, the individual in charge should be completely au fait with the effect of quality on Minnesota Coding and have a degree of competence in over-reading computer based interpretations and codings.

REFERENCES.

1. P.W. Macfarlane, B. Devine, S. Latif, S.C. McLaughlin, D.B. Shoat, M.P. Watts, *Meth. Inform. Med.* **29** (1990) 272-81.
2. P.W. Macfarlane, E.N. Coleman, B. Devine, A. Houston, S.C. McLaughlin, T.C. Aitchison, E.O. Pomphrey, *J. Electrocardiology* **23**(Suppl) (1990) 76-81.
3. R.J. Prineas, R.S. Crow, B. Blackburn, *Minnesota Code Mannual* (1982) John Wright, Bristol.
4. R.S. Crow, R.J. Prineeas, D.R. Jacobs, Blackburn H *Am. J. Cardiol.* **64** (1989) 454-61.
5. P.W. Macfarlane, H.T. Cawood, T.D.V. Lawrie. *Comp. Biomed. Res.* **8** (1975) 189-200.
6. P.W. Macfarlane, M. Podolski. In: *Computerised Interpretation of the ECG XI.* New York. (1986) Eng. Fdtn. 110-13.
7. W.K. Haisty, O. Pahlm, L. Edenbrandt, K. Newman, *Am. J. Card.* (1995) 1450-95.
8. WOSCOPS Study Group. *Lancet* **348** (1996) 1339-42.

BRATISLAVA RESOLUTION

The Workshop on the Standards for Core ECG Laboratories was held as a part of the 24th International Congress of Electrocardiology on Thursday, June 26. At the conclusion of the workshop the participants resolved to request to the Council of the International Society on Electrocadiology for incorporation as one of the society's working groups. The members of this working group would include but would not be restricted to the workshop participants: B. Chaitman, O. Pahlm, L. Bacharova, P. Clemmenssen, P. Macfarlane, R. Selvester, G. Wagner, F. Turazza, P. Rautaharju.

The working group would have the mission of establishing minimum standards for:

- function of ECG core laboratories and their quality control,
- training and certification of the personnel within those laboratories and for the technologists in the individual study sites,
- standardization and quality control of ECG lead locations and training the technologists for using these methods,
- various diagnostic criteria,
- set minimal standards to obtain compatibility between member core labs.

An early goal of the working group would be to write and publish a document "Standards for the Function of an Academic 12-lead Electrocardiographic Core Laboratory" for the purpose of dissemination throughout the international cardiology community. Initially the working group will focus on problems of resting ECG wave morphology. This working group should explore possibilities of meeting during the course of the year when members gather at scientific conferences. There also exists the possibility of using the Internet as a forum for exchange and the working group could potentially be linked to the ICE home page.

One of the members of the working group has offered to look into the accreditation process within the WELAC European standards (Western European Laboratory Accreditation Committee).

One of the members of the group is exploring the possibility for meetings of this working group at future ISCE meetings and planning for on-going workshops at future ICE meetings, including the 1998 meeting in Budapest.

AUTHOR INDEX